Sustainable Healthy Working Life for All Ages—Work Environment, Age Management and Employability

Sustainable Healthy Working Life for All Ages—Work Environment, Age Management and Employability

Editors

Kerstin Nilsson
Clas-Håkan Nygård
Tove Midtsundstad
Peter Lundqvist
Joanne Crawford

MDPI • Basel • Beijing • Wuhan • Barcelona • Belgrade • Manchester • Tokyo • Cluj • Tianjin

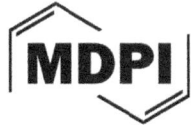

Editors

Kerstin Nilsson
Lund University
Sweden

Clas-Håkan Nygård
Tampere University
Finland

Tove Midtsundstad
Fafo Institute for Labour and
Social Research
Norway

Peter Lundqvist
Swedish University of
Agricultural Sciences
Sweden

Joanne Crawford
Victoria University of
Wellington
New Zealand

Editorial Office
MDPI
St. Alban-Anlage 66
4052 Basel, Switzerland

This is a reprint of articles from the Special Issue published online in the open access journal *International Journal of Environmental Research and Public Health* (ISSN 1660-4601) (available at: https://www.mdpi.com/journal/ijerph/special_issues/Healthy_Working_Life_Ages).

For citation purposes, cite each article independently as indicated on the article page online and as indicated below:

LastName, A.A.; LastName, B.B.; LastName, C.C. Article Title. *Journal Name* **Year**, *Volume Number*, Page Range.

ISBN 978-3-0365-6676-4 (Hbk)
ISBN 978-3-0365-6677-1 (PDF)

© 2023 by the authors. Articles in this book are Open Access and distributed under the Creative Commons Attribution (CC BY) license, which allows users to download, copy and build upon published articles, as long as the author and publisher are properly credited, which ensures maximum dissemination and a wider impact of our publications.

The book as a whole is distributed by MDPI under the terms and conditions of the Creative Commons license CC BY-NC-ND.

Contents

Kerstin Nilsson, Clas-Håkan Nygård, Tove Midtsundstad, Peter Lundqvist and Joanne Crawford
Sustainable Healthy Working Life for All Ages—Work Environment, Age Management and Employability
Reprinted from: *Int. J. Environ. Res. Public Health* **2023**, *20*, 2712, doi:10.3390/ijerph20032712 . . . 1

Kerstin Nilsson and Emma Nilsson
Organisational Measures and Strategies for a Healthy and Sustainable Extended Working Life and Employability—A Deductive Content Analysis with Data Including Employees, First Line Managers, Trade Union Representatives and HR-Practitioners
Reprinted from: *Int. J. Environ. Res. Public Health* **2021**, *18*, 5626, doi:10.3390/ijerph18115626 . . . 7

Kerstin Nilsson and Emma Nilsson
Can They Stay or Will They Go? A Cross Sectional Study of Managers' Attitudes towards Their Senior Employees
Reprinted from: *Int. J. Environ. Res. Public Health* **2022**, *19*, 1057, doi:10.3390/ijerph19031057 . . . 37

Pia Hovbrandt, Per-Olof Östergren, Catarina Canivet, Maria Albin, Gunilla Carlsson, Kerstin Nilsson and Carita Håkansson
Psychosocial Working Conditions and Social Participation. A 10-Year Follow-Up of Senior Workers
Reprinted from: *Int. J. Environ. Res. Public Health* **2021**, *18*, 9154, doi:10.3390/ijerph18179154 . . . 57

Marta Sousa-Ribeiro, Petra Lindfors and Katinka Knudsen
Sustainable Working Life in Intensive Care: A Qualitative Study of Older Nurses
Reprinted from: *Int. J. Environ. Res. Public Health* **2022**, *19*, 6130, doi:10.3390/ijerph19106130 . . . 71

Ellen Jaldestad, Andrea Eriksson, Philip Blom and Britt Östlund
Factors Influencing Retirement Decisions among Blue-Collar Workers in a Global Manufacturing Company—Implications for Age Management from A System Perspective
Reprinted from: *Int. J. Environ. Res. Public Health* **2021**, *18*, 10945, doi:10.3390/ijerph182010945 . 99

Kerstin Nilsson, Anna Oudin, Inger Arvidsson, Carita Håkansson, Kai Österberg, Ulf Leo and Roger Persson
School Principals' Work Participation in an Extended Working Life—Are They Able to, and Do They Want to? A Quantitative Study of the Work Situation
Reprinted from: *Int. J. Environ. Res. Public Health* **2022**, *19*, 3983, doi:10.3390/ijerph19073983 . . . 121

Inger Arvidsson, Ulf Leo, Anna Oudin, Kerstin Nilsson, Carita Håkansson, Kai Österberg and Roger Persson
Should I Stay or Should I Go? Associations between Occupational Factors, Signs of Exhaustion, and the Intention to Change Workplace among Swedish Principals
Reprinted from: *Int. J. Environ. Res. Public Health* **2021**, *18*, 5376, doi:10.3390/ijerph18105376 . . . 139

Sophie Schön Persson, Kerstin Blomqvist and Petra Nilsson Lindström
Meetings are an Important Prerequisite for Flourishing Workplace Relationships
Reprinted from: *Int. J. Environ. Res. Public Health* **2021**, *18*, 8092, doi:10.3390/ijerph18158092 . . . 159

Cicilia Nagel and Kerstin Nilsson
Nurses' Work-Related Mental Health in 2017 and 2020—A Comparative Follow-Up Study before and during the COVID-19 Pandemic
Reprinted from: *Int. J. Environ. Res. Public Health* **2022**, *19*, 15569, doi:10.3390/ijerph192315569 . 173

Saila Kyrönlahti, Subas Neupane, Clas-Håkan Nygård, Jodi Oakman, Soile Juutinen and Anne Mäkikangas
Perceived Work Ability during Enforced Working from Home Due to the COVID-19 Pandemic among Finnish Higher Educational Staff
Reprinted from: *Int. J. Environ. Res. Public Health* **2022**, *19*, 6230, doi:10.3390/ijerph19106230 . . . **193**

Annina Ropponen, Mo Wang, Jurgita Narusyte, Karri Silventoinen, Petri Böckerman and Pia Svedberg
Sustainable Working Life in a Swedish Twin Cohort—A Definition Paper with Sample Overview
Reprinted from: *Int. J. Environ. Res. Public Health* **2021**, *18*, 5817, doi:10.3390/ijerph18115817 . . . **207**

Ella Näsi, Mikko Perkiö and Lauri Kokkinen
The Complexity of Decreased Work Ability: Individuals' Perceptions of Factors That Affect Returning to Work after Sickness Absence
Reprinted from: *Int. J. Environ. Res. Public Health* **2021**, *19*, 113, doi:10.3390/ijerph19010113 . . . **223**

Jianwei Deng, Jiahao Liu, Wenhao Deng, Tianan Yang and Zhezhe Duan
Redefinition and Measurement Dimensions of Sustainable Employability Based on the swAge-Model
Reprinted from: *Int. J. Environ. Res. Public Health* **2021**, *18*, 13230, doi:10.3390/ijerph182413230 . **245**

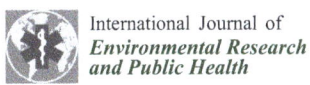

Editorial

Sustainable Healthy Working Life for All Ages—Work Environment, Age Management and Employability

Kerstin Nilsson [1,2,*], Clas-Håkan Nygård [3], Tove Midtsundstad [4], Peter Lundqvist [5] and Joanne Crawford [6]

1. Division of Occupational and Environmental Medicine, Lund University, 221 00 Lund, Sweden
2. Division of Public Health, Kristianstad University, 291 88 Kristianstad, Sweden
3. Department of Health Sciences, Faculty of Social Sciences, University of Tampere, 33014 Tampere, Finland
4. Fafo Institute for Labour and Social Research, 0608 Oslo, Norway
5. Department of People and Society, Swedish University of Agricultural Sciences, 230 53 Alnarp, Sweden
6. School of Health, Victoria University of Wellington, Easterfield Building, Kelburn Parade, Wellington 6140, New Zealand
* Correspondence: kerstin.nilsson@med.lu.se

Citation: Nilsson, K.; Nygård, C.-H.; Midtsundstad, T.; Lundqvist, P.; Crawford, J. Sustainable Healthy Working Life for All Ages—Work Environment, Age Management and Employability. *IJERPH* **2023**, *20*, 2712. https://doi.org/10.3390/ijerph20032712

Received: 10 January 2023
Accepted: 11 January 2023
Published: 3 February 2023

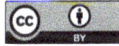

Copyright: © 2023 by the authors. Licensee MDPI, Basel, Switzerland. This article is an open access article distributed under the terms and conditions of the Creative Commons Attribution (CC BY) license (https://creativecommons.org/licenses/by/4.0/).

The proportion of elderly citizens is continuously increasing in most of the industrial world [1–3]. The current demographic trend is characterised by increased longevity and lower fertility rates, resulting in an increasingly ageing population. The retirement age in many countries is being postponed adapting the economic and budgetary implications of increased longevity to the new demographic distribution. Older people are encouraged to continue working and to participate in the labour force for as long as possible [1–3]. The demographic situation stresses the importance of factors that motivate older employees and self-employed individuals to keep working and maintain their employability until an older age, as well as encouraging the organisations and enterprises to care for their employees' employability until an age older than the current retirement age [4–7].

There are a lot of factors that influence risks and problems, as well as employability and a healthy and sustainable working life for all ages at the individual organisational/enterprise and society level. The complexity of these factors has been identified in research. To make this complexity more manageable and comprehensible, the SwAge model has been used to organize these complex factors contributing to a healthy and sustainable working life for all ages in nine different areas of impact and determination. There are nine determinant areas identified in the SwAge-model [4,5], which are: (1) self-rated health, diagnoses, functional diversity; (2) physical work environment; (3) mental work environment; (4) work schedule, work pace, time for recuperation; (5) personal finances, work ability, employability; (6) personal social environment and work–life balance; (7) work social environment, discrimination, leadership and age management; (8) motivation, stimulation and satisfaction with work tasks; (9) knowledge, skills, and competence (Figure 1). This Special Issue will contribute to the development of our theoretical and practical knowledge in the domains that influence people's working life.

This Special Issue aims to collect articles of high academic standard investigating the Sustainable Healthy Working Life for All Ages—Work Environment, Age Management and Employability. Numerous manuscripts were received, of which 13 papers passed the peer-review process and are presented here as reprints.

Conclusion of the new knowledge

This Special Issue includes investigations related to a sustainable working life.

A sustainable working life is hindered by the demographic development, which features more senior workers and the need to work until an older age. The aim of the qualitative study by Nilsson & Nilsson [8] was to investigate organisational measures and suggestions to promote and make improvements for a healthy and sustainable working life for all ages in an extended working life. Based on data from focus group interviews and individual interviews with 145 individuals, the study identifies several measures and actions that might increase employability: to promote a good physical and mental work environment; to promote personal financial and social security; to promote relations, social inclusion and social support in the work situation; and to promote creativity, knowledge development, and intrinsic work motivation. This concept is based on the spheres of determination in the theoretical SwAge-model (sustainable working life for all ages). The authors also present a tool for dialogue and discussion on the work situation and career development of the employee and argue that regular conversations, communication, and close dialogue are needed and are a prerequisite for good working conditions and a sustainable working environment, as well as to be able to manage employees and develop the organisation further. Managers' attitudes to senior workers are important for a healthy and sustainable working life that lasts to an older age. A study by Nilsson & Nilsson [9] therefore evaluated work life factors that managers in the Swedish municipality sector believe are crucial for their employees working or wanting to work until age 65 or older. Based on cross-sectional data from 249 managers, the authors find that more managers believe employees can work (79%) than they believe want to work (58%) until age 65 or older. From the managers' point of view, health, physical work environment, skills, and competence are the factors determining whether employees are able to work until age 65 or older, while insufficient social support at work and a lack of possibilities for relocations are factors that influence their willingness to work until age 65 or older. Hence, the authors concludes that supplementary strategies might be needed to contribute to employees being willing and able to participate in working life until an older age. Hovbrandt et al. [10] investigate the associations between different job types and social participation from a long-term perspective. Based on data from 1098 working respondents aged 55 at baseline and a 10-year follow-up when the respondents were retired, the analyses revealed that social participation varied by job type. Jobs with high decision latitude, as in active and relaxed jobs, seem to predict high social participation, even after cessation of employment. In addition, high social participation during working life is a predictor of high social participation from a long-term perspective, which also promotes healthy aging. Hence, a supportive work environment with possibilities for employees to participate in decision-making may support social participation both prior to as well as after retirement, and thus to healthy aging. A qualitative study by Sousa-Ribeirio et al. [11] conducted among older nurses (aged 55–65 years) aimed to study how they experienced their working life, especially their late career and retirement. The results showed that nurses planned to continue working until the age of 65 and beyond. When reflecting on their late-career decisions, nurses considered nine areas covering individual, work, and organizational factors as central to their ability and willingness to stay. Overall, the nurses had good health and were very satisfied and committed to their job and to the organization. They mentioned having both the professional and personal resources required to cope with the physical and mental job demands, which were perceived as motivational challenges, rather than hindrances. Jaldestadt et al. [12] examined retirement decisions among blue-collar workers in manufacturing across a multi-national company. Taking a systems-level approach, the study identified that at the macro level, national pension systems had an impact, as only one country allowed people to retire earlier and pensions were seen as tough. Factors that influenced early retirement decisions at the meso level were work organisation shift work; at the micro level, the primary concerns were physical work demands and psychosocial work environment and, at the individual level, workers' health and the meaningfulness of their work. At all levels, attitudes towards older workers were crucial in either prolonging work or increasing the risk of retirement. Suggestions from this work include ensuring managers are trained in age management, enabling tailored work, and helping older workers prepare for retirement.

The work environment in the education system is also important for a sustainable working life. School principals' work situation was investigated by two studies. The objective of the study by Nilsson et al. [13] was to increase the knowledge regarding school principals' work situations by examining the associations between various factors and the school principals' assessments of their ability or desire to work until the age of 65 or older. The results showed that about 83% of the school principals stated that they could work and about 50% stated that they wanted to work until 65 years of age and beyond. Their exhaustion symptoms and experiences of an excessive burden, as well as their experiences of support from the executive management in the performance of their managerial duties, were of primary importance for whether the school principals wanted to work until 65 years of age and beyond. The study strengthens the robustness of the theoretical SwAge model regarding the investigated factors related to determinant factors for a sustainable working life and as a basis for developing practical tools for increased employability for people of older ages. Arvidsson et al. [14] investigated to what extent various work environment factors and signs of exhaustion were associated with reported intentions to change workplace among principals working in compulsory schools. The patterns of intended and actual changes in the workplace across two years were described, together with associated changes in occupational factors and signs of exhaustion. Supportive management was associated with an intention to stay, while demanding role conflicts and the feeling of being squeezed between management and co-workers (buffer function) were associated with the intention to change workplace. The principals who intended to change their workplace reported more signs of exhaustion. To increase retention among principals, systematic efforts are needed at the national, municipal, and local level, in order to improve their working conditions. A study by Schön Persson et al. [15] explored prerequisites for flourishing workplace relationships in a municipal healthcare setting for older people. As part of this process, they explored the staff's suggestions as to how work relationships could be improved. Results showed that informal and formal meetings at work were shown to build positively perceived relationships. Suggestions for improving work relationships were also presented. This study contributes to workplace health promotion and has a salutogenic and participatory focus on how to explore workplace relationships as a resource. The flourishing concept shows how workplace relationships can be explored as prerequisites for workplace health promotion.

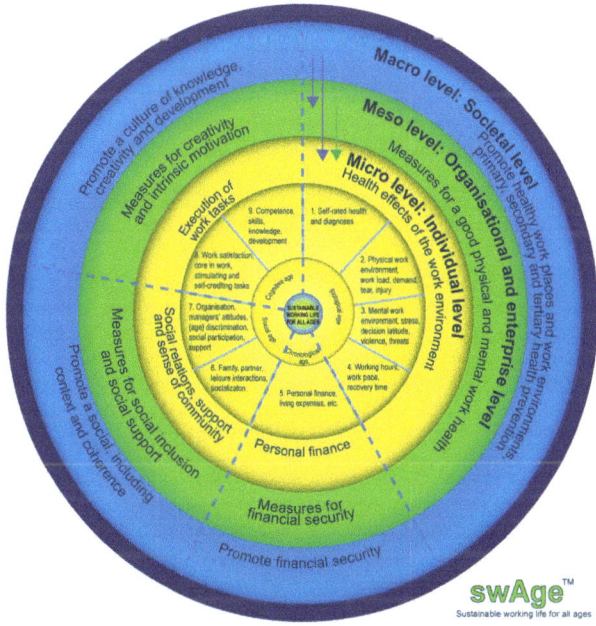

Figure 1. The SwAge-model.

A sustainable working life was stressed by the effects of the COVID-19 pandemic on working life and the work environment. Nagel and Nilsson [16] used a questionnaire to investigate the association between, and the effect of, different factors in nurses' work situations, organised based on the SwAge-model theories of a sustainable working life, associated with nurses' work-related mental health diagnoses, before and during the COVID-19 pandemic. The results showed that lack of joy in the daily work, an increased workload, and lack of support from co-workers had an increased association with work-related mental health diagnoses. Kyrönlahti et al. [17] examined the impact of home working on work ability in a sample of university workers during the COVID-19 pandemic. The study measured at three points after baseline measurements. The results identified that 75% of the sample had stable work ability; 18% of the sample had stable or improved work ability. Analysis identified that this improved work ability was associated with organisational support and significantly less reporting of work-related stress and musculoskeletal disorders. The final group of 8% of the sample had either poor or decreasing work ability. The analysis identified that decreasing work ability was associated with poor ergonomics at the home workplace, low levels of support from the organisation, high stress levels, and high levels of musculoskeletal pain. This highlights the factors that need to be implemented to support continued work ability for those required to work at home.

This Special Issue also includes systematic reviews and discussion papers regarding a sustainable working life. In their study, Ropponen et al. [18] updated information and explored definitions of "sustainable working life" via a systematic literature review and described working life trajectories based on the prevalence of sickness absence, disability pension, and unemployment in a Swedish twin cohort. They found 16 peer-reviewed articles published between 2007 and 2020. The most common definition of "sustainable working life" was the SwAge-model, which included a broad range of factors, e.g., health, physical/mental/psychosocial work environment, work motivation/satisfaction, and the family situation and leisure activities. The annual prevalence across years had a decreasing trend of unemployment over time stated Näsi et al., [19] whereas the prevalence of sickness absence had more variation, with a stable disability pension. They concluded that no consensus exists for a "sustainable working life," meriting further studies. The paper by Deng et al. [20] proposes the development of new ways of measuring sustainable employability. This paper argues for the SwAge-model. By including environmental factors in the measurement of sustainable employability, you can then take into account digital exclusion, intrinsic work value, movement capital, and perceived employability; you can then develop and test measures in this framework. While these are developing concepts, future work can test these factors on the employed and the unemployed.

Conflicts of Interest: The authors declare no conflict of interest.

References

1. OECD. Pensions at a Glance 2019. In *OECD and G20 Indicators*; OECD Publishing: Paris, France, 2019. [CrossRef]
2. WHO. *World Report on Ageing and Health*; World Health Organization: Geneva, Switzerland, 2017. Available online: http://www.who.int/ageing/publications/world-report-2015/en/ (accessed on 1 January 2023).
3. OECD. *Health at a Glance 2019: OECD Indicators*; OECD Publishing: Paris, France, 2019. [CrossRef]
4. Nilsson, K. Conceptualization of ageing in relation to factors of importance for extending working life—A review. *Scand. J. Public Health.* **2016**, *44*, 490–505. [CrossRef] [PubMed]
5. Nilsson, K. A sustainable working life for all ages—The swAge-model. *Appl. Ergon.* **2020**, *103082*, 1–27. Available online: https://www.sciencedirect.com/science/article/pii/S0003687018305313?dgcid=author (accessed on 1 January 2023). [CrossRef] [PubMed]
6. Fleuren, B.P.; de Grip, A.; Jansen, N.W.H.; Kant, I.; Zijlstra, F.R.H. Unshrouding the Sphere from Clouds: Towards a Comprehensive Conceptual Framework for Sustainable Employability. *Sustainability* **2020**, *12*, 6366. [CrossRef]
7. Van der Klink, J.J.L.; Bültmann, U.; Burdorf, A. Schaufeli WB. Zijlstra FRH. Abma FI. BRouwer, S. van der Wilt GJ. Sustainable employability—Definition, conceptualization, and implications: A perspective based on the capability approach. *Scand J. Work Environ. Health* **2016**, *42*, 71–79. [CrossRef] [PubMed]

8. Nilsson, K.; Nilsson, E. Organisational Measures and Strategies for a Healthy and Sustainable Extended Working Life and Employability—A Deductive Content Analysis with Data Including Employees, First Line Managers, Trade Union Representatives and HR-Practitioners. *Int. J. Environ. Res. Public Health* **2021**, *18*, 5626. [CrossRef] [PubMed]
9. Nilsson, K.; Nilsson, E. Can They Stay or Will They Go? A Cross Sectional Study of Managers' Attitudes towards Their Senior Employees. *Int. J. Environ. Res. Public Health* **2022**, *19*, 1057. [CrossRef] [PubMed]
10. Hovbrandt, P.; Östergren, P.-O.; Canivet, C.; Albin, M.; Carlsson, G.; Nilsson, K.; Håkansson, C. Psychosocial Working Conditions and Social Participation. A 10-Year Follow-Up of Senior Workers. *Int. J. Environ. Res. Public Health* **2021**, *18*, 9154. [CrossRef]
11. Sousa-Ribeiro, M.; Petra Lindfors, P.; Knudsen, K. Sustainable Working Life in Intensive Care: A Qualitative Study of Older Nurses. *Int. J. Environ. Res. Public Health* **2022**, *19*, 6130. [CrossRef] [PubMed]
12. Jaldestad, E.; Eriksson, A.; Blom, P.; Östlund, B. Factors Influencing Retirement Decisions among Blue-Collar Workers in a Global Manufacturing Company—Implications for Age Management from A System Perspective. *Int. J. Environ. Res. Public Health* **2021**, *18*, 10945. [CrossRef]
13. Nilsson, K.; Oudin, A.; Arvidsson, I.; Håkansson, C.; Österberg, K.; Leo, U.; Persson, R. School Principals' Work Participation in an Extended Working Life—Are They Able to, and Do They Want to? A Quantitative Study of the Work Situation. *Int. J. Environ. Res. Public Health* **2022**, *19*, 3983. [CrossRef]
14. Arvidsson, I.; Leo, U.; Oudin, A.; Nilsson, K.; Håkansson, C.; Österberg, K.; Persson, R. Should I Stay or Should I Go? Associations between Occupational Factors, Signs of Exhaustion, and the Intention to Change Workplace among Swedish Principals. *Int. J. Environ. Res. Public Health* **2021**, *18*, 5376. [CrossRef] [PubMed]
15. Schön Persson, S.; Blomqvist, K.; Nilsson Lindström, P. Meetings are an Important Prerequisite for Flourishing Workplace Relationships. *Int. J. Environ. Res. Public Health* **2021**, *18*, 8092. [CrossRef]
16. Nagel, C.; Nilsson, K. Nurses' Work-Related Mental Health in 2017 and 2020—A Comparative Follow-Up Study before and during the COVID-19 Pandemic. *Int. J. Environ. Res. Public Health* **2022**, *19*, 15569. [CrossRef]
17. Kyrönlahti, S.; Neupane, S. Nygård, C.-H.; Oakman, J.; Juutinen, S.; Mäkikangas, A. Perceived Work Ability during Enforced Working from Home Due to the COVID-19 Pandemic among Finnish Higher Educational Staff. *Int. J. Environ. Res. Public Health* **2022**, *19*, 6230. [CrossRef]
18. Ropponen, A.; Wang, M.; Narusyte, J.; Silventoinen, K.; Böckerman, P.; Svedberg, P. Sustainable Working Life in a Swedish Twin Cohort—A Definition Paper with Sample Overview. *Int. J. Environ. Res. Public Health* **2021**, *18*, 5817. [CrossRef]
19. Näsi, E.; Perkiö, M.; Kokkinen, L. The Complexity of Decreased Work Ability: Individuals' Perceptions of Factors That Affect Returning to Work after Sickness Absence. *Int. J. Environ. Res. Public Health* **2022**, *19*, 113. [CrossRef]
20. Deng, J.; Liu, J.; Deng, W.; Yang, T.; Duan, Z. Redefinition and Measurement Dimensions of Sustainable Employability Based on the swAge-Model. *Int. J. Environ. Res. Public Health* **2021**, *18*, 13230. [CrossRef] [PubMed]

Disclaimer/Publisher's Note: The statements, opinions and data contained in all publications are solely those of the individual author(s) and contributor(s) and not of MDPI and/or the editor(s). MDPI and/or the editor(s) disclaim responsibility for any injury to people or property resulting from any ideas, methods, instructions or products referred to in the content.

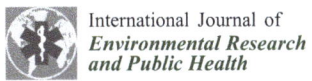

Article

Organisational Measures and Strategies for a Healthy and Sustainable Extended Working Life and Employability—A Deductive Content Analysis with Data Including Employees, First Line Managers, Trade Union Representatives and HR-Practitioners

Kerstin Nilsson [1,2,*] and Emma Nilsson [1]

[1] Division of Occupational and Environmental Medicine, Lund University, 223 81 Lund, Sweden; emma.nilsson.1672@med.lu.se
[2] Department of Public Health, Kristianstad University, 291 88 Kristianstad, Sweden
* Correspondence: kerstin.nilsson@med.lu.se

Citation: Nilsson, K.; Nilsson, E. Organisational Measures and Strategies for a Healthy and Sustainable Extended Working Life and Employability—A Deductive Content Analysis with Data Including Employees, First Line Managers, Trade Union Representatives and HR-Practitioners. *IJERPH* **2021**, *18*, 5626. https://doi.org/10.3390/ijerph18115626

Academic Editors: Paul B. Tchounwou and Albert Nienhaus

Received: 12 March 2021
Accepted: 18 May 2021
Published: 25 May 2021

Publisher's Note: MDPI stays neutral with regard to jurisdictional claims in published maps and institutional affiliations.

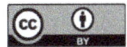

Copyright: © 2021 by the authors. Licensee MDPI, Basel, Switzerland. This article is an open access article distributed under the terms and conditions of the Creative Commons Attribution (CC BY) license (https:// creativecommons.org/licenses/by/ 4.0/).

Abstract: Due to the global demographic change many more people will need to work until an older age, and organisations and enterprises need to implement measures to facilitate an extended working life. The aim of this study was to investigate organisational measures and suggestions to promote and make improvements for a healthy and sustainable working life for all ages in an extended working life. This is a qualitative study, and the data were collected through both focus group interviews and individual interviews that included 145 participants. The study identified several suggestions for measures and actions to increase employability in the themes: to promote a good physical and mental work environment; to promote personal financial and social security; to promote relations, social inclusion and social support in the work situation; and to promote creativity, knowledge development and intrinsic work motivation, i.e., based on the spheres of determination in the theoretical swAge-model (sustainable working life for all ages). Based on the study results a tool for dialogue and discussion on employee work situation and career development was developed, and presented in this article. Regular conversations, communication and close dialogue are needed and are a prerequisite for good working conditions and a sustainable working environment, as well as to be able to manage employees and develop the organisation further. The identified measures need to be revisited regularly throughout the employees' entire working life to enable a healthy and sustainable working life for all ages.

Keywords: employability; ageing; senior; work environment; swAge-model; demography; retirement; global sustainable goal; public health; health promotion; health prevention; empowerment; occupational health care; psychosocial; working hours; recuperation; recovery; private finance; economy; work–life balance; manager; social support; discrimination; motivation; job satisfaction; competence; work ability; creativity; gerontology; older worker; extended working life; age management

1. Introduction

The average life expectancy is above 80 years of age in more than one in three countries on Earth [1–3]. In particular, the ageing of the population is expected to be very rapid in Greece, Korea, Poland, Portugal, Slovakia, Slovenia and Spain, while Japan and Italy are already among the countries with the oldest populations. The proportion of the population active in the labour force is ageing in many countries as well. The population of the labour force in the OECD countries (the Organization for Economic Co-operation and Development) is estimated to decrease by an average of ten percent in 2060 [2]. However, this varies between countries; in Greece, Japan, Korea, Latvia, Lithuania and Poland the proportion of working age population is estimated to decrease by 35 percent or more. With a greater number of pensioners that can no longer contribute to the proportion of hours worked in the countries' economies the average old-age to working-age demographic ratio, computed by keeping age thresholds constant, will result in an increased economic burden for the individuals included in the labour force. In 2080, the number of people older than 65 years of age is estimated to be 58 per 100 people of working age in the OECD countries. To exemplify, this means that 1.7 people of the estimated working age (20–64 years of age) must support each pensioner in a pension system where the retirement age is 65 years of age. This can be compared, for example, with the fact that in 1950 in Sweden the old age dependency burden was about six people of working age (20–64 years of age) who would support every pensioner aged 65 and older. At the same time, the individuals in the labour force must also contribute to other facets in society, such as the support of children and young people who have not yet entered the work force and the individuals aged 20–64 who are not part of working life for other reasons. Rapid ageing of the population contributes to increased pressure on the pension systems in various countries to deliver an adequate and financially sustainable pension system and pensions. The financial crises that have occurred in several countries have also contributed to high public debt and limited scope for manoeuvring the national economy. This increases the risk of widening gaps in society and between countries caused by changes in the working environment, low growth and low interest rates, leading to new challenges for already strained pension systems in several countries. However, low interest rates generate both challenges and opportunities since low interest rates also mean low interest rates for countries' public debt. In contrast, the challenges in ageing societies can also lead to increased benefit payments, which in turn can contribute to higher taxes, lower wage growth, higher unemployment as well as reduced pensions for pensioners. A greater number of people need to keep working to maintain the welfare system in a sustainable financial manner [1–3]. However, in society some hold the attitude that senior workers should quit working and give younger people and the unemployed a chance to enter the labour market. But since the labour market and economy are not static over time, a younger individual cannot automatically take over an older individual's work when the latter retires. With more people staying in the workforce until an older age, purchasing power and demand for goods and services are also expected to increase. Furthermore, a greater number of elderly people will probably increase the need for health promotion efforts and health care since health risks increase with the degeneration of organs and minds, and elderly people make up a large proportion of those in need of care, resulting in increasing the costs of health care in different countries.

To achieve sufficient financial sustainability and to maintain pensions, many countries are postponing the retirement age so that a greater number of people can work for longer and thereby contribute to the national economy. This is because the labour force largely finances the non-working and elderly in the population. However, postponing the retirement age has often proven to be one of the more controversial reforms in many countries, if measures are not promoted at the same time in working life in order to enable a sustainable working life for all ages and to maintain employability. Individuals' employability depends on, for example, their health, competences and ability to function at work but also perceived labour market values. The challenge is how to enable and incentivise people to remain in working life until an older age [1–3]. It is important that individuals maintain good employability until an older age to make it possible and effective to extend working life and postpone the pension age as a measure to promote a sound social economy and to support welfare systems in different countries [4–11].

Earlier studies and a theoretical model on sustainable working life for all ages and employability state nine determinant areas that influence whether people can and want to work and be part of the labour force until an older age, and to promote a healthy and sustainable working life for all ages [5–7,12–15]. The swAge model (sustainable working life for all ages) aims to visualise the complexity, organise and make the connections more understandable. The swAge model is a theoretical model consisting of nine different determinant areas that are significant to a sustainable working life for all ages and that relate to the four spheres of determination regarding employability, the possibility of being able to and willing to be part of working life and different ways of defining age:

A. The health effects of the work environment, which relate to biological age and ageing and include the following areas of determination: (1) Self-rated health, diagnoses and functional diversity, (2) physical work environment with unilateral movements, heavy lifting, risk of accidents, climate, chemical exposure and risk of contagion, (3) mental work environment with risk of stress and fatigue syndrome, threats and violence, and (4) working hours, work pace and the possibility of recuperation during and between work shifts for the employee. A sufficiently sound health is a prerequisite for employability and to be included in working life. However, professional work also affects the biological ageing, the physical and mental health and the need for recovery based on the physical and mental stresses, the wear and tear resulting from work, but also by the strengthening impacts of our work.

B. Economics and financial incentives, which relate to chronological ages' association to society's control of various financial carrots and sticks, for example, through the pension system and social insurance system. Economics and financial incentives include the following determinant area: (5) The personal financial situation's effects on individuals' needs and willingness to work. Professional work contributes to the upkeep of livelihood, food and living expenses, and is often the main source of funding for individuals' lives. Issues with employability due to ill health, lack of support and lack of skills risk causing exclusion from working life and a poorer financial situation for the individual, not least in bad times, e.g., through sick leave, unemployment and early retirement.

C. Relationships, social support and participation, i.e., attitudes in the social context in which the individual finds himself/herself, are considered as well as whether the individual feels included or excluded in the group and receives sufficient social support from the environment when needed, relate to social age and ageing during the life cycle and include the areas of determination: (6) The effects of the personal social environment, with family, friends and leisure context, and (7) the social work environment with leadership, discrimination and the significance of the employment relationship context for individuals' work. Humans are herd animals and working life can contribute to the experience of participation and inclusion in a group, as well as a sense of security. In spite of this, working life can also contribute to the experience of exclusion and neglect, or even discrimination. However, every employee also has a personal life and factors in the environment outside of work, their personal relationships also affect the individual's opportunities and willingness to work. This also affects the employability of the individual.

D. Execution of tasks and activities relate to cognitive age and ageing, intelligence ability, memory, learning and instrumental support, and include the following areas of determination: (8) Motivation, satisfaction and stimulation in the execution of work tasks, and (9) knowledge, competence and the importance of competence development for the individual's work. Working life is constantly changing and employees must be and remain employable in relation to the requirements of knowledge and skills in order to execute the activities and tasks that their work entails. The tasks and activities at work can be a source of motivation, stimulation and joy; we are challenged, learn new things and develop; however, it can also be a source of boredom, dissatisfaction and stagnation from which individuals want to make their exit as soon as possible.

However, the attitudes towards the extension of working life vary according to different levels in the societies. The organisations and enterprises need to implement sustainable measures and strategies to make an extended working life possible for a greater number of individuals [4–16]. It is therefore of great importance to discuss and explore organisational measures with the intent of supporting employability and enabling people to participate in working life for longer, since several countries and societies plan to postpone the retirement age. Hence, the demographic shift and its challenges and opportunities are of special interest to societies, and require the implementation of policies and measures by organisations and enterprises in order to help people stay healthy, active and employable until an older age. Based on prior knowledge and reviewing literature on the subject, there is a limited number of studies and information on how organisations and enterprises can and wish to implement measures and strategies to promote a healthy and sustainable extended working life.

The aim of this study was to investigate organisational measures and suggestions to make improvements for a healthy and sustainable working life for all ages, in an extended working life.

2. Method

The research question, i.e., to investigate organisational measures and suggestions to make improvements for a healthy and sustainable working life for all ages in an extended working life, is one of complexity and involves different contexts in the organisations and enterprises. Therefore, the research design was decided to be qualitative and the data were collected by means of interviews, in order to provide an in-depth investigation of the organisational measures and strategies that can promote a healthy and sustainable working life until an older age.

2.1. Study Population

To maximise the number of participants according to heterogeneity, the recruitment sites included individuals of different sex, different positions and professions, from work domains in both female- and male-dominated workplaces and both from the public as well as the private sector. The total study population consisted of 145 participants, including: first line managers, senior employees (55–72 years of age) in both blue- and white-collar professions, trade union workers, and human resources (HR) personnel (Table 1). The senior employee occupations were nurse, nurse assistant, physician, social worker, medical secretary, carpenter, construction worker, concrete worker, engineer, technician, mechanic, installer, electrician, salesperson and farmer.

Table 1. Distribution of the study population.

Participant Group	Number of Participants			Number of Focus Group Interviews within the Group	Number of Individual Interviews within the Group
	Total	Women	Men		
Employees 55–72 years	87	42	45	14	22
First line managers	45	26	19	8	12
Trade union employees (two of whom were also safety delegates)	6	2	4	3	
Human resources personnel	7	3	4	3	
Total	145	73	72	28	34

The participants were recruited in different ways during the years 2011–2020. A total of 105 of the informants were recruited through a snowball selection at organisations and enterprises. The HR managers at the organisations and enterprises were informed telephonically by the researcher and asked whether the organisation or enterprise was interested in participating in the study. The HR manager in turn directed the request for participation to the management in the organisation and asked for volunteers at different levels in the organisation who were interested in participating in the study. However, the sample of informants was voluntarily collected after the researchers invited the respective workplace to participate in the study and the organisation and the enterprise had accepted. A letter with information about the study was distributed through the contacts at the organisations and enterprises. The contact person informed people with the desired profile of participation and disseminated the information letter. The potential participants then gave their consent to participate or rejected participation. Additionally, 61 participants from an earlier work environment study conducted within the research group, were contacted by mail and received written information about this study with an invitation to participate in the study and to be interviewed. Twenty-two individuals responded and received further information on the study, were asked to participate and accepted and gave consent to participate. Twelve participants from an ongoing intervention study with managers were asked to participate and received further information on the study by phone and were asked to participate. Of those all accepted and gave consent to participate in the interview and in the study. The participants from the trade unions were invited in another way. The researcher e-mailed written information about the study directly to the trade union with an announcement and invitation for interested participants to volunteer for the study. The contact person informed people and disseminated the announcement and the invitation to participate in the study. The sample of voluntary potential participants was identified and subsequently gave their informed consent to participate in the interview and in the study.

2.2. Data Collection

The data were collected by focus group interviews and individual interviews during the years 2011–2020, using semi-structured interview guides with the same basic probing questions to invite the respondents to describe, based on their situation, e.g., what contributed to or would increase the possibility for them or their employees to be able and willing to work until an older age. Some of the collected data has previously been analysed for other purposes, i.e., why some had left working life early and others worked until older age, work motivation, the attitude between managers and employees, and the transfer of knowledge between generations [15–19].

Most of the data were collected through focus group interviews with 111 informants. Focus groups are suitable for obtaining knowledge about perceptions and beliefs regarding a specific topic [20,21]. The purpose of a focus group interview was to stimulate and start a dialogue between the participants to an open discussion within the scope of the study topics [22]. The focus group sessions included 2–7 participants from the same organisation or enterprise. The focus groups consisted of individuals in the distinct positions of first line managers and HR personnel; senior employees (55–72 years of age); and trade unions (Table 1). Two of the trade union workers (one man working at a construction enterprise and one woman working at a health care organisation) were also safety representatives, with the mandate of stopping work immediately if any risk or safety issues occurred in the workplace. The interviews were carried out in neutral and calm surroundings at the respective workplaces. Each interview session lasted $1\frac{1}{2}$–$2\frac{1}{2}$ h and all the discussions were audio recorded and transcribed, although the identities of the interviewees were kept anonymous. However, due to time schedule and logistic issues, the interviews with 34 of the informants were individual interviews. The latter were intended to provide a deeper understanding and knowledge about the individuals' own subjective experience, attitude and perspective of their situation [22]. Twenty-two of the individual interviews took place in the informants' own homes, more specifically at the dinner table in their kitchens. Twelve individual interviews were telephone interviews. Each interview session lasted $1\frac{1}{2}$–2 h and all the discussions were audio recorded and transcribed, but the identities of the interviewees were kept anonymous.

2.3. Analysis

All the interviews were analysed together through a text analysis method, deductive content analysis, to crystallise the relevant parts of the collected data. Deductive content analysis is a suitable choice when an existing theory involves the application of conceptual categories in the analysis of a new context [23]. Deduction can be said to constitute a conclusion from the general to the individual. The deductive content analysis increases the deductive approach by using theories and knowledge from previous research to refine, and possibly extend, a theoretical framework [24]. Additionally, in the content analysis any text that does not fit in the existing theory or the pre-defined categories is assigned new codes and is analysed to verify any new category; hence content analysis also follows an inductive approach.

The analysis in this study was performed in several steps. The analysis started by constructing a formative categorisation matrix with four pre-set categories based on theories and the determinant spheres in the swAge-model [5–7]. In the next step of the analysis, all the interviews were read together as one text to make sense of the whole. So as not to miss anything of importance this was done twice. In the third step of the analysis, specific interesting parts were marked in the text and colour-coded. In the fourth step of the analysis, those colour-coded text parts were put together and given codes. The codes were then grouped and categorised according to their meanings, similarities and differences and linked to the pre-determined categorisations in different themes and sub-themes showing the reappeared basic ideas typical of the participants' descriptions. The presentation of the findings in the following results section of this paper is based on the four pre-determined themes based on the determinant spheres of the theoretical swAge-model [5–7]. Some suggestions of measure activities are related to and supposed to solve issues associated to more than one theme context, to handle this they were sorted into more than one of the four main themes in the end.

3. Results

The result of measures and strategies to highlight in the organisational work, to make improvements for a sustainable extended working life for all ages, are presented under the following themes: Measures for the work environments health effects; Measures for personal financial security; Measures for relation, social support and inclusion; Measures for execution of work tasks.

3.1. Measures for the Work Environments Health Effects

3.1.1. Measures to Consider the Effect of Biological Ageing Related to Employees' Health and Risk Assessments in the Systematic Work Environment Management

The interviewees representing the various occupations participating in this study stated that the areas of importance in terms of decreasing the possibility of an extended working life were physical and mental health problems. The interviewees were of the opinion that a high level of physical and mental demands for many years in a problematic work environment often led to physical health problems, especially in the last year of employment. One participant from HR stated: *"I think that you can perceive a big difference after the age of 60. You lose very much then. Mostly physically. That you cannot be bothered, you are tired. It is hard to work in health care"*. A trade union representative from the construction industry described the health problems associated with increasing age: *"There are many employees who can take two painkillers, both at lunch and breakfast. However, most people go into the bathroom and take them, since most people do not want to show it. I dare not even speculate how large the use of painkillers is. It can range from 50% to 10%. If I must be honest it is very extensive"*. Many interviewees stated the importance of an action plan for organisational measures to examine work environmental risks, take actions and follow up on the measures and actions. A manager stated: *"We need to work with accident prevention all the time, such as to always wear protective goggles, gloves and the like. Such things have of course been an improvement to minor accidents today. But then the second thing, the long process where you work every day in a physically demanding occupation and eventually you will become physically worn out in old age. We have not really come up with how to solve this"*. However, there are actually systems on how to continuously manage these work environmental problems in the day-to-day work. One manager stated: *"If it makes a real impact to work with systematic work environment* management then it is possible that more people can continue to work until an older age, I'd say". Interviewees stated that it is important to systematically work towards making the physical and mental work environments healthier and more sustainable for employees of all ages.

3.1.2. An Organisational Culture That Promotes the Use of Ergonomic Aids

Many of the senior employees in physically demanding work environments described it as problematic to keep working due to the physical work environment. The organisational culture regarding the use of ergonomically correct positions, aids and equipment should be encouraged with the aim of improving physical work health. One manager stated: *"Younger ones just go for it. They hear well, see well and feel good. But when they are around 60 they have tinnitus for not using hearing protections when they were younger. Back pain all the time because when you were 25 you could lift 60 kg, no problem. The back creaked a bit, but it went well. Then it is too late"*. One trade union worker said: *"We have this macho culture: Just go for it!! I have been using the machine every day, year in and year out for ten years and it went well. I cannot feel my arms today, but it does not matter, just go for it. Then the younger guys think: If the senior employees work like that, I should not be weaker. Then they learn the wrong way and the problem continues"*. A manager in health care stated that it was obvious that the use of ergonomic aids can protect and enable the patients, but sometimes the employees were not diligent about protecting themselves and would take their own safety and health for granted. Another manager stated: *"It is important to inform more regularly about accessibility and protection equipment. That it is included as a requirement. We often focus on the patient, when the patient needs an aid we help them so that they understand how to use it. But it is also about our own working environment and health"*. The interviewees stated that it was important to instil a positive attitude to provide a good and safe work environment in the entire organisation. Furthermore, it is not only the managers, HR personnel and trade union representatives who need to be aware of this, the employees must also be educated and take responsibility regarding their own safety so as to enjoy a good work environment.

3.1.3. Rotation, Variation and Change of Duties to Reduce Physical and Mental Demands

Rotation between different work tasks was stated by the interviewees as a measure to reduce health problems from demanding work tasks and situations at work. One senior employee said: *"I am in favour of rotation between different tasks, and I talk from my own experience. You lay slabs and lift the stone, every day. You might lift 7–8 tons a day with your body. It takes a devilish toll on the body, this monotony. Instead, it is better to rotate a little and switch tasks within the work team. It's about planning, to ensure that the conditions to be able to rotate exist"*. One manager said: *"You need to modify the task. When you come up to 60 years, you can't roof a house, you can't make roof trusses. Then there are other tasks. One must plan and structure the workplace. Can we put him in charge of small tasks, or shall we let him handle the logistics?"* To rotate could on the other hand increase fear, insecurity and the experience of more stress, if the senior employee was not used to rotate work tasks but only worked with the same tasks and in the same place. One manager described: *"When I started to work here I introduced the need to rotate on all workstations. Then there were older employees who had difficulty opening the computer at the new table, even though it was exactly the same kind of computer that also looked exactly the same. It was not possible to understand how to do it when they left the table where they had stood for 20 years. Some could not even enter their username. However, after a while it was no problem"*. To rotate work tasks in the workplace was also described as both a barrier and a solution to reduce problems in the mental work environment. It could in some aspects be perceived as stressful to move from a familiar work spot and work tasks to an unknown area, but on the other hand it could be a solution and a possibility to reduce stress and increase the understanding of the total organisation and towards each others' work tasks. A senior employee stated: *"It would have been good to start from the beginning and to really get around. Many of the staff have to move. They have been in one place for 30–40 years. They do not know what it looks like at their neighbouring colleague basically. It is very good to walk around and see what others have it like to appreciate their own, and maybe come back again"*. In other words, a regular rotation between different work tasks seems to be a good measure to promote a healthy and sustainable working life for all ages.

3.1.4. Communication, Information and Participation to Reduce Work Stress

The interviewees described a problematic work situation as when there was a great demand on them to execute their work tasks, even though there were a lot of factors they could not control in their work situation, affecting their ability to execute their work tasks. Additionally, there was organisational development underway that the employees did not understand or perceive as having any possible objective or benefits based on their own position within the organisation. A trade union representative said: *"There are so many reorganisations and we face a lot of new systems. Our members become much stressed if they do not understand why there must be a change or because of the novelty of it. You become frightened and tired of all the new systems [. . .] it could be new and changed monitoring systems, payroll systems, personnel systems, financial systems, planning systems. We need to receive information and be included in what and why these systems are needed. If they are needed"*. The interviewees described that better sharing of information and worker participation in organisational development and changes in work tasks could increase their understanding of what was going on within the organisation. Therefore, they suggested more accurately targeted information about, and participation in, organisational development and work task changes as important measures that could balance the sense of reward and decrease work stress. The senior employees also described how they as employees want to experience a sense of reward for the effort they put into their work tasks. The older employees described how work tasks would not bring fulfilment due to circumstances beyond the employees' control, and that words and actions of appreciation from their managers and organisations could improve their situation, by helping them to better manage their experiences at work and reduce their stress levels.

3.1.5. Reduce Violence and Threats in the Work Situation and Brief Each Other in Support Groups

There are times in the work situation circumstances that can include threats and violence. A senior employee in a health care organisation described: *"There are some patients who are confused and demented and who can become violent and fight. There are also patients with frontal lobe dementia who become completely personality-changed and pull staff down in bed and try to make sexual encounters. They can't help it, but it is our work environment and it is stressful to face this every day and having to defend ourselves"*. Undesirable situations that include violence and threats must be managed properly and reduced so that a higher number of employees of all ages can keep working. An important measure described by the informants was to hold briefing sessions regularly with each other to talk about possible, perceived and experienced situations and issues in the work situation including threats and violence. The possibility of talking about these situations in support groups and with supervisors was described as a much-needed measure to reduce stress and anxiety regarding new situations including threats and violence and on how to handle them.

3.1.6. Work Schedules

Measures regarding the working hours appeared to be important to make working life more sustainable for all ages. An HR practitioner said: *"Many senior employees like to reduce the number of work hours, have shorter work shifts and more flexible working hours to cope and have time to recover"*. Flexibility in the work schedule was stated as important for senior employees' revitalisation and to be able to work until an older age. A manager defined it: *"The possibility of having a little bit more flexible working hours is one of the most important factors for the possibility to keep working in an extended working life, as I perceive it"*. However, many stated that flexibility in working hours was not feasible in many organisations since it would impact the production line. In contrast, others stated that this was not true, because it could be done with better planning and organisation of the work tasks. Another HR practitioner said: *"Many senior people prefer to work fewer hours because they are unable to cope.*

I think younger people would rather work a very long shift and then have time off for two days in the middle of the week. When you are older, you have changed that view and gained the insight to work more often but shorter work shifts to cope. We especially saw this in the workplaces where there was an opportunity to influence working hours and schedule. There you could see that younger people worked much longer work shifts but more rarely. Older people worked more often, though had shorter work shifts, preferably five-hour work shifts". A trade union worker in a construction enterprise stated that many senior employees no longer had the strength needed to work full time and said: *"Those who have come up to 60 years and have physical problems could work part-time, and go down to, say, 75%. If the senior employee had reduced their working hours, by working fewer hours every day, for example from 09:00 to 14:00 (5-h work days), it would not affect the work team and production negatively at all [. . .] In more project-oriented workplaces, for example, the staff could work for three months and then have time off for three months".* However, the trade union worker also mentioned that if senior employees decreased their working hours their pension could be negatively affected, and therefore many senior employees do not consider reduced working hours as a possible choice to have a more sustainable working life.

3.1.7. Work Pace

The senior employees were described to be just as exposed to the demanding mental work environmental problems as the younger ones, i.e., sometimes they experience an insufficient influence of their own decisions and control on their work situation, and some run the risk of being subjected to threats and violence. However, it seems to be especially stressful for the ageing employees with high expectations on their productivity from enterprise/organisation, managers and co-workers when they, due to their biological ageing and health problems, cannot be as productive as before, in some work tasks. A trade union worker described this: *"There are difficulties in the work team when older employees are worn out and cannot perform as well as the other ones. Not to be performing fully anymore and risking dragging down the contracted work in the work team is stressful for the older employees".* The work pace was mentioned when it comes to improving measures for senior employees. One manager stated: *"I feel that those who are 50, 55+, they cannot work at the same work pace of those who are 25–30 years old".* Additionally, many of the senior employees stated that they experienced that work was more stressful these days and that they could not work at such a stressful work pace. Instead, they wanted fewer work tasks; to have the possibility of focusing on fewer tasks, but performing better. Another important measure described by some interviewees was to adapt the work content to the scope of working hours, so that those who work part-time were not expected to perform full-time work in fewer hours. Too many work tasks increase the work pace because it also takes time to switch between different work tasks. A senior employee in elderly care said: *"There are so many work tasks around that have nothing to do with care work at all, and that is stressful. We must document a lot, write a lot and keep contact with relatives. They pull at you from all directions. We must bake, we must get food ready, we must organise activities to the accommodation, and we must pack up diapers. We have to do so many different things, the patients have to wait. The patients complain about that, and then you get yelled at by the manager for not having time to do the care work".* The interviewees stated the importance of good quality in the execution of work tasks, and not to focus as much on quantity. The interviewees described that a measure to achieve this was to have fewer tasks and work at a more comfortable work pace where they could be more considerate and creative in executing their work.

3.1.8. Importance of Self-Care for a Sound (Occupational) Health

The interviewees stated that healthy ageing is about taking care of themselves and their own health. However, it was stated that this was easier with support from the work situation and the organisation. Some interviewees talked about the fact that individual employees have a responsibility of taking care of and managing their own health, but that the prevailing attitude, for example in the workplace, contributed to whether they could and whether they took this responsibility. A manager said: *"There must be a genuine interest in taking care of oneself, because it is not just about exercising, it is also about eating right and sleeping properly and all those other things that affect how we feel in everyday life"*. A senior employee said: *"To get exercise, eat, sleep, and all that influences how we feel in our daily lives is also a part of the working environment"*. Some interviewees spoke of the significance of physical exercise, but also the importance of a healthy diet. The interviewees also stated that people had better eating habits before, when it was possible to get coupons from the enterprise or organisation to exchange for lunch. These days this counts as an income benefit in Sweden and results in increased taxes for the employees, therefore no enterprise or organisation has this system anymore. However, there was a greater concern about the younger generations' possibility of having a sound health. The managers and senior employees pointed out that the younger employees preferred eating fast food instead of maintaining a healthy diet. A manager said: *"We have many people who have a Coca Cola and a chocolate bun for breakfast. I think it would be a good measure to treat the staff to a good breakfast when they come here, so they have the energy to work"*. The manager stated that the young employees of today will be elderly employees one day, and that if they do not change their diet, they will have serious health problems when they get older. The interviewees discussed that physical activity was very important to keep mentally and physically healthy. An occupational health care professional said: *"Fitness in some way is essential for everyone to maintain a sound physical and mental health regardless of desk work or physically demanding work. Exercise either at work or sponsored by work. Exercise at work could be mandatory, not only for police officers and firefighters as it contributes to higher productivity and less sick absence among employees"*. A manager said: *"I don't think there's a chance that you will be able to work until an older age unless you take care of yourself and your body. It can well be stated that a lot of our employees have physically demanding jobs in health care, but who also miscalculate their body if you look at how they maintain their physical exercise and their diet. It's not good. We do what we can there. We provide information, offer lunch and occupational health care and tell about the importance of physical exercise, mental recuperation and a well-balanced diet. That you should exercise even if you have a physically demanding occupation"*. Some interviewees discussed whether measures to develop an organisational culture that promotes self-care and a healthy lifestyle could be a step on the way to a more healthy and sustainable working life, or if it was to violate employee integrity and risk of shaming people.

3.1.9. Physical Activity, 'Maintenance of Functions', to Sustain and Improve Mental and Physical Good Health

Physical activity was stated as an important measure to sustain and improve sound health, both mentally and physically. Organisational support for making it possible and, in addition, compulsory, to exercise at work and as a part of the work schedule, was a measure supposed to support a more sustainable working life until an older age. An HR practitioner stated: *"I come from the police department and also work quite a lot with firefighters. In those occupations physical exercise and maintenance of their body during working hours is mandatory, to score their tests and keep up good physical form in order to do a good job. But it's almost more tiring and demanding to work in health care. Health care professionals need to exercise as much as employees in the police department or fire brigade. It should be equivalent when you save people's lives. I think that all physically demanding service occupations need to get exercise at work, as part of the working hours. It should be a requirement, because it's a safety and work environment issue"*. A senior employee said: *"I think it would be good if they would put fitness exercise in the work schedule. I think many do not want to go away when they get home. They live far from the city where they work. But if they had one hour a week in their working hours I think, if you put it in, many would feel a lot better because of it, it is actually perceivable. We see it in our elderly patients' exercise and raising of their arms every now and then. Just doing that a couple of times a week makes them feel better. Why can't the staff do that, without having to do it in their own leisure time? We get older, as do our shoulders and arms, our bodies shrink, it's really important to exercise. I think most would agree if it was in the working schedule. Don't you too? Now that us co-workers exercise for a few hours, and gently move our arms and shoulders, nothing unusual really, so many have felt good because of it"*.

Another senior employee described that physical activity was not only important for the body but also for the mind. She said: *"You become more alert if you exercise at all, because I know some girls who have started and never done any before, and they say that they are very energetic: I can do more than I did before! And I actually think that you do"*. Physical activity and exercise were highlighted by the interviewees as an important measure to promote a healthy and sustainable working life for all ages.

3.1.10. Occupational Health Services Support to Prevent Work Environment Problems and Increase Good Occupational Health

The interviewees stated the need for measures to make working life healthier for all ages and to make working life more sustainable. Some managers and HR practitioners emphasised the need to place the employees' wellbeing in their systematic work environmental management to handle an extended working life. Someone said: *"When we do our safety rounds and look over tools, activities, etc. we can also look over the employees' physical and mental capacity to work"*. However, the HR practitioners and managers further stated the need for professional help to decide on and implement the measures. An HR practitioner said: *"I think we need to take more action when I see the injuries that employees have today. This will be intensified if we do not begin to take measures in the working environment and work situation now. Measures must be reasonable in some way, if we expect that elderly employees will perform and deliver until an older age in the same way. Perhaps measures for physiotherapeutic rehabilitation. It is not only the somatic part. It is so easy to decide on and take physical action. But it can also be mental. It should not be forgotten. This second part is more difficult to work with. We have occupational health services that we can turn to for help with it, but maybe we also should have something in the administration that we can turn to"*. As the HR practitioner described, the managers have many tasks and responsibilities and they cannot be experts in every field. Therefore, they need to include other professionals and experts to take care of some of the measures in order to make the work situation healthy and sustainable for employees belonging to different age groups.

3.1.11. Summary about Work Environments Health Effects

The participating interviewees stated that an awareness of employees' ageing in their systematic work environment control management and strategy in the daily work at the organisation or enterprise was an important strategy for sustainable working to an older age, i.e., an awareness of ageing in the investigation of working conditions; in the assessing of risks; in the development of an action plan, and when to take action; as well as an awareness of ageing in the follow up of the results. Other measures to promote a good and healthy work environment that supports health and wellbeing, and are of importance for a sustainable working life until an older age, were: an organisational culture that promotes the use of ergonomic aids and tools; rotation and change of work tasks to reduce physical wear; physical activity to maintain bodily functions and keep mentally and physically fit; the importance of a healthy diet for sound (occupational) health; and occupational health care support to promote health and prevent physical and mental injury, illness and stress.

3.2. Measures for Personal Financial Security

3.2.1. Salary and Financial Benefits

One reason to work is to receive salary to finance one´s life. When we asked the senior employees about their reasons to keep working in an extended working life some stated: *"For me it's a financial issue. I am not hypocritical about that"*. A trade union representative said: *"When you work you have reasonably good finances. But, on the other hand, you have less leisure time to do activities than someone in retirement. As a pensioner you will have to live with less money, but much more time to do what you want. It's a balance. When can I leave (for retirement)?"*

The changes in salary and financial benefits are measures that can work both as a carrot and stick for a longer working life.

3.2.2. Measures in the Organisations and Enterprises Work Environment to Promote Continuous Employability

Some interviewees distinguish the need for measures to promote continuous employability, so that senior employees can provide for themselves through continuing to work until an older age. A necessity is that the employee's health is sufficient to work, to be able to participate in working life and to receive a salary. A manager stated: *"Elderly people who are worn out and have a sore neck and shoulders, they get a medical certificate that they cannot lift more than 10 kg. But then we say to that person that we do not have any tasks for them. Because we have not any work tasks where you do not have to lift at least 10 kg. So then there is no possibility of re-employment after their injury and sick absence"*. The interviewees stated that work environment security to reduce risks of occupational diseases, injury, sick absence and disability pension were important for the individual employee's employability and personal finances. A manager said: *"20 years ago, people were unable to work until retirement age in this profession. Because back then you did not have the tools and you did not have the working environment of today. But even today, some are worn out but have to suck it up and work because they have no choice. Otherwise they will have too low pensions and have financial problems"*. Some interviewees stated that the organisations and enterprises were responsible for the working environment, that when the organisation or enterprise chooses not to provide safety aids or tools or does not provide enough people for an activity, they should consider the long-term cost of this since it can cause sickness absence and disability benefits in the long run. A trade union representative said: *"In large workplaces, it is easier to provide more people and protection equipment than in a place where we are two employees, because the price is so bad, we have not considered the cost of that. So, in those workplaces you have to work harder than one would have thought. We also have some smaller workplaces in facility work where we do not have access to the work protection equipment one would need at all times. It is often like that. What to say of the rules of preparation, it is usually included in larger projects, you need this and that, and then it is part of the offer and price, etc. That is where the safety representative should object"*. The interviewees regarded work environment safety representatives at the workplaces and their mandate to stop work if there are any health risks present as an important measure to reduce risks in the workplace that could affect the employees' health, continuous employability and by extension, employee salary and personal finances. Some interviewees, mostly managers, highlighted the importance of safety protection, and how injury and sick absence can cause economic stress for the organisation or enterprise.

3.2.3. Measures to Change the Organisational Culture, to Promote and Increase Responsibility and Employees' Use of Safety Equipment and Assistive Technology in the Workplace

The organisational culture influences how one perceives one's work, tasks, as well as the use of aids, tools etc. Therefore, the organisational culture should promote a responsible and sustainable working life, to prevent employees being worn out physically or mentally. It is also important for the staff that the management shows appreciation for their efforts. A trade union representative stated the importance of taking measures to change the organisational culture: *"We have this macho culture; just go for it! I have used that machine every day for years and years, ten years and it went well. However, I have numbness in my arms today, though that does not matter, just go for it! Now I generalise a little. When the young guys learn, the frail Bengtsson can do it, he is able to, and so am I! Then, for example, we have a young guy today, he is not yet 30 years of age, who must have cortisone pumped into his arms. Not yet 30 years old! It is too weird that it should be like that [. . .] they are 30–35 years old and are starting to have physical problems with knees, back and legs already, and they may not have worked for more than 15 years. After all, it's scary that many of the younger ones can't handle it"*. Many interviewees working in physically demanding workplaces expressed the need to change the organisational culture, to use the aids and tools that were available to avoid being exhausted and unable to work, and subsequently risk financial consequences due to lack of employability. A senior employee who expressed concerns about the organisational culture said: *"Younger people go on just like anyone else. You hear well, look good and feel good. But around 60 you get tinnitus for not using hearing protection, so it is, sore back because when you were 25 you lifted 60 kilos no problem, it creaked a little, but it went well. That's what it is like. Then it's too late"*. Opportunities to maintain employability until an older age and to counteract "macho attitudes" were described as conscious efforts aimed at creating a more favourable organisational culture. The role of the organisational culture in employability at an older age was expressed, above all, by managers in the heavy construction industry. A manager stated: *"There's a huge focus on working environment, actually. [. . .] It was stated by the executive group management that it is not about money, it is about wellbeing at the employees construction site"*. A manager stated that acute injuries were reduced with protection equipment, but that becoming physically worn out seems more difficult to combat using physical means: *"Now we have introduced to always use protection goggles, gloves and the like. Such things have been an improvement to minor accidents today of course. But then in the long run, when you work in a physically demanding profession, you will get worn out eventually"*. Rotation between different work tasks was one measure stated by the informants to reduce health problems in a working environment with heavy physical demands.

3.2.4. Measures to Promote and Increase Employability through Continuous Competence Development

To execute work tasks and activities the employees need appropriate knowledge and competence. Many of the interviewees stated the need for continuous knowledge and competence development for the employees to stay employable. However, some managers, and some senior employees, stated that some of the senior employees do not want to continue developing their knowledge and learn new things. Most organisations and enterprises must undergo continuous development due to the ongoing change in the world and societal circumstances. If an employee does not have the right competence and know-how required for their work tasks, they are not employable. A manager stated: *"When there is change in the organisation, which of course it happens for a bit every now and then, if the employee's competence does not fit the new tasks, they should be placed somewhere else. Then we try to get these employees other tasks and locations. We also need to look at what they bring in competence. Sometimes a senior employee no longer has the right skills and training. They are not as employable anymore"*. Other interviewees stated that with a broad competence and/or special competence it was easier for the employee to change work tasks, workplace or occupation if health issues forced them to do so. The participating interviewees stated that it was of great importance to take measures to promote a continuous improvement of competence, personal development and learning of new skills in order to maintain employees' continuous employability, and in the long term, personal financial security though the possibility to obtain salary from work.

3.2.5. Summary about Personal Financial Security

The interviewees stated that measures to promote personal financial security for senior employees were important to secure their continuous employability. Therefore, measures to ensure work environment security, risk assessment and reduction of work injuries are needed to reduce the risks of health impacts, so that employees can manage an entire working life and not be worn out prematurely and subsequently forced out of working life with less financial benefits through long-term sick leave, disability pension, unemployment or premature retirement. Furthermore, continuous competence development is key, so that senior employees do not risk being laid off due to lack of fitting tasks to workers because their competence is obsolete, or they lack the skills needed and therefore cannot be relocated with continued employability and provide for themselves by participating in working life. Some interviewees also stated the need for a reasonable and sufficient salary regardless of age.

3.3. Measures to Promote Relations, Social Support and Inclusion

3.3.1. Measures to Promote Work–Life Participation by Balancing Working Life and Leisure Time

Employees have a personal life outside their work. The interviewees describe a need for measures in the work situation that utilise individual needs, participation and activities with family, leisure time and hobbies. Many of the senior employees stated that they were much more tired these days. This fatigue affected their leisure time, because they had to prioritise rest and recuperation when they did not work. A senior employee said: *"In the evening when I came home, I did not have the energy to start doing fun things [. . .] I have way too little recuperation. I got a telling-off from my brother last summer; he said that I never call and never come to visit. I replied that I do not have the energy. After work I go home, cook, eat, sit on the couch and then I go to bed. / . . . / Over the years, I feel that the balance has got worse and worse [. . .] We have a little cabin in Falkenberg where we would like to spend some time . . . But we can't, because I don't have time . . . I don't have time to do anything at home"*. Being too exhausted to take part in leisure activities and exercise could cause feelings of embarrassment. A senior employee said: *"It is like you said previously, I am so tired. I am almost ashamed sometimes that I don't have the energy to do anything, anything, other than work and sit in front of the TV. It is like that unless I am off for the whole weekend or something. I don't really do anything during the weeks other than work. It almost feels a little bit embarrassing"*. Many of the interviewed senior employees stated the need for measures to promote senior employees' work schedules and working hours that, other than work, address the need for the individual's participation in a personal social environment, leisure activities, family, hobbies and relaxation. Many state that they would prefer to leave working life due to the lack of content in life besides work, and to have a better possibility of living a full life.

3.3.2. Measures to Promote Social Inclusion in a Team to Increase Participation and Community

The sense of community in the workplace was described as important to create a sustainable extended working life. Difficulties arose if the senior employees sensed feeling like outsiders in their former work team, in which case they would not want to extend their working lives. A trade union worker said: *"There are no guidelines in the enterprise generally saying that when a skilled employee, coming up to 63, 64 years of age, then it should be done like this. They leave it to the team to redistribute responsibilities. There will be an outcry: we should not have him in our work team, because he is worn out! He cannot perform piece work! Actually, piece work is an issue for senior employees"*. All the interviewees stated the importance of the work social environment and measures to promote inclusion of every individual in a reliable team. To be a part of a social group was stated as important to increase the willingness to keep working in an extended working life. An HR practitioner stated: *"Those who appreciate the social life in their work situation and who have a large social network at work tend to work for quite some time"*. A senior employee said: *"I get on well at this job and it feels good. I meet many nice colleagues and managers who appreciate the effort, so there is no hard consideration to keep working"*.

Another senior employee said: *"One thing that makes you want to come here and work is that you have a lot of friends and acquaintances. People you meet every day, talk and hang out with"*. An organisational culture with sustainable values allows customisation of the work situation. The sense of participating in something larger than oneself and working with colleagues were stated as important factors to keep working in an extended working life.

3.3.3. Measures to Increase the Senior Employees' Status in an Occupation and a Work Team

The interviewees describe that it is key to feel that work tasks and activities are perceived as important and needed for the productivity and the organisation. Having appropriate resources and equipment to execute the work tasks was seen as important in order to experience appreciation from the organisation and the manager. Some production and professional groups included in the study had received new work uniforms and were offered training days, which assisted in raising the status and value of the employees to the organisation. A senior employee describes: *"It was Anna (a manager) who introduced it. She cared a lot about raising the status of their careers. So they got uniforms that say 'Cleaning Department' on them, and they all got training. A whole week of training. It cost a lot of money, but I think it made them feel more appreciated"*. However, the participants described that male-dominated occupations and work tasks have a higher status within the organisation and are more appreciated than female dominated occupations. A participant stated: *"Men have higher status in organisations. All who needed got work uniforms that were paid for by the organisation, and they do not have to take them home to wash themselves. They have full time work, and also have a higher salary for the same work tasks"*. Some participants implied that this difference in status was part of the fact that more women left working life earlier than men. They stated it as an important measure to promote and increase the status of female-dominated occupations and work tasks to increase their willingness to remain in an extended working life.

3.3.4. Social Support to Promote and Increase the Senior Employees' Self-Esteem in the Organisation

Social support was described as a measure to increase the older employees' willingness to stay in working life for longer. One manager stated that many senior employees had to change their own self-image by themselves too, and said: *"It is often the general idea in society that individuals are not interested in the labour market when they are over 55. This is in many people's heads. If you do not believe in yourself then it will be tough"*. Another manager said: *"I have employees who basically have the same chronological age, but where one has decided to work until 67 and the other to work until 65. I think many start to dip down when they begin to see the end of working life in any way. Then, it is a lot about motivation, and I discovered that it determines quite a lot and that's pretty much about it. Attitude and motivation affect a lot"*. Some interviewees stated that because of old age, health problems or personality, some employees do not want to be in the front line. They want to take it easy, have enough time to recover and do a good job at their own pace. Therefore, a means to keep a larger number of senior employees within the organisation until an older age was to make it possible to have different positions based on the senior employees' own needs. However, they need to have the ability to know that they are good enough and to feel included in the social participation despite not being able to keep up with a fast work pace. A manager said that they have made agreements within the work team to make it possible for everyone to get best, or at least good enough, fitted tasks: *"There was an agreement and this elderly nurse has since then expressed that she feels very calmed by it. She does a satisfactory job, but she does not need to do this to be in the front line. [. . .] She avoided the stress, she has expressed that; now I know what I should do, I will do what I must. For it is not fair that one should leave a long working life with a sense of failure; I'm not good enough. Then it is better to have taken that into consideration"*. Measures to promote and increase an employee's self-esteem in the organisation, irrespective of the employee being the most productive worker or not, were said to be important in remaining in an extended working life.

3.3.5. Measures to Promote and Increase the Attitude of Employees as a Productivity Investment

The interviewees stated that it was an important measure to feel included in a social group and to be seen as a unique individual to make work–life more sustainable until an older age.

All the respondents stated the importance of different age groups at the workplace because it takes time to build experience from life. One of the trade union workers said: *"It takes such a long time to build up experience that some older key people are worth gold to the organisation"*. Senior employees were described as a resource offering valuable assets for organisations and companies. Measures to take care of and promote the senior employees' experience-based knowledge were needed both for the acknowledgement of the senior employees and for the prosperity of the organisation. Some managers described that they included senior employees in development meetings for the business and new projects even though the employees were older and did not have much time left before retirement. A manager stated: *"It is very valuable to have a senior employee in the production and in the work team, they know what to do and have been through most problems so they keep calm in the most difficult and problematic situations"*. Having mixed age groups strengthens creativity, growth and flourishing because experience and knowledge meet and can be exchanged. To highlight and promote the senior employees' value to the work team and the production was described as an important measure in the quest for creating a healthy and sustainable extended working life. Some of the respondents also described how customers and patients who themselves were elderly preferred to turn to senior employees with their requests. This is probably because they perceived it to be easier to meet in a common reference framework and historic familiarity with someone in the same age group that facilitates the communication.

3.3.6. Measures and Actions to Decrease Negative Attitudes and (Age) Discrimination

Managers, HR practitioners, trade union representatives and senior employees stated that it was important not to generalise, not to hold stereotypes that all senior employees are the same and take actions and measures to eliminate negative attitudes toward ageing, victimisation and age discrimination because of effects on work ability related to biological and cognitive ageing. The attitude towards senior employees held by managers, co-workers and organisations influences the senior employees' experience of motivation to work. However, in the analysis it was possible to determine some negative attitudes towards senior employees in the work organisation. A manager stated: *"To put it bluntly: it is a fact that you want to invest in the younger employees, they've got many years left. Now we have laws and regulations that govern us and control us to not make any difference because of age"*. Another manager described how older employees' productivity was not as high as the younger employees': *"I may, as supervisor, not expect the same productivity of a 65-year-old employee that I can of a 30-year-old. But is it okay that older employees are not as effective? Is it okay if they cannot do the same things? That they cannot produce at the same level? Can we justify that we expect different things at different ages from our employees? For it is like that in reality"*. Some senior employees indicated that they felt discriminated against because of their age, and that it was important to change this perception. One senior employee said: *"I heard at some point that when you as an older employee continue and work for longer, you do not make place for younger generations. I do not know how to understand this because it is not really true. It is not a matter of a generational switch. It is about competence. You should see us more as individual employees with different competences, instead of a certain age"*. The participants stated that it was important to eliminate negative age-related attitudes and to acknowledge individuals instead of generalising about individual employees based on their chronological age and on stereotypically negative attributed characteristics of the social age group elderly employee, i.e., to age discriminate.

3.3.7. Summary about Relations, Social Support and Inclusion

The interviewees stated that measures to promote social inclusion, participation, coherence and social support in the work situation by considering whether all employees were included in the work social environment and in the work team are of great importance. They also stated the importance of measures to decrease negative attitudes and (age) discrimination, and to increase social support and the senior employees' self-esteem in the organisation. As well as to appreciate the senior employees' mentoring, (working) life experience and calming effect on the work team as an important productivity investment. Additionally, employees have a personal life outside work and senior employees, due to their biological ageing, need more time for recuperation, the work schedules need to pay attention to individual needs for social participation outside work and activities with family, leisure time and hobbies.

3.4. Measures for Execution of Work Tasks

3.4.1. Measures to Increase Motivation and Work Satisfaction

At work people must perform work tasks and activities to receive their salaries. Many interviewees describe that their work tasks and the content of their work activities were very important to them. This was especially the case with older employees with work tasks and activities involving problem-solving, where they could utilise their abilities and skills in a way that they could not do outside of work, who stated that they did not want to retire from working and that it was of great importance for them to stay in working life. However, other older employees stated that their work tasks and activities lacked meaning and were a reason for them to leave working life. One senior employee stated the need for measures in working life to make the work interesting, motivating, meaningful and stimulating, the employee put it like this: *"If you go to the same place and do the same thing for 40 years, then it is not as much fun. We receive new challenges when we get into new projects, with new people, and in making sure that it works"*. To sometimes declare and highlight the employees' work roles, tasks and activities in the bigger picture of the workplace, to the production and in society, was described as a measure that would increase the experience of the tasks and work activities as motivating, meaningful and appreciated within the organisation, enterprise and society. Measures to promote the experience of work tasks as interesting, meaningful and stimulating, or the experience of activities together with co-workers as stimulating and meaningful, were described as important in order to keep working until an older age. The feeling of importance when performing work tasks was described as meaningful and stimulating by one senior employee older than 65 years, who stated: *"I still feel curious, I am not fed up by what I am doing at work, but find stimulation in it all the time"*. Another senior employee said: *"I would not have kept working if I had not been stimulated. It applies to conditions and everything"*. Many participants stated that the experience of importance in work tasks constituted a preference to remain in an extended working life.

3.4.2. The Rotation and Change of Work Tasks in Order to Increase Motivation and Work Satisfaction

Some interviewees described the rotation between different work tasks to be a measure that motivates and stimulates employees to remain in an extended working life. One manager stated: *"I think we need to have rotation. It should be mandatory to work in different places and to move around at work. Between different tasks, within their own workplace or in another department. Because I have seen when we have forced people to move around, at first it is only disastrous for this person. They believe that working life is over. Six months later, when you ask them, they say it's quite amazing, really good: "I have had to learn again, I have seen new things and met new people" they say. I have never heard anyone say that it was a disaster when it's been a while. In the beginning of the change many are paralysed by fear, but then after a while it is only positive"*. One senior employee described how she got a new job after a reorganisation, including rotation between work tasks within the work team, she stated: *"I love the contacts, the meetings you have with new people, it doesn't matter if they are older or younger. There are always new meetings, new challenges; how do I solve this? And then the wellbeing of the team. A bunch that always stand up for each other, you have problems and crises within the team that you always have, so you can sit down, nurses and manager and everything, so it is a great concept and great manager, it helps a lot. The manager, she trusts the work team. It is a security for us"*. However, some of the interviewees stated that to make rotation possible the employees had to have the skills needed for various work tasks. One manager said: *"Rotation is important. But the skills issue is very important at that. It's about people who think that it might be good to go on and widen their views and their areas of expertise, otherwise it will not work. To participate in knowledge development, or to read up on their skills by themselves"*. This manager also described how it was his issue to motivate the employees to develop. Individual development and broader know-how from the rotation of work tasks was also described as an important measure for the employees' employability and possibility to keep working in a changing work organisation and working life. However, the interviewees also stated that not all employees could rotate and do every work task in the workplace due to functional variation in physical or mental capabilities.

3.4.3. Measures to Highlight the Employees' Abilities

Some of the participants stated that in work and at the workplace, the individual employee sometimes becomes anonymous and assumes the role of an employee to perform the assigned tasks and activities at work. The individual's unique abilities run the risk of becoming invisible and of not coming to fruition. To experience oneself as a replaceable cog in the organisation's machinery was described as having a draining effect on the motivation. The meaning of their own individual efforts was experienced as non-existent by employees. Some of the senior interviewees who had left working life at an early age, i.e., before 64 years of age, stated that they had experienced work as a barrier to do more meaningful and satisfying things with their life and that they would have gladly stopped working even earlier if their personal finances had allowed it. One interviewee who felt that he did not receive any appreciation at work stated: *"I was quite skilled at finding problems in the energy system and solving these problems so that the organisation could save a lot of money. But, they never thanked me for that. I sold myself cheap at that job and never got any credit for my commitment"*. Another senior interviewee said: *"New managers, who were economists and did not know anything about the work tasks and how to do things, changed the organisation. You and your work team couldn't decide on how to execute the work tasks anymore and there was much more stress"*. One interviewee made this statement: *"I put so much into that work but nobody cared and no-one appreciated me anymore. My manager frankly did not give a damn. It was no fun anymore [...] if someone cares and appreciates what you do, you want to do it even better, but if no-one cares you stop caring too"*. This type of experience caused frustration and made work feel dull and uninteresting. Therefore, many of the participants stated the importance of paying attention to the employees' individual skills and specialities and to highlight them as unique individuals, important to the functionality and productivity of the organisation or enterprise. Some managers described how they had made their employees responsible for different areas and tasks to increase the motivation and the employees' experience of being needed and required by the organisation. Some managers also described how they had noticed some employees' leisure interests and utilised those skills in new work tasks for the employee in the workplace, which had been a success for both the enterprise and to the employees' motivation to work.

3.4.4. Measures to Promote Competence Development in Order to Enable Continued Employability

To execute their work tasks the employees need to have the appropriate knowledge, competence and skills. Some interviewees stated that competence development needs to be continuous to address the changes in work, tasks, as well as to meet changes in the world and technology development. An HR practitioner stated: *"As long as you work you need to have the right skills to do the job. That is pretty simple. The day you stop training is, well, on the day you go home"*. That the staff has the appropriate knowledge and abilities lies not least in the interests of the enterprise and the organisation. It is costly to lose competence and to have to recruit new employees. A manager said: *"Retaining and developing staff is important for the work and business. It is true that hiring a new mechanic, it costs about a million before they are up and running and fully productive. And if you let go of a mechanic who worked here, you must start all over again. We continuously train a huge amount here in the workplace as well. And we did not have to dismiss anyone for that reason"*. It was described as an important measure both to the employees and to the organisation that employees are enabled to continue their employability.

3.4.5. Competence Development Regardless of Age

Cognitive ageing affects individuals' reactions, memory and ability to store knowledge, this was described by some of the interviewees. A manager said: *"Elderly may need more* time to learn new things that are not in line with their previous knowledge. But I have not worked with someone who had to leave his post because he could not handle the new technology. But it's just giving them different durations of time". Unfortunately, there were managers who indicated that they did not really see the benefit of training and developing the competence of senior employees who would be leaving working life soon. A manager said: *"To be completely honest, it is the younger employees that we want to invest in. The elderly are already on their way out of here"*. But there were also managers who, on the contrary, saw it as more important to invest new knowledge and competence development in the senior employees because they already had extensive knowledge, therefore they could add more value to the business directly. *"I can see it almost in the way that in younger employees you have to invest a lot of money. You must educate. You must make sure they go on. But then when people are over 50, then you can harvest. Then you get the return! You don't have to keep them going. They know their stuff! They are self-sufficient! They take their own development initiatives to the extent needed! You get a lot of stuff. It's harvest time!"* Many of the participants stated that an important measure to enable employees to continue working until an older age was that they continued to develop their competence and skills until the day they ended their working life.

3.4.6. Organisational Culture That Acknowledges and Utilises (Senior) Employees' Experience and Knowledge

On having lived a long life, a person accumulates many positive and negative experiences and generic skills that can be added to book learning from formal education. The use of this experience-based knowledge was highlighted by several different interviewees. The participants described how measures to enable the senior employee's experience-based knowledge to be utilised in the work tasks were valuable for the senior employee, being able to use and get access to this experience-based knowledge, which also contributed to their experience of feeling valuable, and that this experiential knowledge was a valuable asset for organisations and enterprises. A senior employee said: *"It is important to utilise skills. Leave us the freedom to do our job based on our expertise. So that we can help and support if you need to discuss something, and at the same time that there is a possibility for us to have support if we need support at work"*. Measures to transfer and exchange knowledge and competence between the generations were identified as a significant investment to both new employees, the senior employees and to the work organisation. A manager said: *"It is important to have the opportunity of utilising the elderly's competence and commitment. They may practise some sort of mentoring and transfer their knowledge to different teams"*. Furthermore, senior employees who possessed special skills were more interesting for the employer to retain and they gladly met these employees' demands for adaptation of work tasks, just to be able to keep these employees until an older age. A trade union representative said: *"It takes a long time to build experience, so some people with what they have gone through are worth gold to the organisation./ . . . / I think it makes you a little bit special to the enterprise and you have better opportunity in negotiations. Maybe that you can work three days a week, then we make this deal. Then these people (senior employees) feel a little bit like, a little proud, you see"*. Measures to promote and increase an organisational culture where the employees' knowledge, no matter if it is experience-based knowledge or knowledge from education, is utilised and considered important to the organisation, seem to motivate and stimulate senior employees to keep working until an older age according to several of the interviewees.

3.4.7. Summary about the Execution of Work Tasks

Measures to promote knowledge, competence development, creativity and intrinsic motivation in the performance of work tasks were described by the interviewees as an important strategy to enable employees to participate in a sustainable working life until an older age. Furthermore, that the organisational culture lets older employees have the possibility of developing skills and be included in the development and new projects in the workplace regardless of age. Rotation of work tasks could be a way to learn new skills and abilities to keep employees employable in the organisation, but also in the case of reorganisations and change in the production. Rotation of tasks, e.g., changing occupation and activities within the organisation and switching work tasks was also suggested to make change of duties, to reduce monotony in tasks, and to increase motivation and job satisfaction. To utilise the senior employees' experience-based knowledge by asking them to mentor new employees is a way of exchanging knowledge between generations and was described as a measure to increase the motivation and meaningfulness at work, but also to increase the employees' employability and total know-how within the organisation.

4. Discussion

The population is ageing in many countries, therefore the aim of this study was to investigate organisational actions and proposals that promote an extended working life and maintain employability. The results of the conducted interviews in this study presented several organisational measures and suggestions to make improvements and to promote a healthy and sustainable working life for all ages in an extended working life, which also aligns with the nine determinant areas in the swAge-model [5–7]. The findings from this study contribute to strengthening the robustness of the theoretical implications and content of the swAge-model, theories on employability and how to promote a sustainable extended working life.

The results collected from the interview data were organised into four main themes based on the four spheres of determination in the theoretical swAge-model, and with a number of extracted sub-themes of organisational measures and suggestions for a healthy and sustainable extended working life. The four main themes were: Measures for health effects associated with working environment; Measures for personal financial security; Measures for social inclusion and social support in the work situation; Measures for creativity and intrinsic work motivation. These themes are also closely related to the research on what people consider in the decision whether to keep working for some years or to retire, i.e., the consideration of: (i) their own health in relation to the work situation and work environment versus retirement; (ii) their personal financial situation in employment versus retirement; (iii) the opportunities of social inclusion in working life situations versus retirement; (iv) and the opportunities for meaningful and self-crediting activities in working life versus retirement [5,6,15].

The research results supported by theories of sustainable working life for all ages and employability [4–16] can hopefully help narrow the gap between theory and practice through the implications to be used as a toolbox to be applied by practitioners, managers and employees in their dialogue and discussion on employability and employee career development. Some measure activities and suggestions are sorted into more than one of the four main themes due to the context in the theme, e.g., rotation was described to be a good measure for different reasons. Therefore, some measure activities are described repeatedly in different themes based on separate reasons. However, the fact that a measure suggestion occurs based on different reasons in different themes shows the usefulness of this action to increase employability and for a sustainable extended working life.

4.1. Measures for Health Effects Associated with Working Environment

The health effects of the work environment affect employees' ability and willingness to work and participate in working life and thus also their employability [5,6]. Systematic work environment management is a part of the EU regulations (89/39/EEG) and is compulsory in all the participating countries in the EU. Employers, according to this, must systematically examine the workplace on a regular basis to eliminate risks in the work environment and to prevent employees from suffering ill health and injuries caused by work. According to a recent study, a proper systematic work environment management in the workplace is statistically significant and associated with employees being able to work until an older age [25]. Many interviewees in this study stated that an awareness of employee ageing was needed in their systematic work environment control scheme, because the risks differ in different age groups. The biological ageing, as well as a higher risk of developing chronic diseases associated with an older age also increase the risks in the work environment, additionally, senior employees in general have declining hearing, sight, reaction ability and speed, which increase the risks of injury in this age group [5,6,26–28]. The interviewees in this study stated that, to reduce the risk of developing health problems because of the working environment, the organisational culture needs to promote the use of ergonomic aids; rotation and change of work tasks to reduce tear and strain; regular physical activity to maintain bodily functions and to stay mentally and physically healthy; the importance of diet for (occupational) health. Additionally, they suggest a better use of the occupational health care to support and promote health and to prevent physical and mental injury, illness and stress. However, a recent study in Sweden stated that the occupational health care accessible through the workplace nowadays is not statistically significant and associated with whether the employees are able to work until 65 years of age or beyond, but that there was a potential to change this, if occupational health care starts focussing on the age perspective in the workplaces [25]. In a healthy and sustainable working life for all ages awareness of this is important, as well as to implement measures to promote the work environments' health effects.

4.2. Measures for Personal Financial Security

Employability is important for the individuals' opportunity to maintain sound personal finances; however, personal finances in turn affect whether the individual can and wants to work and participate in working life [5,6]. It is much better for employees' wellbeing if they work because they want to, and not because they cannot afford to leave the workplace [29]. In this study many interviewees stated that employees who were injured or had a disease and were not fully productive, also had problems with their employability if they could no longer execute their work tasks, if they could not be moved to another part of the organisation and enterprise or if they could not be re-employed within a reorganisation. Additionally, the interviewees stated that employees were not as employable if their skills and knowledge were dated or they did not keep up with the technology developments or did not have the latest knowledge, resulting in not being able to execute their duties and tasks as expected or to be relocated within their organisation. Earlier studies also state the need for employees to stay employable in the objective of being able to participate in an extended working life and provide for themselves [30,31]. Likewise, earlier studies state the necessity for organisations and enterprises to implement actions and measures to help the employees stay employable on the basis of ethics and humanity, and because risk prevention and competence development for the employees mean less expenses for the organisation compared to recruitment and new hiring [30,32]. In a healthy and sustainable working life for all ages it is important to have awareness and measures to promote personal financial security.

4.3. Measures to Promote Social Inclusion, Participation, Coherence and Social Support in the Work Situation

The social support and social inclusion that the employees experience affect their ability and willingness to work and participate in working life, as well as their employability [5,6]. Many interviewees stated the importance of measures to promote social inclusion and social support in the work situation by considering whether all employees were included in the work social environment and in the work team. Additionally, earlier research states the importance of social inclusion, participation, coherence and social support in the work situation [15,33,34]. An important part in this area is the leadership. The manager needs to know that the employee needs to acknowledge his/her unique personal situation based on his/her: health, physical and mental working environment, need for recuperation, personal social/family situation, need for skills and knowledge, in relation to his/her work tasks, etc. Different employees need different social support and level of participation in the work situation. No employee can experience wellbeing or be able to produce at his/her best level if they feel excluded or discriminated against based on their age or other factors. Several interviewees describe the importance of actions and measures to decrease negative attitudes and (age) discrimination, and to promote and increase social support and senior employees' self-esteem in the organisation. Many manager interviewees participating in this study stated that the older employees who were also mentors had a calming effect on the work team, which was an important productivity investment. Furthermore, earlier studies state the older employees' experience and calming effect as important [28,33]. However, in order to increase the willingness to participate in an extended working life the senior employees also need to know they are valued, feel appreciated and have the possibility of participating and being included in a social context in the organisation. In a healthy and sustainable working life for all ages it is important to be aware of and take actions and measures to promote social inclusion, participation, coherence and social support in the work situation.

4.4. Measures to Promote Knowledge, Development, Creativity and Intrinsic Motivation in the Performance of Work Tasks

Whether employees are able to perform their work duties and activities or not affects their ability and willingness to work and participate in working life, as well as their employability [5,6]. According to many of the interviewees, motivation and skills were important in order to stay at work and in employment until an older age. Earlier studies also state the importance of skills, knowledge development, stimulation, meaningfulness and motivation in the work tasks for the employees' willingness to work [35,36]. Additionally, earlier research states that the employees' skills and knowledge are especially important to maintain their employability [30,31,36]. However, the organisational culture should afford older employees' the possibility of developing skills and be included in the development and in new projects at the workplace, regardless of age, and to fuel the employees' ability to keep up to date on their knowledge and experience of stimulation in work tasks. Measures and activities such as rotation of work tasks, e.g., changing occupation and activities within the organisation and switching work tasks, could be a way to reduce monotony in work tasks, to learn new skills and work tasks and to increase motivation and job satisfaction to retain employees in the organisation or within reorganisations and changes in production. Some interviewees suggested, and some had also tried, to utilise the older employees' knowledge and experience through the possibility of being a mentor to new employees, by having responsibility for work areas, and by participating in activities such as discussions groups to exchange knowledge between generations of employees and increase the work teams' common knowledge. In a healthy and sustainable working life for all ages it is important to be aware of and take measures to promote knowledge, development, creativity and the employees' experience of intrinsic motivation in the performance of work tasks.

4.5. Limitations

A limitation of interview studies might be the established context, since researchers could approach the data with bias simply by their personality and body language in the interview situation [22]. However, the researchers who conducted these interviews are very used to interviewing and this limitation is therefore probably not an issue that affects the results. Additionally, there might be a risk that in direct content analysis the findings are more supportive rather than non-supportive of the pre-defined categories. However, in the present study, the pre-defined categories from the theoretical swAge-model were not used to guide data collection or probe questions during the interviews. The pre-defined categories were only applied during the analytical process. In terms of trustworthiness, the quality of a content analysis depends on the availability of extensive and appropriate data [37]. These findings represent different work domains, different occupational groups and professions, from different hierarchical positions within the organisations. However, findings from qualitative studies could not be stated to be transferable to all other cultural contexts. Regarding the transferability of the findings, it could be said that the themes are relevant to many others in similar workplaces. The findings were also well-aligned with those of earlier studies about employability and senior employees' problems and possibilities regarding whether they can and want to participate in an extended working life, and thereby add to the accumulation of results regarding senior employees' possibility of working in an extended working life [33].

4.6. Implications

The implications of the findings in this study, based on the interviewees' own words, are that there are many possible measures to implement, which can be improved in organisations and enterprises to make circumstances in working life healthier and more sustainable for employees of all ages and to increase employability. One management tool to investigate what measures the individual employees primarily need to stay employable is through recurring individual career development discussions with employees. The manager and employee can systematically use a matrix together at the development discussion, where the needs are mapped and followed up at the subsequent development discussion (see Appendix A). The suggestions for organisational measures based on the findings in this study are:

4.6.1. Measures to Promote a Sound Physical and Mental Work Environment for Employees by Considering to

- Establish an organisational culture that promotes the use of technical and ergonomic aids.
- Establish reduced work stress, balanced workload, duties and responsibilities.
- Establish increased effort/reward balance.
- Establish good communication, information and participation to reduce work stress.
- Establish safety activities to reduce violence and threats in the work situation.
- Establish rotation, variation and change of duties and work tasks to reduce physical demand, static workload, wear and tear. As well as to reduce mental demands, stress, vulnerability and threatening situations.
- Establish work schedules that allow for sufficient recovery through breaks during work and time for recuperation between work shifts.
- Establish work pace at a reasonable rate so the employees can cope physically and mentally, if there are shifts with a faster work pace these should be complemented by shifts with a slower work pace.
- Establish physical activity for maintenance of the body, and to sustain and improve mental and physical good health.
- Establish the importance of a healthy diet for a good (occupational) health.
- Establish access to occupational health services and support to prevent work environment problems and increase good occupational health.

4.6.2. Measures to Promote Personal Financial and Social Security by Considering to

- Establish salary and financial benefits responding to a reasonable personal financial security and sufficient wellbeing.
- Establish work environmental security management and risk assessment to reduce the risk of health problems causing decreased employability and to reduce the risk of less financial benefits by sick leave, disability pension and unemployment.
- Establish measures for competence development and continued employability to make senior employees able to provide for themselves by working until an older age.

4.6.3. Measures to Promote Social Inclusion and Social Support in the Work Situation by Considering to

- Establish situational- and age-adapted leadership with a focus based on employees' needs; these should be adapted for the best possible support of the work and development.
- Establish activities for social inclusion in the work team and to build a community and sense of security to increase the attraction of extended employment.
- Establish risk assessment and activities to reduce negative attitudes, victimisation, scapegoat mentality and (age) discrimination in the workplace.
- Establish social support to increase the senior employees' self-esteem, sense of acknowledgement, sense of security and inclusion in the organisation.

- Establish access to a balanced level of information regarding ongoing activities and changes in the organisation.
- Establish participation in decisions that affect the employees' work tasks and work situation.
- Establish activities to pay attention to individual employees as an important productivity investment, e.g., mentoring and calming effect on the group as well as entrepreneurship and ideas.
- Establish working schedules (with a balance between shorter and longer work shifts and time for recuperation between work shifts) that take into consideration and utilise the employees' individual needs, participation and activities with family, leisure time and hobbies.

4.6.4. Measures to Promote Creativity and Intrinsic Work Motivation by Considering to

- Establish activities to increase motivation, stimulation and meaningfulness in work tasks.
- Establish the possibility for professional development, and new knowledge and competence development regardless of the employees' age and position in the organisation.
- Establish an organisational culture that enables employees' opportunities and skills (outside work as well) to be part of or to be involved in problem-solving, organisational development and new projects.
- Establish an organisational culture that takes into consideration and appreciates (senior) employees' experience and knowledge as a production asset.
- Establish activities and an organisational culture that state the need for the employees' continuous development of knowledge and skills to maintain their ongoing employability.
- Establish possibilities for the employees to take care of and manage larger or smaller work areas with the intention of stimulating, paying significance to and instilling motivation in the work tasks as well as increasing the individuals' employability.
- Establish possibilities of rotation and change of duties and work tasks to reduce boredom and increase motivation and job satisfaction.

5. Conclusions

The demographic changes in society place strain on organisations and enterprises. The need for an extended working life, and the simultaneous higher average age among employees increase the need for measures to enable a healthy and sustainable working life for all ages. This study has identified various proposals for measures and actions that could increase the employees' employability and ability to cope in working life until an older age. The identified issues are explained in association to each of the four themes' context based on the spheres of determination in the theoretical swAge-model [5–7]. The results state that some needed measure activities and suggestions could be applied to more than one theme and issue, since working life is complex and the areas of determination associated with employability until an older age have some overlapping domains. However, to some extent, all nine determinant areas are associated with the four spheres of determination in the swAge-model and need to be considered in work places and societies that want working life to be satisfying and sustainable for employees of all ages in the work force. Employability is often perceived as a society's and employer's considerations of an employee's ability to execute work tasks; however, it also regards whether employees want to and are able to work. Regular conversations, communication and close dialogue are needed and are prerequisites for good working conditions and a healthy working environment, as well as to be able to manage employees and develop the organisation further. The implication of the "tools for dialogue and discussion on employability and employees' career development" (Appendix A) was based on the analysis of the interviews and findings in this study, and will hopefully be useful for organisations and enterprises in order to consider and implement needed measures with the intention of contributing to the employees' employability in a sustainable working life for all ages. These measures should not only be applied to senior employees since all employees, hopefully, will become older employees some day and their health and skills need to be taken care of throughout their entire working life.

A healthy and sustainable working life for all ages is highlighted as significant and needed around the world [1–4]. Additionally, the United Nations' Sustainability Goal Agenda-2030 describes the need of decent work for all to enable a sustainable future [38]. The developed suggestions for measures and tools for dialogue and discussion in this study are intended to be implemented in workplaces. This study resulted in measure suggestions and a tool was developed based on the Swedish context, though hopefully the results can be usefully implemented and evaluated in depth in intervention studies of other countries' work force context to develop a more sustainable working life for all ages.

Author Contributions: The authors K.N. and E.N. completed the analysis, K.N. authored the paper, and K.N. and E.N. approved the final manuscript. All authors have read and agreed to the published version of the manuscript.

Funding: This study was funded by the Swedish Research Council for Health, Working Life and Welfare (Forte) and AFA insurance. The financiers were not involved or had any role in the design of the study, the data collection, the analysis, the interpretation of data or in the writing of this paper.

Institutional Review Board Statement: The study was conducted according to the guidelines of the Declaration of Helsinki, and approved by the Swedish Ethical Review Authority (Dnr. 2013:722).

Informed Consent Statement: Informed consent was obtained from all subjects involved in the study.

Data Availability Statement: The data used in this study are managed by the authors. To access these data please contact the authors.

Conflicts of Interest: The authors declare no conflict of interest.

Appendix A

Tools for dialogue and discussion on employability and employees' career development-swAge^{TM}-model

Date:
Employee: ....
Manager: ....

Before the implementation of the career development discussion:

The conversation is based on mutual trust where both parties have a shared responsibility for the conversation. Allocate time for all steps to be taken.

During the career development discussion, the employee's work situation is discussed, as well as their individual goals, furthermore a competence development plan is drawn up.

Conduct your career development discussion from different perspectives:

- Follow up and provide feedback on what has happened since the last career development discussion by going through last year's goals and competence development plan together.
- Discuss the employee's current position to tune in to what the present situation looks like and possible wishes for change or development.
- Talk about the future in order for you and your employee to create a common view of the employee's work tasks and how these should be prioritised, as well as goals and development areas.
- Furthermore, make sure to reflect on the age of the employee, i.e., the biological age, the chronological age, the social age and the cognitive age, as well as gender.

Documentation of the career development discussion:

The career development discussion must be documented to make it easier to follow up on what the manager and employee have agreed on. In the event of a change of manager, the document provides support to avoid any ambiguity regarding the employee's individual goals and career development. Sensitive information should not be documented in these discussion templates since the documentation from the development discussion is considered a public document. Questions of a private nature, rehabilitation issues, neglect, etc. are more appropriately addressed in an employee meeting not focused on career development, the documentation is then to be kept in a different manner appropriate for the purpose, for example in agreement on tests and written admonishment.

The career development discussion must be documented and signed or confirmed by both the manager and the employee so that there is a consensus on what has been said and documented, as well as confirmation that both agree on what has been discussed and agreed upon during the career development discussion. The documentation provides the basis for the subsequent development discussion.

To keep in mind during the career development discussion:

- Keep phones turned off.
- Treat the development discussion as a conversation in confidence and make an agreement if or when something needs to be passed on.
- Listen actively and ask counter-questions for clarification and to make sure you have reached an understanding.
- Respect each other's perceptions or experiences even if they are not unanimous.
- Do not promise anything that cannot be done.
- Do not forget to address if there are any specific requests or if there are previously agreed issues to discuss during the development discussion.
- Issues that are not related to the career development discussion are to be taken in a different context.
- End the career development discussion by evaluating the conversation together, what has been good and what can be improved until next time.

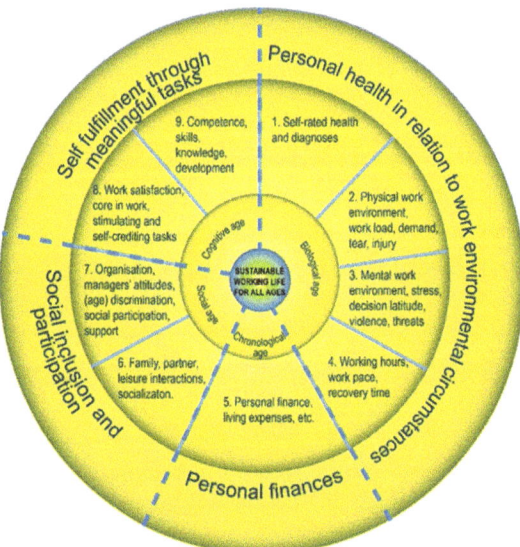

Figure A1. The micro level of the swAge™-model—Sustainable working life for all ages. Available online: https://swage.org/en.html (accessed on 1 March 2021).

The matrix for dialogue and discussion on employability and employees' career development

How does the employee experience their work situation? Fill in the matrix and document the employee's experience of their work situation based on the nine determination areas for a healthy and sustainable working life for all ages (see Figure A1 above):	
1. Their health, wellbeing, functional diversity, diagnoses in relation to the work situation?	
2. Physical work environment (promotive and preventive factors, demanding factors, workload, vibrations, repetitive motions or strain, ergonomic and technical aids and tools, climate, chemical health risks)?	
3. Mental work environment (promotive and preventive factors, demanding factors, stress, demand and control, threats, violence)?	
4. Work hours, work pace, breaks, schedule, time for recuperation?	
5. Finances—the extent of the employment, appointments procedure, employment security? (Salary and salary benefits are primarily to be discussed during a salary negotiation meeting)	
6. Balance between personal social environment and work?	
7. Work social environment, participation, social support, community, sense of security in work team, leadership, informal leaders, co-workers, co-operation, discrimination?	
8. Experience of possibility to work satisfaction, motivation, stimulation with work tasks and activities, core tasks at work, percentage distribution and balance between different work tasks?	
9. Knowledge, competence, possibility of using skills, too hard/too easy work tasks, developing work tasks?	

Individual goals and competence development: Start with the organisations' objectives. Break these down so that they provide a basis for the individual's goals and the purpose of the employee's work tasks to the organisation. The goals should be concrete and possible to implement and follow up.				
Individual goals. What can and should be developed?	How will it happen?	When	Responsible	When follow-up
Competence Development Short term goals of development (about 1 year)	How will it happen?	When	Responsible	When follow-up
Competence Development Long term goals of development (about 3 years)	How will it happen?	When	Responsible	When follow-up

Other notes and comments: ....

References

1. World Economic Forum. Global Agenda Council on Ageing. 2016. Available online: https://www.weforum.org/communities/global-agenda-council-on-ageing/ (accessed on 11 April 2020).
2. OECD. *Pensions at a Glance 2019: OECD and G20 Indicators*; OECD Publishing: Paris, France, 2019. [CrossRef]
3. OECD. *Health at a Glance 2019: OECD Indicators*; OECD Publishing: Paris, France, 2019. [CrossRef]
4. Eurofound. *Sustainable Work over the Life Course: Concept Paper*; Publications Office of the European Union: Luxembourg, 2015.
5. Nilsson, K. A sustainable working life for all ages—The swAge-model. *Appl. Ergon.* **2020**, *86*, 103082. [CrossRef]
6. Nilsson, K. Conceptualization of ageing in relation to factors of importance for extending working life—A review. *Scand. J. Public Health* **2016**, *44*, 490–505. [CrossRef]
7. Nilsson, K. To Work or Not to Work in an Extended Working Life? Factors in Working and Retirement Decision. Ph.D. Thesis, Lund University, Lund, Sweden, 18 January 2013.
8. de Wind, A.; Geuskens, G.A.; Ybema, J.F.; Bongers, P.M.; van der Beek, A.J. The role of ability, motivation, and opportunity to work in the transition from work to early retirement—Testing and optimizing the Early Retirement Model. *Scand. J. Work Environ. Health* **2015**, *41*, 24–35. [CrossRef]
9. Van der Klink, J.J.L.; Bültmann, U.; Burdorf, A.; Schaufeli, W.B.; Zijlstra, F.R.H.; Abma, F.I.; BRouwer, S.; van der Wilt, G.J. Sustainable employability—Definition, conceptualization, and implications: A perspective based on the capability approach. *Scand. J. Work Environ. Health* **2016**, *42*, 71–79. [CrossRef] [PubMed]
10. Fleuren, B.P.I.; van Amelsvooort, L.G.P.M.; de Grip, A.; Zijlstra, F.R.H.; Kant, I. Time takes us all? A two-wave observational study of age and time effects on sustainable employability. *Scand. J. Work Environ. Health* **2018**, *44*, 475–484. [CrossRef] [PubMed]
11. Fleuren, B.P.; de Grip, A.; Jansen, N.W.H.; Kant, I.; Zijlstra, F.R.H. Unshrouding the Sphere from Clouds: Towards a Comprehensive Conceptual Framework for Sustainable Employability. *Sustainability* **2020**, *12*, 6366. [CrossRef]

12. Nilsson, K.; Rignell-Hydbom, A.; Rylander, L. Factors influencing the decision to extend working life or to retire. *Scand. J. Work Environ. Health* **2011**, *37*, 473–480. [CrossRef]
13. Nilsson, K. Vem kan och vill arbeta till 65 år eller längre? En studie av anställda inom hälso-och sjukvården. [Who can and want to work until 65 years or beyond? A study with employed in health and medical care]. *Arbete Hälsa* **2005**, *14*, 1–35. (In Swedish)
14. Nilsson, K. *Förlängt Arbetsliv—En Litteraturstudie Av Faktorer Med Betydelse För Förlängt Arbetsliv Som Alternativ till Tidig Pensionsavgång. [Extended Working Life—A Literature Review on Factors Important to an Extended Working Life as an Alternative to Early Retirement]*; Swedish National Institute of Working life: Malmö, Sweden, 2003. (In Swedish)
15. Nilsson, K. Why work beyond 65? Discourse on the decision to continue working or retire early. *Nordic J. Work. Life Stud.* **2012**, *2*, 7–28. [CrossRef]
16. Ilmarinen, J. *Toward a Longer Working Life: Aging and Quality of Working Life in the European Union*; Finnish Institute of Occupational Health: Helsinki, Finland, 2006.
17. Nilsson, E.; Nilsson, K. Time for Caring? Senior care employees' occupational activities in the cross draft between their work priorities, "must-do's" and meaningfulness. *Int. J. Care Coord.* **2017**, *20*, 8–16. [CrossRef]
18. Nilsson, K. Active and healthy ageing at work—A qualitative study with employees 55–63 years and their managers. *Open J. Soc. Sci.* **2017**, *5*, 13–29. [CrossRef]
19. Nilsson, E.; Nilsson, K. The transfer of knowledge between younger and older employees in the health and medical care: An intervention study. *Open J. Soc. Sci.* **2017**, *5*, 71–96. [CrossRef]
20. Krueger, R.; Casey, M. *Focus Groups: A Practical Guide for Applied Research*, 4th ed.; Sage: Thousand Oaks, CA, USA, 2009.
21. Then, K.L.; Rankin, J.A.; Ali, E. Focus group research: What is it and how can it be used? *Can. J. Cardiovasc. Nurs.* **2014**, *24*, 16–22. [PubMed]
22. Kvale, S. *Den Kvalitativa Forskningsintervjun. [The Qualitative Research Interview]*; Studentlitteratur: Lund, Sweden, 2001. (In Swedish)
23. Hsieh, H.-F.; Shannon, S.E. Three approaches to qualitative content analysis. *Qual. Health Res.* **2005**, *15*, 1277–1288. [CrossRef] [PubMed]
24. Assarroudi, A.; Heshmati Nabavi, F.; Armat, M.R.; Ebadi, A.; Vaismoradi, M. Directed qualitative content analysis: The description and elaboration of its underpinning methods and data analysis process. *J. Res. Nurs.* **2018**, *23*, 42–55. [CrossRef]
25. Nilsson, K. When is work a cause of early retirement and are there any effective organisational measures to combat this? A population-based study of perceived work environment and work-related disorders among employees in Sweden. *BMC Public Health* **2020**, *20*, 1–15. [CrossRef]
26. Ahola, K.; Sirén, I.; Kivimäki, M.; Ripatti, S.; Aromaa, A.; Lönnqvist, J. Work-Related Exhaustion and Telomere Length: A Population-Based Study. *PLoS ONE* **2012**, *7*, e40186. [CrossRef]
27. von Bonsdorff, M.E.; Kokko, K.; Seitsamo, J.; von Bonsdorff, M.B.; Nygård, C.-H.; Ilmarinen, J.; Rantanen, T. Work strain in midlife and 28-year work ability trajectories. *Scand. J. Work Environ. Health* **2011**, *6*, 455–463. [CrossRef]
28. Fridriksson, J.F.; Tómasson, K.; Midtsundstad, T.; Sivesind Mehlum, I.; Hilsen, A.I.; Nilsson, K.; Albin, M.; Poulsen, O.M. *Working Environment and Work Retention*; Nordiska Ministerrådet TemaNord: Copenhagen, Denmark, 2017; Volume 559, 121p.
29. Wang, M.; Shultz, K.S. Employee Retirement: A Review and Recommendations for Future Investigation. *J. Manag.* **2010**, *36*, 172–206. [CrossRef]
30. Gratton, L.; Scott, A. *The Corporate Implications of Longer Lives. MIT Sloan Management Review*; Massachusetts Institute of Technology: Cambridge, MA, USA; Springer: Medford, MA, USA, 2017; Available online: http://mitsmr.com/2mFYyU9 (accessed on 11 April 2020).
31. Lent, R.W.; Lopez, A.M.; Lopez, F.G.; Sheu, H.B. Social cognitive theory and the prediction of interests and choice goals in the computing disciplines. *J. Vocat. Behav.* **2008**, *73*, 52–62. [CrossRef]
32. Dengler, P. *Lifelong Employability Thriving in an Ageing Society*; Springer Gabler: Zürich, Switzerland, 2018.
33. Nilsson, K. Managers' attitudes to their older employees—A cross-sectional study. *Work* **2018**, *59*, 49–58. [CrossRef] [PubMed]
34. Mykletun, R.; Furunes, T. The Ageing Workforce Management Programme in Vattenfall AB Nordic, Sweden. In *Older Workers in a Sustainable Society. Labor, Education & Society*; Ennals, R., Salomon, R.H., Eds.; Peter Lang Verlag: Frankfurt, Germany, 2011; pp. 93–106.
35. Hovbrandt, C.; Håkansson, C.; Karlsson, G.; Albin, M.; Nilsson, K. Prerequisites and driving forces behind an extended working life among older workers. *Scand. J. Occup. Ther.* **2017**, *28*, 1–13. [CrossRef] [PubMed]
36. Salthouse, T. Aging and measures of processing speed. *Biol. Psychol.* **2000**, *54*, 35–54. [CrossRef]
37. Willig, C. *Introducing Qualitative Research in Psychology*; McGraw-Hill Education: London, UK, 2013.
38. United Nations. Agenda-2030, Goal 8, Employment, Decent Work for All and Social Protection. Available online: https://sdgs.un.org/topics/employment-decent-work-all-and-social-protection (accessed on 16 April 2021).

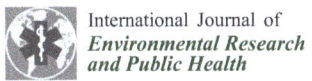

Article

Can They Stay or Will They Go? A Cross Sectional Study of Managers' Attitudes towards Their Senior Employees

Kerstin Nilsson [1,2,*] and Emma Nilsson [1]

1. Division of Occupational and Environmental Medicine, Lund University, 223 81 Lund, Sweden; emma.nilsson.1672@med.lu.se
2. Department of Public Health, Kristianstad University, 291 88 Kristianstad, Sweden
* Correspondence: kerstin.nilsson@med.lu.se or Kerstin.Nilsson@Hkr.Se

Citation: Nilsson, K.; Nilsson, E. Can They Stay or Will They Go? A Cross Sectional Study of Managers' Attitudes towards Their Senior Employees. *IJERPH* **2022**, *19*, 1057. https://doi.org/10.3390/ijerph19031057

Academic Editors: Paul B. Tchounwou and Toni Alterman

Received: 9 November 2021
Accepted: 15 January 2022
Published: 18 January 2022

Publisher's Note: MDPI stays neutral with regard to jurisdictional claims in published maps and institutional affiliations.

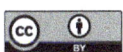

Copyright: © 2022 by the authors. Licensee MDPI, Basel, Switzerland. This article is an open access article distributed under the terms and conditions of the Creative Commons Attribution (CC BY) license (https://creativecommons.org/licenses/by/4.0/).

Abstract: A larger amount of older people need to participate in working life due to the global demographic change. It is the employer, through the manager, who enables employees to have access to measures in the workplace that facilitate and enable a sustainable extended working life. The aim of this study was to evaluate work life factors associated with managers believing their employees can work versus wanting to work until age 65 or older. This cross-sectional study included 249 managers in the Swedish municipality sector. Logistic regression analysis was used to investigate associations between different univariate estimates and in data modelling using the SwAge-model. The result stated that 79% of managers believed their employees 'can' work and 58% of managers believed their employees 'want to' work until age 65 or older. Health, physical work environment, skills and competence are associated the strongest to managers believing employees 'can' work until age 65 or older. Insufficient social support at work and lacking possibilities for relocations associated the strongest to managers believing employees would not 'want to' work until age 65 or older. Though, several countries (especially in Europe) have included in their social policy measures that retirement age be increased after 65, proposing ages approaching 70. When these proposals become laws, through obligation, people will have no choice (if they want to or if they can continue working). However, people's attitudes to work may be different (especially after the COVID-19 pandemic), and this analysis of the participating managers' attitudes showed there is a difference between why employees 'can' versus 'want' to work respectively. Therefore, different strategies may be needed to contribute to employees both being able to and willing to participate in working life until an older age. These findings on managers' perspectives, regarding whether they believe employees would be able to versus would want to work and the SwAge-model, will hopefully contribute to an increased understanding of organisational actions and measures in the process of creating a sustainable extended working life and to increase senior employees' employability.

Keywords: employability; ageing; work environment; swAge-model; demography; retirement; work–life balance; social support; discrimination; work ability; older worker; senior worker; extended working life; age management

1. Introduction

Retirement is a valid and socially acceptable way for an employee to withdraw from working life, e.g., from a physically and mentally demanding work situation, depending on whether their personal financial situation will be sufficient with a pension, whether they do not want to continue working due to the social situation and environment in the workplace, their skills not being utilized in the work tasks or that they do not experience motivation and stimulation in their work tasks [1,2]. However, the proportion of senior citizens is continuously increasing in most of the industrial world [3]. Longevity and lower fertility rates characterise the current demographic trend and result in an increasingly ageing population. A consequence analysis carried out by the Organization for Economic

Cooperation and Development (OECD) compared the senior boom to have economic and budgetary implications like the social effects resulting from natural disasters [3]. The increasing senior population entails a larger amount of people in the pension system, and the demographic change will result in an increased old-age dependency ratio when fewer citizens active in the workforce must provide for an increasing number of senior citizens. Retirement ages in many countries are being postponed as a way of adapting to the new demographic distribution. Senior citizens are encouraged to continue working and participating in the labour force for as long as possible [3–6]. This demographic situation stresses the importance of factors motivating senior employees to experience that they can and want to work until an older age. However, in the workplace, it is the employer, through the manager, who enables employees to have access to measures that facilitate labour force participation. Therefore, the manager's attitudes towards senior employees are important to investigate in relation to enabling a sustainable longer working life.

Previous studies state that some managers hold negative and stereotypical attitudes towards senior employees, such as having more difficulties in adjusting to change, working slower, being less educated as well as holding negative attitudes towards or being frightened of new technology [7]. Perceiving senior employees as stagnant and as an obstacle to organisational development pushes people out of working life early [8–12]. Managers have a key role in the work organisation and on how to motivate and make measures in the work situation to enable employees to extend their working lives. Previous research states that some managers hold negative attitudes towards their senior employees and identify age discrimination [1,7,13–17]. Furthermore, there is published research identifying nine determinant areas connected to employability and whether individuals work or not [1,2,7–44]. These nine areas are also described in the theoretical swAge-model (sustainable working life for all ages) [1] and are: (1) self-rated health and diagnoses; (2) physical work environment; (3) mental work environment; (4) working hours, work pace, time for recuperation; (5) personal financial situation; (6) personal social environment; (7) work social environment; (8) stimulation and motivation in work tasks; (9) competence development, skills, knowledge. Though, to our knowledge, and after further searches in the databases Scopus and PubMed, there appears to be a lack of scientific, published studies and knowledge of managers' attitudes and beliefs towards why their employees would be able to versus would want to work in an extended working life.

The hypothesis in the discussion about a longer working life is that everyone should work to an older age, but we want to investigate whether it is possible to detect a difference between what contributes to wanting to work versus being able to work. Working in the public sector has been associated with early withdrawal from working life in previous studies [33–35,44]. However, more information is needed on the managers' attitudes towards determinant factors for their employees' workforce participation and for a sustainable working life. To better understand how managers can motivate employees and make working life healthier and sustainable until an older age, it is of particular interest to examine whether the managers believe that their employees 'can' and 'want to' work until an older age, associated with the nine determinant areas.

The aim of this study was to evaluate the main factors associated with whether managers believe their employees want to, versus being able to, work until 65 years of age or older in their workplace.

2. Materials and Methods

The research design was quantitative, and by a cross-sectional survey investigating factors associated with whether managers believe their employees would be able to or would want to work in an extended working life. The surveys' objective was specifically to examine whether municipality managers believed their employees would be able to or would want to work, managers' attitudes towards their senior employees and factors of interest for work participation and retirement.

2.1. Study Population

As previously described, working in the public sector has been associated with early withdrawal from working life in earlier studies [33–35,44]. The study population in this study consisted of managers in one of the largest municipalities in Sweden. The subjects were identified by the personnel register of employed and there was a total investigation including all the 456 employed managers in the municipality. Therefore, the study population additionally all had the same employer, i.e., the same municipality employer, and the same policies regarding employment conditions, rehabilitation and retirement [45].

The study design of the data collection was a web survey in 2018. The individuals in the present study were sent a questionnaire through their work electronic mail. After two reminders, 249 individuals answered the questionnaire. This corresponded to a response rate of 54.6% and constituted the final study population.

The gender distribution of survey respondents was 29% male managers and 71% female managers. The age distribution in the study group was 27–65 years of age, with a median age of 50 years. Survey respondents, the final study population, generally corresponded with the gender distribution of the managers in the participating municipality, i.e., 30% male and 70% female managers, aged 27–65 years with a median age of 50 years. Additionally, 96% of managers responding to the survey worked 40 h/week (full-time), and 90% were managers in a full-time position. However, we did not have any figure of the distribution of managers working full-time or part-time in the entire municipality.

2.2. The Questionnaire

The questions in the questionnaire have been tested and previously used in other studies [7,14,16,19]. The selected statements were based on previous studies executed by our research group [46–48], a literature review [15], and other surveys [49–52]. The questionnaire was tested in a group of 15 individuals (i.e., managers in our own surroundings and other researchers familiar with questionnaires and qualitative investigations) who responded to the web questionnaire and left comments. They comment both on the questions themselves as cognitive testing and readability of items, and on the process, i.e., how it worked to receive information letters and the questionnaire via e-mail as well as how they experienced responding to the online questionnaire. The evaluation of this pilot process resulted in the reformulation of a few question statements before it was distributed to the study population.

Most studies in this research field examine one or a few areas with significance for a sustainable longer working life and employability. The SwAge model is a theoretical model that intends to take a holistic approach and embrace most of all the different aspects and factors that in working life affect the ability to be able and willing to work. We, therefore, used the SwAge model as a model to examine all the areas of influence for a sustainable working life and employability in our intention to contribute to an increased understanding and knowledge in the research area. Accordingly, the questionnaire's statements included factors associated with employees work situation subdivided into the nine theoretical themes of the SwAge-model [1], i.e.,: (1) health; (2) physical work environment; (3) mental work environment; (4) working hours, work pace, time for recuperation; (5) the personal financial situation; (6) personal social environment; (7) work social environment; (8) work tasks, stimulation and motivation; (9) competence development, skills, knowledge.

The statements' response options in the nine areas of the SwAge-model were dichotomised from four to two variables, i.e., from highly agree and partly agree to just 'agree', and from partly disagree and highly disagree to just 'disagree'. In the analysis, we were interested in the managers' answers to these different statements regarding their employee's work situations and how these were associated with the outcome of two specific questions. The first question was whether the responding managers thought their employees would want to work until 55–59, 60–64, 65 or 66 years of age or older, and the second question was whether the responding managers thought their employees would be able to work until 55–59, 60–64, 65 or 66 years of age or older. The response options were dichotomised at 65 years of age (i.e., working until <65 years of age and ≥65 years of age respectively).

Furthermore, the questionnaire included questions regarding at what age managers identified their female and male employees as senior employees; in which business area they were managers and how long they believed to be able to work themselves and at what age they wished to retire themselves.

2.3. Statistical Analysis

The analyses were conducted by the statistical software program IBM SPSS Statistics 25. Regarding the aims of the study, we used the statistical method of logistic regression analysis to investigate the associations between different factors in the work situation measured by statements and the two outcomes in this study, i.e., whether the managers believe that their employees 'want to work until 65 years of age or older' and 'are able to work until 65 years of age or older'. Logistic regression analysis generated odds ratios (OR), as well as 95% confidence intervals (CI) and p-values, for the statement's association with the two outcomes. For each of the two outcomes, we used the following analytical strategy:

(1) Analysis of each of the nine areas in the SwAge-model: We started with univariate analysis, i.e., we evaluated the associations for one statement at a time. In the second step, we kept the statement with the lowest p-value (if $p < 0.05$) and tentatively included all other statements, one at a time. In the third step, we kept the two statements with the lowest p-values (if both $p < 0.05$) and tentatively included the remaining statements, one at a time. This procedure continued for as long as the p-values for all included statements were <0.05.

(2) Analysis including all nine areas in the SwAge-model: The multivariate model for all determinant areas together started by including syntaxes of the selected statements from area (1) and area (2), etc., to build a multivariate model. The statements with p-values < 0.05 were kept in the model in the next step, in which we also included the selected statements from the next area. This procedure continued until all nine areas were included in a final model. After that, the discarded statements from the nine areas were tested, one at a time, against the final model, to investigate whether the model was robust once more.

3. Results

The managers stated different ages to be the possible general retirement age for their employees, i.e., until what age they believed their employees would be able to work and would want to work in general. The proportion of managers who stated that most of their employees would be 'able work until 65 years of age or older' was 77%. The proportion of managers who stated that most of their employees would 'want to work until 65 years or older' was 58%.

3.1. Statements Associated with Managers Believing That Their Employees in General 'Cannot Work until 65 Years of Age or Older'

The statements from the nine determinant areas were analysed with logistic regression analysis to identify the association between the statements and managers believing that their employees in general **could not work until 65 years of age or beyond** (Table 1). In the first step, the univariate estimates were analysed. The ones that were statistically significant in the next step of the analysis were included in the multivariate model within the determinant area.

Both statements in the determinant area *Self-rated health and diagnoses* were statistically significant and associated with whether the managers believed that their employees could not work until 65 years of age or older, i.e., "The majority of my employees have some kind of diagnosis or chronic disease", "The majority of my employees do not seem to experience well-being in their daily life".

Of the seven statements in the area *physical work environment*, only two statements proved to be statistically significant and included in the multivariate model of the area, i.e., "I experience that my employees in general have many tasks involving a physically demanding work load and heavy lifting" and "I do not experience that my employees have a reasonable physical work load".

The area *the personal financial situation* consists of only one statement that proved to be statistically significant to whether the managers believed that their employees could not work until 65 years of age or older, i.e., "I experience that my employees in general feel pressured by their personal financial situation".

In the area *work social environment,* two of seven statements proved to be statistically significant, and accordingly included in the multivariate model, i.e., "My employees in general do not receive sufficient support from me to be able to work until the normal retirement age", "I am not satisfied with the extent of support that I offer my employees for them to be able to cope with their work tasks".

Three of seven statements in the area *stimulation and motivation in work tasks* proved to be statistically significant. However, only one of the statements in this determinant area proved to be statistically significant in the final multivariate model, i.e., "I do not experience it being possible to adjust work tasks to senior employees in my organisation".

In the determinant area *competence development, skills, knowledge,* three of seven statements proved to be statistically significant. However, only two statements, "I do not experience that my employees have access to sufficient technical support" and "I do not experience it important to keep senior employees in the organization based on their competence", proved to be statistically significant and included in the final multivariate modelling.

There were no statistically significant associations in the areas *Mental work environment, Working hours, work pace and time for recuperation* and *Personal social environment* with whether the managers believed that their employees would not be able to work until 65 years of age or older.

The final step of the analysis, regarding determinant areas associated with whether the managers believed that their employees would be able to work, was a multivariate model of all the determinant areas combined. Five statements proved to be statistically significant and associated with whether the managers believed that their employees would not be able to work until 65 years of age or older (Table 1). The statements belonged to three of the nine determinant areas. One statement belonged to the area *Self-rated health and diagnoses,* two statements belonged to *Physical work environment* and two statements belonged to the area *Competence development, skills, knowledge*. The strongest observed association in the multivariate model was for the statement "I do not experience that my employees have a reasonable physical work load" followed by "I experience that my employees in general have many tasks involving a physically demanding work load and heavy lifting", "I do not experience it being important to keep senior employees in the organisation based on their competence", "I do not experience that my employees have access to sufficient technical support", and "The majority of my employees have some kind of diagnosis or chronic disease".

Table 1. Distributions regarding whether the managers believe their employees' 'can work' outcome for the statements included in the univariate and final multivariate model of each determinant area and in total for all nine determinant areas. The corresponding odds ratios (OR), significant value (P) and 95% confidence intervals (CI) obtained from logistic regression. ORs indicate the statements' relation to the managers' belief whether their employees' cannot work until 65 years of age or older.

Determinant Sphere	Determinant Areas	Statement	The Managers' Belief Whether Their Employees' Cannot Work until 65 Years of Age or Older								
			Univariate Estimates			Multivariate Model in Each Determinant Area			Multivariate Model Including All Nine Determinant Areas		
			OR	P	95% CI	OR	P	95% CI	OR	P	95% CI
Health impacts of the work environment	Self-rated health and diagnoses	The majority of my employees do not seem to experience wellbeing in their daily life	4.381	0.006	1.51–12.68	4.238	0.009	1.43–12.57	2.725	0.033	1.086–6.841
		The majority of my employees have some kind of diagnosis or chronic disease	3.035	0.005	1.41–6.54	3.126	0.005	1.42–6.89			
	Physical work environment	I experience that my employees in general have many tasks involving a physically demanding work load and heavy lifting	7.014	<0.001	3.05–16.15	5.366	<0.001	2.239–12.860	4.660	0.002	1.779–12.209
		I do not experience that my employees have a reasonable physical work load	7.130	<0.001	2.65–19.16	4.719	0.004	1.632–13.644	4.832	0.008	1.526–15.361
		I experience that my employees in general run the risk of occupational injury and occupational disease based on the physical work environment	4.332	0.004	1.59–11.84						
		I experience that my employees in general have many physically unilateral work tasks	2.090	0.049	1.00–4.35						
		I do not experience that there is sufficient ergonomic support and aids for my employees work	1.632	0.341	0.60–4.48						
		I do not experience that my employees in general are good at using ergonomic support and aids	1.063	0.87	0.51–2.20						
	Mental work environment	I do not experience that there is a general balance between the demands put on my employees in their work, and the control they have in executing their work tasks	1.813	0.115	0.865–3.800						
		I experience that my employees run the risk of being subjected to violence and threats in their work	1.368	0.319	0.739–2.535						
		I experience that my employees in general run the risk of occupational injury and occupational disease based on the mental work environment	1.338	0.404	0.675–2.655						
		I experience that my employees in general are too stressed in their work due to current circumstances in the work place	1.306	0.408	0.694–2.461						
		I experience that my employees in general are too stressed in their work due to political decisions and circumstances in society	1.225	0.507	0.672–2.233						

Table 1. Cont.

Determinant Sphere	Determinant Areas	Statement	The Managers' Belief Whether Their Employees' Cannot Work until 65 Years of Age or Older									
			Univariate Estimates			Multivariate Model in Each Determent Area			Multivariate Model Including All Nine Determent Areas		
			OR	P	95% CI	OR	P	95% CI	OR	P	95% CI
	Working hours, work pace and time for recuperation	I do not experience that my employees in general have sufficient opportunity of taking breaks when working	2.066	0.059	0.972–4.390	2.066	0.059	0.972–4.390			
		I do not experience that my employees in general have a good work schedule that enables recuperation between work shifts"	2.003	0.118	0.838–4.784						
		I experience that it can be a problem to keep the work activities running due to lack of temp workers when employees are off work	1.276	0.431	0.696–2.341						
		I experience that my employees in general have too many work tasks due to lack of employees	1.239	0.528	0.636–2.415						
Financial incentives	Personal financial situation	I experience that my employees in general feel pressured by their financial situation (i.e., having difficulty getting by on their salary, health insurance and/or other social security systems)	3.269	<0.001	1.619–6.601	3.269	<0.001	1.619–6.601			
Social inclusion, relations and participation	Personal social environment	I do not experience that my employees in general have sufficient opportunity of combining work with their leisure activities and social relations in their leisure time.	2.472	0.062	0.956–6.390	2.472	0.062	0.956–6.390			
		I do not experience that my employees in general have sufficient opportunity of combining work with their family situation, partner, children, grandchildren, etc.	1.964	0.205	0.692–5.572						
	Work social environment	My employees in general do not receive sufficient support from me to be able to work until ordinary retirement age	5.451	0.005	1.656–17.946	4.158	0.023	1.212–14.268			
		I am not satisfied with the extent of support that I offer my employees for them to be able to cope with their work tasks	2.415	0.017	1.169–4.989	2.290	0.035	1.060–4.948			
		I do not experience that my employees in general receive sufficient support to be able to cope with their work tasks from their co-workers, others in the organization and supporting organizations	1.833	0.190	0.740–4.540						
		I am not satisfied with the quality of the support that I offer my employees for them to be able to cope with their work tasks	1.652	0.333	0.598–4.568						
		I experience that my senior employees are subjected to discrimination/disregard by others in the workplace (co-workers, patients, clients, etc.)	2.115	0.488	0.255–17.569						
		I do not experience that my employees in general have reasonable opportunity to participate in decisions regarding work organisation	1.150	0.780	0.433–3.054						

Table 1. Cont.

Determinant Sphere	Determinant Areas	Statement	The Managers' Belief Whether Their Employees' Cannot Work until 65 Years of Age or Older							Multivariate Model Including All Nine Determent Areas		
			Univariate Estimates			Multivariate Model in Each Determent Area					
			OR	p	95% CI	OR	p	95% CI	OR	p	95% CI
Execution of work tasks	Stimulation and motivation in work tasks	I do not experience leadership to be crucial for senior employees' considerations to keep working after 65 years of age	1.016	0.960	0.558–1.849						
		I do not experience it being possible to adjust work tasks to senior employees in my organization	3.900	<0.001	2.053–7.408	3.900	<0.001	2.053–7.408			
		In my experience it is hard to find work tasks to relocate employees who experience their work environment as too physically demanding	2.621	0.004	1.36–5.05						
		In my experience it is hard to find work tasks to relocate employees who experience their work environment as too mentally demanding	2.230	0.030	1.081–4.600						
		I do not experience that my employees in general have reasonable opportunity of participation in decisions regarding their work tasks	3.720	0.070	0.899–15.400						
		I do not experience that my employees in general are satisfied in their daily work	2.400	0.086	0.883–6.520						
		I do not experience that my employees in general have work tasks that they experience as stimulating and meaningful	2.302	0.368	0.375–14.138						
	Competence development, skills, knowledge	I do not experience that my employees have access to sufficient technical support	3.468	0.003	1.547–7.772	3.539	0.003	1.557–8.043	2.834	0.030	1.109–7.244
		I do not experience it being important to keep senior employees in the organization based on their competence	2.322	0.022	1.128–4.778	2.497	0.016	1.188–5.25	3.572	0.002	1.603–7960
		I do not experience that my senior employees have the right knowledge and experience for their work tasks	2.536	0.035	1.069–6.015						
		I do not experience that my senior employees in general have opportunity of continuous competence development	2.131	0.132	0.796–5.702						
		I do not experience that my senior employees in general have the knowledge and experience that enable them to find a job in the eventuality of re-organization and changes	1.469	0.220	0.795–2.713						
		I do not experience that my employees in general have work tasks where they feel they can use their skills and knowledge	1.741	0.653	0.155–19.565						
		I do not experience that my employees in general have knowledge and experience that enables them to be reallocated in our organization	1.055	0.860	0.581–1.915						

3.2. Statements Associated with Whether Managers Believed That Their Employees in General 'Do Not Want to Work until 65 Years of Age or Older'

To identify the association between the statements from the nine determinant areas and whether the managers believed their employees in general **would not want to work until 65 years of age or older**, the association was analysed through logistic regression analysis following the same steps as described above (Table 2). In the determinant area *Self-rated health and diagnoses*, one of the two statements proved to be statistically significant, i.e., "The majority of my employees have some kind of diagnosis or chronic disease", and included in the final multivariate model in the area.

In the determinant area *Physical work environment*, one of seven statements proved to be statistically significant, i.e., "In my experience it is hard to find work tasks to relocate employees who experience their work environment as too physically demanding", and included in the final multivariate model.

In the determinant area *Mental work environment*, i.e., the impact on the individual's mental health caused by the work environment, one of six statements proved to be statistically significant and associated with whether the managers believed that their employees would not want to work until 65 years of age or older, i.e., "I do not experience that there is a general balance between the demands put on my employees in their work, and the control they have in executing their work tasks".

In the determinant area *Working hours, work pace and time for recuperation*, two of four statements proved to be statistically significant to whether the managers believed that their employees would not want to work until 65 years of age or older. However, only the statement "I do not experience that my employees in general have sufficient possibilities to take breaks when working" proved to be statistically significant and included in the modelling of the final multivariate model for the determinant area.

In the determinant area *Work social environment*, one of seven statements proved to be statistically significant and associated with whether the managers believed that their employees would not want to work until 65 years of age or older, and therefore, included in the multivariate model, i.e., "My employees in general do not receive sufficient support from me to be able to work until ordinary retirement age".

One of four statements belonging to the determinant area *Stimulation and motivation in work tasks* proved to be statistically significant and associated with whether the managers believed their employees would not want to work until 65 years of age or beyond, i.e., "I do not experience it being possible to adjust work tasks to senior employees in my organisation".

In the determinant area *Competence development, skills, knowledge* one of seven statements proved to be statistically significant, i.e., "I do not experience that my employees have access to sufficient technical support", and included in the final model after the multivariate modelling.

No statements belonging to the determinant areas *Personal financial situation* and *Personal social environment* showed statistically significant associations with whether the managers believed their employees would not want to work until 65 years of age or older.

In the final multivariate model of all determinant areas combined, two statements proved to be statistically significant and associated with whether the managers believed that their employees would not want to work until 65 years of age or older (Table 2). The statements belonged to two of the nine determinant areas. One statement belonged to the determinant area *Work social environment*, and one statement belonged to the determinant area *Stimulation and motivation in work tasks*. The statement included in the multivariate model that proved the strongest observed association to whether the managers believed their employees would not want to work in an extended working life was "My employees in general do not receive sufficient support from me to be able to work until ordinary retirement age", followed by "In my experience it is hard to find work tasks to relocate employees who experience their work environment as too physically demanding".

Table 2. Distributions regarding whether the manager believe their employees' 'want to work' outcome for the statements included in the univariate and final multivariate model of each determinant areas and in total for all nine determinant areas. The corresponding odds ratios (OR), significant value (P) and 95% confidence intervals (CI) obtained from logistic regression. ORs indicate the statements' relation to whether the managers believe their employees do not want to work until 65 years of age or beyond.

| Determinant Sphere | Determinant Areas | Statement | The Managers Believe Their Employees' Not Want to Work until 65 Years of Age or Beyond ||||||||
| | | | Univariate Estimates ||| Multivariate Model in Each Determinant Area ||| Multivariate Model Including All Nine Determinant Areas |||
			OR	P	95% CI	OR	P	95% CI	OR	P	95% CI
Health impacts of the work environment	Self-rated health and diagnoses	**The majority of my employees seem not to experience wellbeing in their daily life**	2.989	0.052	0.990–9.027	2.989	0.052	0.990–9.027			
		The majority of my employees have some kind of diagnosis or chronic disease	1.563	0.234	0.750–3.260						
	Physical work environment	I experience that my employees in general run the risk of occupational injury and occupational disease based on the physical work environment	2.661	0.062	0.951–7.448						
		I experience that my employees in general have many tasks involving a physically demanding work load and heavy lifting	1.744	0.168	0.791–3.847						
		I do not experience that my employees in general have a reasonable physical work load	1.601	0.326	0.626–4.093						
		I do not experience that my employees in general are good at using ergonomic support and aids	1.289	0.422	0.694–2.394						
		I experience that my employees in general have many physically unilateral work tasks	1.303	0.445	0.660–2.573						
		I do not experience that there is sufficient ergonomic support and aids for my employees work	1.192	0.709	0.475–2.990						
	Mental work environment	**I do not experience that there is a general balance between the demands put on my employees in their work, and the control they have in executing their work tasks**	2.054	0.037	1.043–4.045	2.054	0.037	1.043–4.045			
		I experience that my employees in general are too stressed in their work due to political decisions and circumstances in society	1.601	0.070	0.963–2.664						
		I experience that my employees in general run the risk of occupational injury and occupational disease based on the mental work environment	1.698	0.083	0.932–3.093						
		I experience that my employees in general are too stressed in their work due to current circumstances in the work place	1.362	0.245	0.809–2.291						
		I experience that my employees run the risk of being subjected to violence and threats in their work	1.112	0.699	0.649–1.905						

Table 2. Cont.

			The Managers Believe Their Employees' Not Want to Work until 65 Years of Age or Beyond								
			Univariate Estimates			Multivariate Model in Each Determent Area			Multivariate Model Including All Nine Determent Areas		
Determinant Sphere	Determinant Areas	Statement	OR	P	95% CI	OR	P	95% CI	OR	P	95% CI
	Working hours, work pace and time for recuperation	I do not experience that my employees in general have sufficient possibilities to take breaks when working	2.376	0.017	1.164–4.851	2.376	0.017	1.164–4.851			
		I do not experience that my employees in general have a good work schedule that enables recuperation between work shifts	2.493	0.032	1.081–5.747						
		I experience that it can be a problem to keep the work activities running due to lack of temp workers when employees are off work	1.157	0.574	0.696–1.922						
		I experience that my employees in general have too many work tasks due to lack of employees	1.037	0.902	0.583–1.845						
Financial incentives	Personal financial situation	I experience that my employees in general feel pressured by their financial situation (i.e., having difficulty getting by on their salary, health insurance and/or other social security systems)	1.140	0.698	0.588–2.213						
Social inclusion, relations and participation	Personal social environment	I do not experience that my employees in general have sufficient opportunity of combining work with their leisure activities and social relations in their leisure time.	2.225	0.093	0.875–5.658						
		I do not experience that my employees in general have sufficient opportunity of combining work with their family situation, partner, children, grandchildren, etc.	2.067	0.155	0.760–5.624						
	Work social environment	My employees in general do not receive sufficient support from me to be able to work until ordinary retirement age	4.582	0.025	1.208–17.380	4.582	0.025	1.208–17.380	4.972	0.022	1.263–19.574
		I am not satisfied with the extent of support that I offer my employees for them to be able to cope with their work tasks	1.671	0.136	0.846–3.300						
		I do not experience that my employees in general receive sufficient support to be able to cope with their work tasks from their co-workers, others in the organization and supporting organizations	1.462	0.378	0.629–3.397						
		I am not satisfied with the quality of the support that I offer my employees for them to be able to cope with their work tasks	1.237	0.666	0.470–3.259						
		I experience that my senior employees are subjected to discrimination/disregard by others in the workplace (co-workers, patients, clients, etc.)	1.394	0.644	0.340–5.708						
		I do not experience that my employees in general have reasonable opportunity of participation in decisions regarding work organization	1.460	0.404	0.600–3.557						

Table 2. Cont.

Determinant Sphere	Determinant Areas	Statement	The Managers Believe Their Employees' Not Want to Work until 65 Years of Age or Beyond								
			Univariate Estimates			Multivariate Model in Each Determinant Area			Multivariate Model Including All Nine Determent Areas		
			OR	P	95% CI	OR	P	95% CI	OR	P	95% CI
Execution of work tasks	Stimulation and motivation in work tasks	I do not experience leadership to be crucial for senior employees consideration to keep working after 65 years of age	1.417	0.181	0.851–2.359						
		In my experience it is hard to find work tasks to relocate employees who experience their work environment as too physically demanding	2.836	<0.001	1.657–4.855	2.836	<0.001	1.657–4.855	2.812	<0.001	1.621–4.872
		I do not experience it being possible to adjust work tasks to senior employees in my organization	1.867	0.017	1.116–3.123						
		In my experience it is hard to find work tasks to relocate employees who experience their work environment as too mentally demanding	1.721	0.057	0.983–3.013						
		I do not experience that my employees in general have reasonable opportunity of participation in decisions regarding their work tasks	1.204	0.802	0.281–5.158						
		I do not experience that my employees in general are satisfied in their daily work	1.861	0.208	0.708–4.893						
		I do not experience that my employees in general have work tasks that they experience as stimulating and meaningful	2.226	0.386	0.365–13.577						
	Competence development, skills, knowledge	I do not experience that my employees have access to sufficient technical support	2.622	0.018	1.180–5.828	2.622	0.018	1.180–5.828			
		I do not experience it being important to keep senior employees in the organization based on their competence	1.588	0.178	0.810–3.112						
		I do not experience that my senior employees have the right knowledge and experience for their work tasks	1.853	0.147	0.805–4.266						
		I do not experience that my senior employees in general have opportunity of continuous competence development	1.584	0.337	0.620–4.048						
		I do not experience that my senior employees in general have the knowledge and experience that enable them to find a job in the eventuality of re-organization and changes	1.128	0.654	0.665–1.914						
		I do not experience that my employees in general have work tasks where they feel they can use their skills and knowledge	2.792	0.404	0.250–31.212						
		I do not experience that my employees in general have knowledge and experience that enables them to be reallocated in our organization	1.040	0.878	0.627–1.726						

4. Discussion

In a workplace, it is the employer who, through the manager, enables employees to have access to measures that facilitate labour force participation. Therefore, the manager's attitudes are important to investigate in relation to the facilitation of an extended, sustainable working life. There are some areas that determine whether individuals can versus want to work respectively. Furthermore, these determinant areas are important to the individual's retirement and retirement planning [1,2,14–16,19]. In an organisation or enterprise, it is mainly the manager who makes decisions regarding these determinant areas. The investigation analysis regarded which determinant area was the most important to the managers' belief that their employees can versus want to work in an extended working life. The multivariate model stated that three areas were statistically significant and associated with managers believing that their employees **could not work until 65 years of age or older**, i.e., *Self-rated health and diagnoses*, *Physical work environment* and *Competence development, skills, knowledge*. Furthermore, the results of the multivariate model stated that two of these areas were statistically significant and associated with managers believing that their employees would **not want to work until 65 years of age or older**, i.e., *Work social environment* and *Stimulation and motivation in work tasks*. In order to analyse determinant areas of work life participation in this study, the swAge-model was used to structure the analysis. The swAge-model includes nine areas determinant to participation in working life (see the Introduction paragraph). The discussion below follows the structure of the swAge-model and investigates the nine determinant areas associated with the managers believing that their senior employees can versus want to work respectively.

4.1. Self-Rated Health and Diagnoses

Individuals' health situation, i.e., the area *Self-rated health and diagnoses*, is significant to whether individuals can participate in working life at all [1,2,14–20]. However, in this study, the managers considered the employees who currently participated in working life, and most of the managers (93%) believed their employees to experience sound well-being and health status in their daily lives. Still, the results of the multilevel model in the logistic regression analysis stated that well-being and diagnosed health status among employees were of great importance to whether employees would be able to work until an older age. In the multivariate models, only the employees' own experience of well-being proved to be statistically significant to both whether employees were able to work as well as whether employees wanted to work until 65 years of age or older. Furthermore, self-rated health and wellbeing being a better predictor for employees' extended working life than diagnoses have been stated in one earlier study [19]. Therefore, activities and measures to increase employees' own experience of well-being appear to be important factors in order to increase employability and the possibility of an extended working life.

4.2. Physical Work Environment

The results from this study state the physical work environment is of great importance to whether managers believe that their employees would not be able to work in an extended working life. However, the physical work environment did not prove to be statistically significant to whether the manager believed that their employees did not want to work until 65 years of age or older. A poor physical work environment and work conditions increase the risk of work accidents, leave people worn out and push them to leave working life prematurely [1,2,14–16,21–23]. If so, they would not be able to work and would have difficulties remaining employable. Therefore, taking measures to reduce the risks in the physical work environment appears to be of great importance to employees' ability to work in an extended working life.

4.3. Mental Work Environment

Mental work conditions, stress and lack of control when executing work tasks have also been mentioned as important predictors for employees' sickness absence and retirement planning [1,2,14–16,24–26]. In these analyses of this survey, it emerged that the managers did not consider the mental work environment to be of any statistically significant importance to whether their employees would not be able to work beyond the age of 65. However, a statistically significant association was proven with whether their employees would want to work until an older age, i.e., the mental work environment determinant "demands and control" at work. However, this did not prove to be statistically significant in the multivariate model for neither being able to nor wanting to work. Since the mental strain from the work environment accounts for a large proportion of sickness absence from work, managers may need to take the mental work environment more seriously.

4.4. Working Hours, Work Pace and Time for Recuperation

The determinant area *Working hours, work pace and time for recuperation* proved to be statistically significant and especially related to managers believing their employees would not want to work until an older age in the univariate model in this study. Some studies highlight a moderate work pace and working hours as important to facilitate sufficient time for rest and recuperation, as well as for employability and the mental and physical ability to execute work tasks [1,2,14–16,27–29]. Furthermore, different work schedules have been stated as a statistically significant, successful tool to increase employees' possibility of working until an older age. The manager probably needs to consider that senior employees, in general, need more time for rest and recuperation. Therefore, working hours, work pace and sufficient time for recuperation are important factors for the ability to work in an extended working life.

4.5. Financial Incentives

The determinant area *Financial incentives* included research regarding whether the risk of poverty keeps employees in the workforce or whether it is possible to quit working with sufficient personal financial well-being [1,2,14–16,30–32]. However, financial incentives did not prove to be statistically significant to whether the managers believed their employees would be able to or want to work until 65 years of age or beyond in the final models.

4.6. Personal Social Environment

The personal social environment and attitudes in surrounding society also influence withdrawal from working life, for example through marital status, whether the life partner is working or whether the senior employee wants to spend more time with relatives and leisure pursuits [1,2,14–16,33–35]. The determinant area *Personal social environment* did not prove to be statistically significant in this study. Perhaps the managers primarily focus on the work situation and not as much on the fact that employees also have a personal life outside working life that influences whether they can or want to work.

4.7. Work Social Environment

What the management and leadership in the organisation are like, whether the attitudes are positive towards and between employees, whether workers are included in the organisation, or whether there is a stereotypical idea of senior employees as stagnant and an encumbrance [1,2,7,14–16,36,37]. Actually, the employees not receiving sufficient support from their manager, a statement belonging to the determinant area *Work social environment*, proved to be the most important, i.e., had the highest statistically significant OR, in the multivariate model of all determinant areas associated with whether the managers believed their employees would not want to work in an extended working life. The manager has a very important role and decision power regarding measures, norms and strategies in the workplace and to enable individual employees to work in an extended working life [1,2,14–16,26,36,37]. Therefore, it is important that managers' attitudes towards their senior employees are positive if society wants a larger amount of people to have the possibility to participate in working life until an older age, due to the demographic development where a larger number of senior citizens need to earn a living.

4.8. Stimulation and Motivation in Work Tasks

Individuals need activities. According to previous studies, motivating and simulating tasks have an impact on employees and increase their activity, employability and participation in an extended working life [1,2,14–16,38–40]. The determinant area *Stimulation and motivation in work tasks* proved to be statistically significant to whether the managers believed their employees both would not be able to and would not want to work until 65 years of age or older. However, in the multivariate model, it only proved significant to whether the managers believed their employees would not want to work until 65 years of age or older. This is in line with earlier studies of employees' own experiences and wishes to work in an extended working life or not [14,16,34]. Managers, organisations and companies need to take steps to enable the experience of motivation and stimulation in work tasks in order to make employees want to participate in working life until an older age.

4.9. Competence Development, Skills, Knowledge

Statements in the determinant area *Competence development, skills, knowledge* proved to be statistically significant to managers believing their employees both would be able to and would want to participate in an extended working life in this study. Competence development, skills, knowledge were stated as a high predictor of whether the manager believed their senior employees would be able to work until an older age in the multivariate model. This is consistent with previous studies that state that the level of education, competence and the possibility of developing skills, but also whether employees are able to utilize their skills in their work tasks, to be important factors to extended work life participation [1,2,14–16,41–43]. Therefore, it is important that managers and the organisation contribute to enabling the development of competence, skills and knowledge for all employees irrespective of age if the employees should remain employable until an older age.

4.10. Limitations and Strength of the Study

The study design is cross-sectional and has limitations since it only shows the result from one point in time. However, this study is the baseline measurement in a longitudinal study regarding factors affecting an extended working life. This baseline investigation will be followed up when employees leave working life, as well as with their health and sickness absence during working life. This entire project will provide a good possibility to investigate the effect of the managers' attitudes and whether they believe that their employees can and want to work respectively, as well as their attitudes towards measures and action proposals with the aim of enabling a sustainable extended working life, when their employees retire from working life.

The Swedish municipality studied has a larger number of female employees, which corresponded with that most of the study population and the respondents were women.

Although the municipal community included in the study was the eighth largest in Sweden with 456 managers identified to participate in the study, a potential weakness was that 46,4% of the managers in the original study population did not participate. However, the participation rate was 54.6%, compared to other studies this was an expected and normal participation rate of surveys. Additionally, the average age was 50.4 with a range of 25–67, therefore, most managers appear to be in the later stage of their career. Perhaps a study population with a larger proportion of younger managers would have given different results. However, on average, in Swedish working life and in the municipal sector, the average age of managers is high, as in most industrial countries, therefore, the study population corresponds to the general composition of the labour force [3–5].

A strength of this study is that it is a total sampling including all the managers in the municipality, and all participation managers work in the same municipality and had the same employer, which minimised the risk of different employment conditions, rehabilitation policies and retirement policies [45].

One strength of this study was the possibility to examine differences between determinant areas and whether managers believe that their employees can or want to extend their working life beyond 65 years of age. All nine determinant areas in the analysis are included in the swAge-model and have been identified in previous studies as very important to retirement and retirement planning [1,2,14–16], however, all areas have not previously been included in the same study regarding managers' attitudes towards their employees' possibility to work in an extended working life. The results of this study strengthen the theories of the swAge-model.

The questionnaire was sent out after a review of the theoretical basis in the area, the swAge-model, and the majority of the statements in the questionnaire have previously been validated and used in previous studies.

Furthermore, to the best of our knowledge, no previous studies have analysed the distinction between whether managers believe their employees 'can' and 'want to' work, respectively, in an extended working life.

5. Conclusions, Theoretical Contribution and Practical Implications

Work is an important part of an individuals' life. However, in the workplace, it is the employer, through the manager, who enables employees to have access to measures that facilitate labour force participation. Therefore, the manager's attitudes are important to investigate in relation to enabling a sustainable extended working life. Since several countries (especially in Europe) have included in their social policy measures from government plans through that the retirement age to be increased after 65, proposing ages approaching 70. When these proposals become laws, through obligation, people will have no choice despite if they do not want to or if they cannot continue working! However, the new situation, generated by the COVID-19 pandemic, changed a lot of the perceptions among managers and employees related to the work processes. To force all people to extend their working life without any organisational work environment activities could be problematic. This study and analysis of the participating managers' attitudes showed there is a difference between why employees 'can' versus 'want' to work, respectively. Different determinant areas of work life participation are associated with whether managers believe that their employees are able to work versus that their employees want to work until 65 years of age or older. The results of this study show that health, physical work environment, skills and competence were areas of particular importance to managers believing that their employees **can work until 65 years of age or older**. The results also stated that the well-being, work social environment and stimulation and motivation in work tasks were the most important to managers believing that their employees **want to work until age 65 or older**. These results strengthen the theoretical framework of the SwAge-model [1,5] and could hopefully contribute to a better understanding and development of measure activities that need to be conducted to perform a more sustainable extended working life.

Different strategies may be needed to both contribute to the employees being able to and wanting to participate in working life until an older age. To create a more sustainable working life for all ages, as well as to increase the possibilities to extend working life, organisational measures and activities are needed throughout the entire working life. Individuals' employability until an older age depends on the nine determinant areas included in the four determinants spheres: health impacts of the work environment; the financial situation; social inclusion, relations and participation; execution of work tasks [1,2,15,53]. To increase the sustainability of working life, and to promote work life participation until an older age, managers must know what measures need to be taken for their ageing employees. One tool that managers could use is to investigate the workplace with support from the nine determinants of the SwAge model, to find out what activities and measures are needed, for example using the template available for this task [1,2,53].

The results from this study will hopefully contribute to the understanding of the process of extended working life. Additionally, the study's contribution of knowledge can hopefully be used in workplace interventions and future research for a sustainable working life until an older age.

Author Contributions: K.N. and E.N. have completed the analysis, authored the paper and approved the final manuscript. All authors have read and agreed to the published version of the manuscript.

Funding: This study was funded byAFA Insurance (Sweden): 170298. The financiers were not involved or had any role in the design of the study, the data collection, the analysis, the interpretation of data or in the writing of this paper.

Institutional Review Board Statement: The study was conducted according to the ethical codes and principles expressed in the Declaration of Helsinki and was approved by The Regional Ethical Review Board in Lund (no 2018/27).

Informed Consent Statement: Informed consent to participate was collected from the participants in the survey.

Data Availability Statement: The data used in this study is managed by the authors. To access this data please contact the authors.

Conflicts of Interest: The authors declare no conflict of interest.

References

1. Nilsson, K. A sustainable working life for all ages–The swAge-model. *Appl. Ergon.* **2020**, *86*, 103082. [CrossRef] [PubMed]
2. Nilsson, K.; Nilsson, E. Organisational Measures and Strategies for a Healthy and Sustainable Extended Working Life and Employability—A Deductive Content Analysis with Data Including Employees, First Line Managers, Trade Union Representatives and HR-Practitioners. *Int. J. Environ. Res. Public Health* **2021**, *18*, 5626. [CrossRef] [PubMed]
3. OECD. *Pensions at a Glance 2017: OECD and G20 Indicators*; OECD Publishing: Paris, France, 2017. [CrossRef]
4. Eurostat. *Active Ageing and Solidarity between Generations–A Statistical Portrait of the European Union 2012*; Publications Office of the European Union: Luxembourg, 2011.
5. European Commission. *Demography Report*; (Short analytical web note; 3/2015); Publications Office of the European Union: Luxembourg, 2015.
6. Hess, M. Rising preferred retirement age in Europe: Are Europe's future pensioners adapting to pension system reforms? *J. Aging Soc. Policy* **2017**, *29*, 245–261. [CrossRef] [PubMed]
7. Nilsson, K. Managers' attitudes to their older employees-A cross-sectional study. *Work* **2018**, *59*, 49–58. [CrossRef]
8. Nilsson, K. Attitudes of managers and older employees to each other and the effects on the decision to extended working life. In *Older Workers in a Sustainable Society. Labor, Education & Society*; Ennals, R., Salomon, R.H., Eds.; Peter Lang Verlag: Frankfurt, Germany, 2011; pp. 147–156.
9. Oakman, J.; Wells, Y. Retirement intentions: What is the role of push factors in predicting retirement intentions? *Ageing Soc.* **2013**, *33*, 988–1008. [CrossRef]
10. Johnston, D.W.; Wang-Sheng, L. Retiring to the good life? The short-term effects of retirement on health. *Econ. Lett.* **2009**, *103*, 8–11. [CrossRef]
11. Ilmarinen, J. *Toward a Longer Working Life: Aging and Quality of Working Life in the European Union*; Finnish Institute of Occupational Health: Helsinki, Finland, 2006.
12. Saurama, L. Experience of early exit. In *A Comparative Study of the Reasons for and Consequences of Early Retirement in Finland and Denmark in 1999–2000*; Finnish Centre for Pension Studies: Helsinki, Finland, 2004.
13. Stypinska, J.; Konrad Turek, K. Hard and soft age discrimination: The dual nature of work-place discrimination. *Eur. J. Ageing* **2017**, *14*, 49–61. [CrossRef] [PubMed]
14. Nilsson, K.; Rignell-Hydbom, A.; Rylander, L. Factors influencing the decision to extend working life or to retire. *Scand. J. Work Environ. Health* **2011**, *37*, 473–480. [CrossRef]
15. Nilsson, K. Conceptualization of ageing in relation to factors of importance for extending working life–A review. *Scand. J. Public Health* **2016**, *44*, 490–505. [CrossRef] [PubMed]
16. Nilsson, K. The Influence of Work Environmental and Motivation Factors on Seniors' Attitudes to an Extended Working Life or to Retire. A Cross Sectional Study with Employees 55–74 Years of Age. *Open J. Soc. Sci.* **2017**, *5*, 30–41. [CrossRef]
17. McGoldrick, A.E.; Arrowsmith, J. Discrimination by age: The organizational response. In *Ageism in Work and Employment*; Glover, I., Branine, M., Eds.; Ashgate Publishing Ltd.: Stirling, Scotland, 2001; pp. 75–96.
18. Pietiläinen, O.; Laaksonen, M.; Rahkonen, O.; Lahelma, E. Self-rated Health as a Predictor of Disablility Retirement–The Contribution of Ill-Health and Working Conditions. *PLoS ONE* **2011**, *6*, e25004. [CrossRef] [PubMed]
19. Nilsson, K.; Rignell-Hydbom, A.; Rylander, L. How is self-rated health and diagnosed dis-ease associate with early or deferred retirement: A cross sectional study with employees aged 55–64. *BMC Public Health* **2016**, *16*, 886. [CrossRef]

20. Börsch-Supan, A.; Brugiavini, A.; Croda, E. The role of institutions and health in European patterns of work and retirement. *J. Eur. Soc. Policy* **2009**, *19*, 341–358. [CrossRef] [PubMed]
21. Karlsson, N.E.; Carstens, J.M.; Gjesdal, S.; Alexandersson, K.A.E. Work and Health. Risk fac-tors for disability pension in a population-based cohort of men and women on long-term sick leave in Sweden. *Eur. J. Public Health* **2008**, *18*, 224–231. [CrossRef]
22. Sauré, P.; Zoabi, H. Retirement Age across Countries: The Role of Occupations, Swiss National Bank Working Papers 6/2012, Zurich. 2011. Available online: http://papers.ssrn.com/sol3/papers.cfm?abstract_id=1940452 (accessed on 10 March 2020).
23. von Bonsdorff, M.E.; Rantanen, T.; Törmäkangas, T.; Kulmala, J.; Hinrichs, T.; Seitsamo, J.; von Bonsdorff, M.B. Midlife work ability and mobility limitation in old age among non-disability and disability retirees: A prospective study. *BMC Public Health* **2016**, *16*, 154–161. [CrossRef]
24. Kunze, F.; Reas, A.M.L. It Matter How Old You Feel: Antecedents and Performance Consequences of Average Relative Subjective Age in Organizations. *J. Appl. Psychol.* **2015**, *100*, 1511–1526. [CrossRef] [PubMed]
25. Hovbrandt, P.; Carlsson, G.; Nilsson, K.; Albin, M.; Håkansson, C. Occupational balance as described by older workers over the age of 65. *J. Occup. Sci.* **2019**, *26*, 40–52. [CrossRef]
26. Canivet, C.; Choi, B.K.; Karasek, R.; Moghaddassi, M.; Staland-Nyman, C.; Östergren, P.-O. Can high psychological job demands, low decision latitude, and high job strain predict disability pensions? A 12-year follow-up of middle-aged Swedish workers. *Int. Arch. Occup. Environ. Health* **2013**, *86*, 307–319. [CrossRef] [PubMed]
27. Mykletun, R.; Furunes, T. The Ageing Workforce Management Programme in Vatenfall AB Nordic, Sweden. In *Older Workers in a Sustainable Society. Labor, Education & Society*; Ennals, R., Salomon, R.H., Eds.; Peter Lang Verlag: Frankfurt, Germany, 2011; pp. 93–106.
28. Furunes, T.; Mykletun, R. Managers' Decision Latitude for Age Management: Do Managers and Employees have the same (implicit) Understanding. In *Older Workers in a Sustainable Society. Labor, Education & Society*; Ennals, R., Salomon, R.H., Eds.; Peter Lang Verlag: Frankfurt, Germany, 2011; pp. 107–116.
29. Laaksonen, M.; Metsä-Simola, N.; Martikainen, P.; Pietiläinen, O.; Rahkonen, O.; Gould, R.; Partonen, T.; Lahelma, E. Trajectories of mental health before and after old-age retirement and disa-bility retirement: A register-based study on purchases of psychotropic drugs. *Scand. J. Work Environ. Health* **2012**, *38*, 409–417. [CrossRef] [PubMed]
30. Cobb-Clark, D.A.; Stillman, S. The Retirement Expectations of Middle-aged Australians. *Econ. Rec.* **2009**, *85*, 146–163. [CrossRef]
31. Brenes-Comacho, G. Favourable changes in economic well-being and self-rated health among the elderly. *Soc. Sci. Med.* **2011**, *72*, 1228–1235. [CrossRef]
32. Nilsson, K.; Östergren, P.-O.; Kadefors, R.; Albin, M. Has the participation of older employ-ees in the workforce increased? Study of the total Swedish population regarding exit working life. *Scand. J. Public Health* **2016**, *44*, 506–516. [CrossRef]
33. Hanson Frieze, I.; Olson, J.E.; Murrell, A.J. Working Beyond 65: Predictors of Late Retirement for Women and Men MBAs. *J. Women Aging* **2011**, *23*, 40–57. [CrossRef]
34. Gyllensten, K.; Wentz, K.; Håkansson, C.; Nilsson, K. Older assistant nurses' motivation for a full or extended working life. *Ageing Soc.* **2019**, *39*, 2699–2713. [CrossRef]
35. Friis, K.; Ekholm, O.; Hundrup, Y.A.; Obel, E.B.; Grønbaek, M. Influence of health, lifestyle, working conditions, and sociodemog-raphy on early retirement among nurses: The Danish Nurse Cohort Study. *Scand. J. Public Health* **2007**, *35*, 23–30. [CrossRef] [PubMed]
36. Jensen, P.H.; Juul Møberg, R. Age Management in Danish Companies: What, How and How Much? *Nord. J. Work. Life Stud.* **2012**, *2*, 49–65. [CrossRef]
37. Cheung, F.; Wu, A.M.S. An investigation of predictors of successful aging in the workplace among Hong Kong Chinese older workers. *Int. Psychogeriatr.* **2012**, *24*, 449–464. [CrossRef]
38. Jokela, M.; Ferrie, J.E.; Gimeno, D.; Chandola, T.; Shipley, M.J.; Head, J.; Vahtera, J.; Westerlund, H.; Marmot, M.G.; Kivimäki, M. From Midlife to early Old Age. Health trajectories Associated With Retirement. *Epidemiology* **2010**, *21*, 284–290. [CrossRef] [PubMed]
39. Oude Hengel, K.; Blatter, B.M.; van der Molen, H.F.; Bongers, P.M.; van der Beek, A.J. The effectivness of a construction worksite prevention program on work ability, health, and sick leave: Results from a cluster randomized controlled trial. *Scand. J. Work Environ. Health* **2013**, *39*, 456–467. [CrossRef] [PubMed]
40. Hovbrandt, C.; Håkansson, C.; Karlsson, G.; Albin, M.; Nilsson, K. Prerequisites and driving forces behind an extended working life among older workers. *Scand. J. Occup. Ther.* **2019**, *26*, 171–183. [CrossRef]
41. Mather, M. Aging and cognition. *Cogn. Sci.* **2010**, *1*, 346–362. [CrossRef]
42. Backes-Gellner, U.; Schneider, M.R.; Veen, S. Effect of Workforce Age on Quantitative and Qualitative Organizational Performance: Conceptual Framwork and Case Study Evidence. *Orgaisational Stud.* **2011**, *32*, 1103–1121. [CrossRef]
43. Doyle, Y.G.; McKee, M.; Sherriff, M. A model of successful ageing in British populations. *Eur. J. Public Health* **2012**, *22*, 76–77. [CrossRef] [PubMed]
44. Forma, P.; Tuominen, E.; Väänänen-Tomppo, I. Who wants to continue at work? Finnish pension reform and the future plans of older workers. *Eur. J. Soc. Secur.* **2005**, *7*, 227–250. [CrossRef]
45. Li, C.-Y.; Sung, F.-C. A review of the healthy worker effect in occupational epidemiology. *Occup. Med.* **1999**, *49*, 225–229. [CrossRef]
46. Bengtsson, E.; Nilsson, K. *Äldre Medarbetare. [Older Worker.]*; Swedish National Institute of Working Life: Malmö, Sweden, 2004.

47. Nilsson, K. Äldre medarbetares attityder till ett långt arbetsliv. Skillnader mellan olika yrkesgrupper inom hälso- och sjukvården. [Older workers attitude to an extended working life. Differences between occupations in health and medical care]. *Arbetsliv Omvandl.* **2006**, *10*, 1–74.
48. Nilsson, K. Vem kan och vill arbeta till 65 år eller längre? En studie av anställda inom hälso- och sjukvården. [Who can and want to work until 65 years or beyond? A study with employed in health and medical care]. *Arb. Hälsa* **2005**, *14*, 1–35.
49. Karasek, R.; Theorell, T. Healthy Work. In *Stress, Productivity and the Reconstruction of Working Life*; Basic Books: New York, NY, USA, 1990.
50. Torgén, M.; Stenlund, C.; Ahlberg, G.; Marklund, S. *Ett hållbart arbetsliv för alla åldrar. [A Sustainable Working Life to All Ages.]*; Swedish National Institute of Working life: Stockholm, Sweden, 2001.
51. Jönsson, S.; Tranquist, J.; Petersson, H. *Mellan Klient och Organization. Psykosocial Arbets-miljö i Arbete Med Människor. [Between Client and Organization. Mental Work Environment in Human Service Work.]*; Swedish National Institute of Working Life: Malmö, Sweden, 2003. (In Swedish)
52. Antonovsky, A. *Unreveling the Mystery of Health-How People Manage Stress and Stay Well*; Jossey-Bass Publishers: San Francisco, CA, USA, 1987.
53. swAge-Model. Available online: https://swage.org/en.html (accessed on 11 June 2021).

Article

Psychosocial Working Conditions and Social Participation. A 10-Year Follow-Up of Senior Workers

Pia Hovbrandt [1,2,*], Per-Olof Östergren [3], Catarina Canivet [3], Maria Albin [1,4], Gunilla Carlsson [5], Kerstin Nilsson [1] and Carita Håkansson [1]

[1] Division of Occupational and Environmental Medicine, Department of Laboratory Medicine, Lund University, 22363 Lund, Sweden; Maria.Albin@med.lu.se (M.A.); kerstin.nilsson@med.lu.se (K.N.); carita.hakansson@med.lu.se (C.H.)
[2] Occupational Therapy and Occupational Science Research Group, Department of Health Sciences, Lund University, 22100 Lund, Sweden
[3] Division of Social Medicine and Global Health, Department of Clinical Sciences in Malmö, Lund University, 22213 Malmö, Sweden; per-olof.ostergren@med.lu.se (P.-O.Ö.); catarina.canivet@med.lu.se (C.C.)
[4] Unit of Occupational Medicine, Institute for Environmental Medicine, Karolinska Institute, 17177 Stockholm, Sweden
[5] Active and Healthy Ageing Research Group, Department of Health Sciences, Lund University, 22100 Lund, Sweden; gunilla.carlsson@med.lu.se
* Correspondence: pia.hovbrandt@med.lu.se

Abstract: Social participation is important for health, and it is well known that high strain jobs impact negatively on mental and physical health. However, knowledge about the impact of psychosocial working conditions on social participation from a long-term perspective is lacking. The purpose of this study was to investigate the associations between different job types and social participation from a long-term perspective. A comprehensive public health questionnaire "*The Scania Public Health Survey*", was used, and psychosocial working conditions were measured with a Swedish translation of the Job Content Questionnaire. Based on data from 1098 working respondents aged 55 at baseline and a 10-year follow-up when the respondents were not working, the analyses revealed that social participation varied by job type. Jobs with high decision latitude, as in active and relaxed jobs, seem to predict high social participation, even after cessation of employment. Besides that, the result suggests that high social participation during working life is a predictor of high social participation from a long-term perspective which promotes healthy aging. Incentives for working longer are strongly related to good working conditions. A supportive work environment with possibilities for employees to participate in decision making, i.e., high control, is vital for a sustainable working life. This may contribute to an extended working life and may also support social participation prior to retirement as well as after retirement and thus to healthy aging.

Keywords: aging; extended working life; decision latitude; health promotion; life-course perspective; work-life balance; retirement; self-rated health; social activities; sustainable working life; work environment

1. Introduction

The demographic change with an increased number of older people is an important factor for public health. Previous findings show for example that experiencing greater enjoyment in life may predict more years in good health [1]. However, the findings are still inconsistent, and it is crucial to find predictors for healthy aging. The concept of "healthy aging" concerns several determinants such as personal and behavioral factors and the social as well as the physical environment [2]. Specifically, the importance of having a life-course perspective is emphasized since aging is a lifelong process [3]. Although social participation patterns remain relatively stable through people's life course, factors in working life might also impact on opportunities for social participation in very old age [4].

Thus, investigating social participation, which may contribute to health and well-being in old age, from a long-term perspective, is important.

Social participation is a broad concept including leisure activities or meeting with friends and consists of interactions with others in society or the community [5]. Several studies have also found how important social participation is for life satisfaction and healthy aging [6–8]. Moreover, social participation contributes to both cognitive and physical health in old age [9–13]. Additionally, formal social participation seems to predict higher levels of quality of life and lower levels of depressive symptoms among older people [14]. What older people value and choose to be engaged in often depends on what they have done in the past, according to the Continuity Theory of Aging [15]. Continuity means an adaptive strategy for change in the aging process, promoted by personal preferences and social behavior based on earlier activities. Supporting the continuity theory, a longitudinal study focusing on age-related changes in leisure, including social participation, showed that participation earlier in life was a strong predictor of participation in leisure activities also in late life [16]. Consequently, it could be important to have a repertoire of activities from the past to choose from in old age, when, for example, work tasks must be replaced with other activities [17,18]. Furthermore, social participation contributes to a sense of being included in a social context [17,19,20], and, among very old people, social participation was shown to be preferable and of special importance for their well-being [21]. However, to the best of our knowledge the influence of working conditions on social participation from a long-term perspective beyond working life has not yet been explored.

The Job Strain Model (JSM) explains the psychosocial aspects of work and proposes four types of psychosocial job exposure: high strain, relaxed, active, and passive [22]. These four job types are combinations of high and low levels of psychosocial job demands and decision latitude. JSM postulates that high strain (high job demands and low decision latitude) increases the risk of ill health, and empirical support for this has been shown in epidemiological studies of, e.g., coronary heart disease, stroke, diabetes, depression, and neck and shoulder disorders (for recent reviews see [23–25]. Job strain has also been related to poor survival in a long-term follow-up after retirement [26].

Among people aged 45–64 years, associations between psychosocial work conditions and social participation using the Job Strain Model have been shown [22,27]. More specifically, Lindström [27] found that passive and high strain jobs were negatively associated with social participation, and that active and relaxed jobs were associated with higher levels of social participation. Work stressors among working adults aged 57–65 was also found to be predictors of limited physical functioning 20 years later [28]. Thus, there may be factors in working life that also have effects on social participation in later life.

Summing up, several studies found that social participation is important for health [6,8,11,13,29], and that high strain jobs impact negatively on mental and physical health [24,25]. However, knowledge about the impact of job strain on social participation from a long-term perspective is lacking. The Scania Public Health Cohort, with 10-year follow-up data, provides a unique opportunity to assess social participation and earlier work-related determinants. In line with previous findings in a cross-sectional study design [27], we hypothesize that there are associations between psychosocial work conditions and social participation from a longitudinal perspective. More precisely, our hypothesis is that low decision latitude, passive job, and job strain are negatively associated with high social participation, and that high decision latitude, active job, and relaxed job are associated with higher levels of social participation.

The purpose of the current study was to investigate the associations between psychosocial working conditions and social participation from a long-term perspective. More specifically the study aimed

- to investigate whether psychosocial demands and their combinations predict social participation among 55-year or older working people in a 10-year follow-up when they were not working.

- to investigate if high decision latitude was associated with social participation at baseline and predicted high social participation at follow-up.

2. Material and Methods

2.1. Sample and Settings

Comprehensive public health questionnaires, "*The Scania Public Health Survey*", were sent out, by post, in 2000, 2005, and 2010 to a non-proportional geographically stratified sample of inhabitants in 33 municipalities of the county of Scania in the south of Sweden [30]. These individuals were randomly selected from the population register, such that equal representation was achieved from all 33 municipalities in the region of Scania, Sweden. Details according to design have been described elsewhere [30]. In total, 24,922 subjects born 1919–1981 (age 18–80) were asked to participate in 2000 and of these 13,604 responded (58% response rate). In 2010, an identical questionnaire was sent out to the 12,117 respondents from the first wave who were still alive and living in Scania, which was responded to by 9103 subjects (75% response rate).

In the present study we included respondents who were 55+ and still working at least 10 h/week at baseline in 2000 and who did not work at follow-up in 2010. The final cohort ended up being 1098 respondents of whom 51% were men and 49% were women (Figure 1).

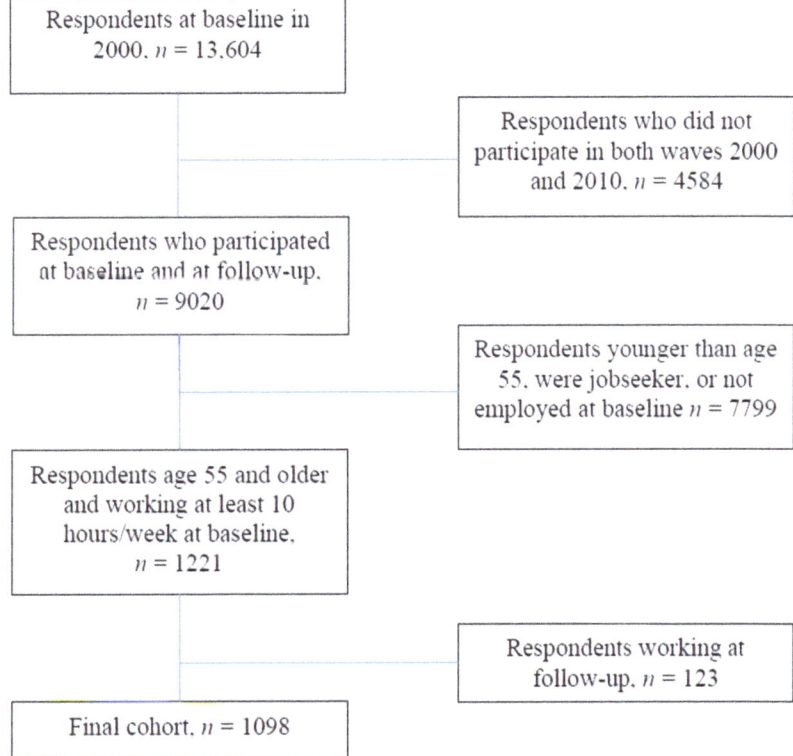

Figure 1. Flow chart of the study sample.

2.2. Outcome Variables

Social participation (during the past year) describes how actively a person has taken part in activities in society. The social participation variable consisted of 13 items: participation in study circle/course at work, study circle/course at leisure time, union meeting, meeting of other organization, theatre/cinema, arts exhibition, church, sports event, had written letter to editor of a newspaper/magazine, demonstration of any kind, visited public event (night club, dance or similar), larger family gathering, or been at a private party. Items were dichotomized (yes/no) and summed up, and if three or less were indicated, the social participation of that person was classified as low, and if four or more were indicated, the social participation of that person was classified as high [31]. This question has been used in Sweden since 1960s and has been validated in an earlier study [32].

2.3. Exposure Variable

Psychosocial working conditions were measured with a Swedish translation of the original Job Content Questionnaire (JCQ) [33]. JCQ is based on the JSM [34] and was further developed [22] with a focus on psychosocial demands and control. High demands refer to intensive or rapid work where the employee may experience conflicting demands. Job control refers to the degree of decision-making authority and skill discretion of the employee, i.e., decision latitude. The JCQ items consist of 14 statements where respondents were asked to either agree or disagree on a four level Likert scale (1–4). Thus, the answer is based on the individual's own experience of demands and control in the working environment. Consequently, there could be variations in the same profession. Two continuous variables reflecting psychosocial job demands and decision latitude were thus created, and both were dichotomized at the median level. Following the demand-control model, four different job types were defined by combining psychosocial demands and decision latitude. That is, high strain job is a combination of high demands and low decision latitude, *relaxed* job is a combination of low demands and high decision latitude, *active* job is a combination of high demands and high decision latitude, and passive job is a combination of low demands and low decision latitude.

2.4. Other Baseline Characteristics

Demographic characteristics considered sex, married/cohabitating versus single, and length of education (dichotomized into 12 years and less, corresponding to primary and secondary school, vs. 13 years or more corresponding to university).

Financial stress was captured by the question "How often during the past 12 months have you had difficulties paying your bills (rent, electricity, telephone, mortgage, insurance, etc.)?" with response alternatives "Every month", "About half of the months", "A few times" and "Never". The answer was considered as financial stress if the respondent had answered "Every month" or "About half of the months", and as "No financial stress" if the answer was "A few times" or "Never".

To capture the family situation the question was posed, "Do you have any old or sick relative that you need to help, refer to or care for?" with the response alternatives yes or no.

Physical activity was measured by a single question asking about leisure time activity (household work excluded) with the response alternatives: mostly sedentary leisure time activities, moderate leisure time physical activities, regular exercise, hard or competitive sports/training regularly or several times a week. Answers were dichotomized, as physically active (last three alternatives) vs. Not physically active (first alternative).

Self-rated health was measured with the question, "In general, how do you rate your current health status" with five response alternatives "Excellent", "Good", "Fair", "Bad", and "Very bad" [35–37]. This single question is considered to be the most reliable and valid item estimate of the self-rated health status [38]. Answers were dichotomized as "Good self-rated health" if the respondent had answered "excellent" and "good", and Poor self-rated health if the answer was "fair", "bad", and "very bad" in any of the two waves 1999 and 2010.

2.5. Statistical Analysis

Kruskal Wallis test was used to detect differences between the four job types (high strain, relaxed, active, and passive) in social participation rates at baseline and McNemar's test to detect within each job type group changes in social participation rates between baseline and follow-up 10 years later. Bivariate logistic regression was used to test whether the potential confounders, sex, self-rated health, marital status, not caring for a sick relative, education level, financial stress, and physical activity at baseline, were associated with social participation at follow up. Thereafter, a stepwise multivariate logistic regression analysis was performed to test if high decision latitude at baseline was associated with high social participation at baseline and follow-up. The model was adjusted for the confounders, whose p-values in the bivariate logistic regression analyses were <0.10, i.e., good self-rated health, not caring for a sick relative, high educational level, and physically active. Low decision latitude with the lowest social participation rates was selected as the reference category.

To test for a possible effect modification, i.e., the effect of having two factors worse than additive, a synergy index (SI) was calculated as proposed by Rothman [39]. The following algorithm was used where SI = 1 meant no additive effect, SI > 1 meant a signified synergistic effect, and SI < 1 meant an antagonistic effect.

$$SI = \frac{RR(AB) - 1}{[RR(Ab) - 1] + [RR(aB) - 1]}$$

RR = risk ratio; Ab = exposed to one of the factors; aB = exposed to the other factor; AB = exposed to both factors.

The two factors included in this calculation were self-rated health and educational level at baseline. The level of statistical significance was set at $p < 0.05$. The statistical analyses were conducted with SPSS, version 24 (IBM Corp., Armonk, NY, USA).

2.6. Ethics

The study was conducted in accordance with the Helsinki Declaration and The Regional Ethical Review Board in Lund approved the study (2016/720).

3. Results

3.1. Descriptive Results

The mean age of the respondents was 58 years and the oldest individual, who still was working, was 76 years of age at baseline. As shown in Table 1, more than 80% of the respondents in the study were married or cohabiting. Notably, very few of the respondents reported financial stress during the past 12 months. Additionally, very few reported that they were helping a sick or old relative. More than half of the respondents reported good self-rated health, and a quite high proportion reported that they were physically active in their leisure time. Regarding job type, about one third in this study had a passive job (low demands/low decision latitude), almost one fifth of the respondents had a relaxed job (low demands/high decision latitude), an active job (high demands/high decision latitude), or a high strain job (high demands/low decision latitude), respectively.

Table 1. Sociodemographic variables, and psychosocial working conditions at baseline, $n = 1098$.

Characteristics	n of Respondents (Missing)	%
Sex		
Men	563	51
Women	535	49
Married/cohabitating	16	2
Yes	894	81
No	188	17
Education	34	3
12 years or less	653	60
13 years or more	411	37
Financial stress	11	1
Yes	19	2
No	1068	97
Self-rated health	(11)	1
Good	669	61
Poor	418	38
Helping old or sick relative	(18)	2
Yes	287	26
No	793	72
Physical activity	(31)	3
Yes	934	85
No	133	12
Job type	(166)	11
Passive	363	33
Relaxed	204	19
Active	227	20
High strain	188	17

3.2. Variations in Social Participation between Different Job Type

As can be seen in Table 2, social participation varied by job type. At baseline, high social participation was most common in the active group (91%), followed by 89% in the relaxed group, 82% in the high strain group, and 78% in the passive group; differences between groups were statistically significant ($p < 0.001$). Regarding the within-group evolution in social participation levels between baseline (year 2000) and follow-up (year 2010), social participation decreased in all groups (p-levels varying between 0.004 and <0.001). Differences between job type and high social participation at follow up were statistically significant between active and high strain group ($p < 0.001$), active and passive group ($p < 0.001$), relaxed and passive group ($p < 0.001$), and relaxed and high strain group ($p < 0.001$) but not between any other groups.

Table 2. Social participation at baseline and follow-up, in four job type groups, p values for change in social participation between 1999 and 2010, $n = 982$.

	Passive, $n = 363$ (%)		p Value	Relaxed, $n = 204$ (%)		p Value	Active, $n = 227$ (%)		p Value	High Strain, $n = 188$		p Value
	2000	2010		2000	2010		2000	2010		2000	2010	
High	282 (78)	227 (62)	<0.001	181 (89)	162 (79)	0.004	206 (91)	177 (78)	<0.001	155 (82)	119 (63)	<0.001
Low	81 (22)	136 (38)		23 (11)	42 (21)		21 (9)	50 (22)		33 (18)	69 (37)	

3.3. Associations between Potential Confounders and High Social Participation

As can be seen in Table 3, the baseline variables associated with high social participation at follow-up were good self-rated health, not caring for sick relative, high educational level, and physically active. Moreover, the strongest predictor of high social participation at follow-up was high social participation at baseline, OR 8.37 (5.84–11.99) (not in tables).

Table 3. Associations between potential confounders, measured at baseline, and high social participation at the 10-year follow up.

Potential Confounders	OR (95% CI)
Female gender	1.14 (0.88–1.48)
Good self-rated health	**2.11 (1.62–2.74)**
Married/cohabiting	1.25 (0.90–1.75)
Not caring for a sick relative	**1.44 (1.06–1.96)**
High education level	**3.48 (2.56–4.73)**
Financial stress	0.60 (0.24–1.52)
Physically active	**2.40 (1.66–3.48)**

Note: Variables associated with high social participation at follow-up in bold text.

High decision latitude, physically active, as well as high educational level were associated with high social participation in all models at baseline (Table 4).

Table 4. Associations between high decision latitude at baseline, as defined by the demand-control model, and high social participation at baseline and at the 10-year follow up, respectively (n = 982).

Variables	Model 1 OR (95% CI)	Model 2	Model 3	Model 4	Model 5	Model 6
2000						
High decision latitude	2.29 (1.58–3.33)	2.24 (1.53–3.27)	2.12 (1.45–3.10)	1.59 (1.06–2.38)	1.58 (1.05–2.37)	
Physically active		2.44 (1.55–3.86)	2.23 (1.39–3.58)	2.08 (1.27–3.39)	2.08 (1.27–3.41)	
Good self-rated health 1999			1.32 (0.90–1.94)	1.20 (0.80–1.80)	1.22 (0.81–1.84)	
High educational level				3.08 (1.93–4.92)	3.01 (1.88–4.81)	
Not caring for a sick relative					1.11 (0.72–1.70)	
2010						
High decision latitude	2.18 (1.64–2.91)	2.13 (1.59–2.86)	2.01 (1.49–2.70)	1.53 (1.12–2.10)	1.49 (1.09–2.05)	1.37 (0.98–1.91)
Physically active		2.38 (1.58–3.58)	1.96 (1.29–2.99)	1.79 (1.16–2.78)	1.78 (1.15–2.77)	1.51 (0.94–2.42)
Good self-rated health 1999–2010			1.90 (1.41–2.55)	1.90 (1.40–2.58)	1.94 (1.42–2.64)	1.92 (1.38–2.66)
High educational level				3.01 (2.14–4.26)	2.98 (2.11–4.21)	2.50 (1.74–3.58)
Not caring for a sick relative					1.43 (1.01–2.03)	1.44 (0.99–2.08)
High social participation at baseline						6.29 (4.15–9.54)

High decision latitude at baseline predicted high social participation at 10-year follow-up. In this model, physically active, good self-rated health at both occasions, high educational level, and not caring for a sick relative were also significant. However, when adjusting for high social participation at baseline high decision latitude, physically active and not caring for a sick relative were no longer significant. High social participation became then the most significant predictor in the model.

We also examined the synergistic effect between latitude at work and self-rated health and educational level on social participation respectively. Not surprisingly, the prevalence of social participation was highest among workers with high decision latitude and good self-rated health and lowest among workers with low decision latitude and poor self-rated health (Table 5). The synergy index between high decision latitude at work and self-rated health on social participation was 2.1, which means that the positive factors reinforce each other's effect.

Table 5. Interaction analysis with synergy index, regarding latitude at work and self-rated health, both measured at baseline in 1999 and social participation in 2010. Scania Public Health Cohort, n = 975.

Decision Latitude and Self-Rated Health in 2000	n	% Cases with High Social Participation	OR [a]	95% CI [b]	SI [c]
Low latitude and poor health	176	53	1		
Low latitude and good health	369	68	1.4	0.9–2.1	
High latitude and poor health	90	64	1.7	0.9–3.3	
High latitude and good health	340	82	3.2	1.9–5.4	2.1
	975				

[a] OR, odds ratio; [b] CI, confidence interval; [c] SI, synergy index.

Workers with high decision latitude and high educational level showed the highest prevalence of social participation although they did not differ much from workers with low decision latitude and high educational level (Table 6).

Table 6. Interaction analyses with synergy index, regarding latitude at work and level of education, both measured at baseline in 1999 and social participation in 2010. Scania Public Health Cohort, n = 961.

Decision Latitude and Educational Level in 2000	n	% Cases with High Social Participation	OR [a]	95% CI [b]	SI [c]
Low latitude and low educational level	386	56	1		
Low latitude and high educational level	149	83	5.2	2.6–10.6	
High latitude and low educational level	195	71	2.1	1.3–3.3	
High latitude and high educational level	231	85	4.5	2.6–7.9	0.66
	961				

[a] OR, odds ratio; [b] CI, confidence interval; [c] SI, synergy index.

According to educational level the synergy index was 0.66 indicating no additive effect between the positive factors, i.e., high decision latitude and high educational level. This means that the presence of both high decision latitude and high educational level reduced the risk of their separate effects on high social participation.

4. Discussion

4.1. Main Findings

In this study, we investigated the associations between psychosocial working conditions and social participation from a long-term perspective. We firstly tested whether psychosocial demands and their combinations predicted social participation among 55-year or older working people in a 10-year follow-up when they were not working. The result showed that social participation varied by job type, which supports our hypothesis that high decision latitude, active job, and relaxed job should be associated with higher levels of social participation. Thus, it seems like high decision latitude predicts high social participation, even after cessation of employment.

Our findings additionally showed that an unwanted effect of low decision latitude was low social participation. Decision latitude has increasingly been shown to also predict other behavioral patterns of importance for health and well-being, i.e., to be a cause behind the causes [40]. The status syndrome points to the social ingredients of health and that *"the major determinants of health are social"* ([40] p. 1103). Although work gives structure in daily life and contributes to both physical and mental well-being, work may also be stressful. Specifically, circumstances without control in erratic situations, without social support, and without recovery can be very stressful and thus have a negative impact on health [40]. This leads to leisure time physical activity declining among those with low job control [41]. The chance for developing a healthy lifestyle was more likely among those with high decision latitude than for those with low decision latitude [42].

Moreover, when we adjusted for social participation at baseline, this was the strongest predictor of social participation at follow-up. This may be understood based on the Continuity Theory [15,43], suggesting that older people are motivated to use their past experiences that worked well to shape their future life course. Thus, older people conceptualize their past as a great resource that influences adaptations to new situations. That is, those with high social participation during working life in the present study could more easily adapt to a situation as retired with continuing social participation. However, in the present study, only the amount of social participation the respondents participated in was included. Regardless, this is in line with previous studies testing the Continuity Theory, which tended to focus on older people's activity patterns over time [16,44]. These studies also lack information on how respondents value different activities. Among older workers it was found that high workload, i.e., high strain earlier in middle-age, hindered them from valuable activities such as social participation [20]. A balanced life with possibilities for a mix of different activities besides work seems to be important for a sustainable working life that may also contribute to healthy aging.

Since continuity is not only about what older people do but also and, maybe more importantly, about the meaning behind their participation [45], further studies are needed to explain associations between work-related factors and the meaning in social participation for older people to connect the results more fully to Continuity Theory.

In line with previous findings, our study confirms how the risk associated with passive and high strain job in midlife also impacts negatively on health factors in old age. For example, longitudinal studies suggested that midlife work stressors were associated with more musculoskeletal pain and mobility problems [28,45–48] and dementia after retirement age [49]. In a recent study with a focus on passive jobs and high strain jobs in late midlife, it was found that high strain jobs among women and passive jobs among men were associated with decreased physical functioning 20 years later [28]. Thus, it is obvious that psycho-social work conditions such as passive and high strain jobs have negative consequences from a long-term perspective and the present study confirms that this is also true according to social participation. To our knowledge, the current study is the first to show how work-related factors, i.e., especially decision latitude, predicted high social participation in a long-term perspective. Consequently, to strive for a sustainable working life, it is of vital concern to also consider factors in the work environment that may have a positive effect on healthy aging.

4.2. Methodological Considerations

The strength in the present study is the longitudinal design in a national large population with respondents from midlife to old age, and the use of an established psychosocial work condition model, i.e., JSM [33]. Some limitations should also be noted. First, we did not study men and women separately, which should be done in future research. Second, although there is an agreement in research that higher levels of social participation are associated with positive outcomes [50], to count the number of activities is just one aspect of social participation. The number of activities does not say anything of experience of social participation, which is important since it is the meaning of activities that appears to promote health [51]. Future research with qualitative or mixed methods might be applicable to investigate how social participation more deeply might be related to the Continuity Theory of aging. Nevertheless, the findings in the present study gave a picture of how much the respondents participated in the included activities and therefore made it possible to analyze associations with, and predictions of, psychosocial work conditions. Furthermore, another important issue is the possible causality between the variable health and social participation [52]. It may be so that healthier people are more prone to participate in social activities, or the reverse causality that social participation has positive effects on health, or that both social participation and health influence each other [53]. Maybe not very surprisingly, a synergistic effect was found between high decision latitude at work and self-rated health on social participation, while an antagonistic effect between high decision latitude and high educational level was found.

4.3. Possible Implications

This study adds valuable information on the role that midlife psychosocial work environment plays in late life, such as within social participation. For instance, the findings could be used to improve midlife interventions aimed at promoting social participation later in life. Good psychosocial working conditions in a supportive work environment with possibilities for decision making is beneficial not only in working age but also after retirement. Thus, it is of vital concern that both policy makers and employers take actions for a sustainable working life that prevent work injuries and support a balanced working life.

Considering an aging population in many European countries, an extended working life is of vital concern [54] and, therefore, pension reforms are changing to both restrict early retirement and raise the standard retirement age. However, incentives for working longer are strongly related to good working conditions [55,56] and work strain is also an important risk factor for work ability from a long-term perspective [57–59]. Although a previous study showed no associations between physical and psychosocial working conditions and workability [60], another study found that job resources, such as job control, predicted longer time in working life [61]. More and more people actually work beyond the retirement age already today [62], but a large proportion still retires before the statutory retirement age due to work-related risk factors [54,63]. Consequently, an extended working life is only possible with measures that contribute a sustainable working life [64]. Thus, a life-course perspective with measures for a sustainable working life with possibilities for, for example, social participation, is important. A starting point for such a measure could be the theoretical swAge-model [65,66], focusing measurements on health effects associated with working environment, for personal financial security, for social inclusion and social support in the work situation, and for creativity and intrinsic work motivation [67]. A supportive work environment with an organization that encourage employees to participate in decision making, i.e., high control, are vital for a sustainable working life. This may contribute to an extended working life and may also support social participation prior to retirement as well as after retirement, which is an important factor for healthy aging.

5. Conclusions

Previous research with long term perspectives has mainly focused on physical functioning and not on other aspects of daily life, such as social dimensions, that are important for healthy aging. In particular, high decision latitude predicted higher levels of social participation while low decision latitude may reduce the chances for active aging. This study adds valuable information on the role that midlife psychosocial work environment plays in late-life, here social participation. For instance, it could potentially be used to improve midlife interventions aimed at promoting social participation later in life.

Author Contributions: Conceptualization, P.H., P.-O.Ö., M.A., G.C., K.N. and C.H.; formal analysis, P.H., C.C. and C.H.; writing—original draft preparation, P.H. and C.H.; writing—review and editing, all authors. All authors have read and agreed to the published version of the manuscript.

Funding: This study was funded by the Swedish Research Council for Health, Working Life, and Welfare (Ref. 2012–1696).

Institutional Review Board Statement: The study was conducted according to the guidelines of the Declaration of Helsinki and was approved by The Regional Ethical Review Board in Lund (720/2016).

Informed Consent Statement: Our study is based on comprehensive public health questionnaires "The Scania Public Health Survey", that were sent out, by post, in 2000, 2005, and 2010 to a non-proportional geographically stratified sample of inhabitants in Scania. In total, 24,922 subjects born 1919–1981 (age 18–80) were asked to participate in 2000 and, of these, 13,604 responded (58% response rate). In 2010, an identical questionnaire was sent out to the 12,117 respondents from the first wave who were still alive and living in Scania, 9103 of which responded (75% response rate), as shown in Figure 1. In both the invitation letter and the cover letter, information was provided about the purpose of the study and that participation was voluntary and also that all information from the questionnaire would be handled regarding confidentiality and personal integrity during storage, analysis, and publication. Information was also given that each participant has the right to obtain the information available regarding him/her when desired, and that this information must be deleted upon on request. Before the analysis for this study, we also advertised in the daily press in Scania to inform participants about the procedure and that they could contact P-O Östergren by mail or phone if they did not wish to participate in this survey. All information given was in accordance with approval by The Regional Ethical Review Board in Lund. For this kind of study, we cannot meet the respondents for oral information and by the respondents answering the questionnaire they gave their consent to participate.

Data Availability Statement: The dataset used and analysed during the current study is available from the corresponding author on reasonable request.

Acknowledgments: With permission, the authors would like to thank Anna Oudin, Statistician at Division of Occupational and Environmental Medicine, Lund University, for valuable support with the statistical analyses.

Conflicts of Interest: The authors declare no conflict of interest.

References

1. Zaninotto, P.; Steptoe, A. Association Between Subjective Well-being and Living Longer Without Disability or Illness. *JAMA Netw. Open* **2019**, *2*, e196870. [CrossRef]
2. WHO. Decade of Healthy Ageing: Baseline Report. *Geneva*. Available online: https://www.who.int/publications/i/item/9789240023307 (accessed on 26 August 2021).
3. WHO. World Report on Ageing and Health. *Geneva*. Available online: https://www.who.int/publications/i/item/9789241565042 (accessed on 26 August 2021).
4. Hovbrandt, P.; Fridlund, B.; Carlsson, G. Very old people's experience of occupational performance outside the home: Possibilities and limitations. *Scand. J. Occup. Ther.* **2007**, *14*, 77–89. [CrossRef] [PubMed]
5. Levasseur, M.; Richard, L.; Gauvin, L.; Raymond, E. Inventory and analysis of definitions of social participation found in the aging literature: Proposed taxonomy of social activities. *Soc. Sci. Med.* **2010**, *71*, 2141–2149. [CrossRef] [PubMed]
6. Gibson, H.J.; Singleton, J.F. *Leisure and Aging: Theory and Practice*; Human Kinetics: Champaign, IL, USA, 2012.
7. Huxhold, O.; Miche, M.; Schüz, B. Benefits of having friends in older ages: Differential effects of informal social activities on well-being in middle-aged and older adults. *J. Gerontol. Ser. B-Psychol. Sci.* **2014**, *69*, 366–375. [CrossRef] [PubMed]
8. Klugar, M.; Cáp, J.; Klugarová, J.; Marecová, J.; Roberson, D.; Kelnarova, Z. The personal active ageing strategies of older adults in Europe: A systematic review of qualitative evidence. *JBI Database Syst. Rev. Implement. Rep.* **2016**, *14*, 193–257. [CrossRef]
9. Bourassa, K.J.; Memel, M.; Woolverton, C.; Sbarra, D.A. Social participation predicts cognitive functioning in aging adults over time: Comparisons with physical health, depression, and physical activity. *Aging Ment. Health* **2017**, *21*, 133–146. [CrossRef]
10. He, Q.; Cui, Y.; Liang, L.; Zhong, Q.; Li, J.; Li, Y.; Lv, X.; Huang, F. Social participation, willingness and quality of life: A population-based study among older adults in rural areas of China. *Geriatrics Gerontol. Int.* **2017**, *17*, 1593–1602. [CrossRef]
11. Hughes, T.F.; Flatt, J.D.; Fu, B.; Chang, C.C.; Ganguli, M. Engagement in social activities and progression from mild to severe cognitive impairment: The MYHAT study. *Int. Psychogeriatr.* **2013**, *25*, 587–595. [CrossRef]
12. Li, C.; Jiang, S.; Li, N.; Zhang, Q. Influence of social participation on life satisfaction and depression among Chinese elderly: Social support as a mediator. *J. Community Psychol.* **2018**, *46*, 345–355. [CrossRef]
13. Paillard-Borg, S.; Fratiglioni, L.; Xu, W.; Winblad, B.; Wang, H.-X. An Active Lifestyle Postpones Dementia Onset by More than One Year in Very Old Adults. *J. Alzheimer's Dis.* **2012**, *31*, 835–842. [CrossRef]

14. Santini, Z.I.; Jose, P.E.; Koyanagi, A.; Meilstrup, C.; Nielsen, L.; Madsen, K.R.; Koushede, V. Formal social participation protects physical health through enhanced mental health: A longitudinal mediation analysis using three consecutive waves of the Survey of Health, Ageing and Retirement in Europe (SHARE). *Soc. Sci. Med.* **2020**, *251*, 112906. [CrossRef]
15. Atchley, R.C. A Continuity Theory of Normal Aging. *Gerontologist* **1989**, *29*, 183–190. [CrossRef] [PubMed]
16. Agahi, N.; Ahacic, K.; Parker, M.G. Continuity of leisure participation from middle age to old age. *J. Gerontol. Ser. B* **2006**, *61*, S340–S346. [CrossRef] [PubMed]
17. Nilsson, K. Why work beyond 65? Discourse on the Decision to Continue Working or Retire Early. *Nord. J. Work. Life Stud.* **2012**, *2*, 7–28. [CrossRef]
18. Nilsson, K. The ability and desire to extend working life. In *Healthy Workplaces for Men and Women in All Ages Knowledge Compilation*; V.E. Swedish Work Environment Authority: Stockholm, Sweden, 2016; pp. 36–59.
19. Christiansen, C.; Townsend, E. The occupational nature of social groups. In *Introduction to Occupation: The Art and Science of Living, International Edition*, 2nd ed.; Christiansen, C., Townsend, E., Eds.; Pearson Education, Inc.: Upper Saddle River, NJ, USA, 2010; pp. 175–210.
20. Hovbrandt, P.; Carlsson, G.; Nilsson, K.; Albin, M.; Håkansson, C. Occupational balance as described by older workers over the age of 65. *J. Occup. Sci.* **2018**, *26*, 40–52. [CrossRef]
21. Nilsson, I.; Löfgren, B.; Fisher, A.G.; Bernspång, B. Focus on Leisure Repertoire in the Oldest Old: The Umeå 85+ Study. *J. Appl. Gerontol.* **2006**, *25*, 391–405. [CrossRef]
22. Karasek, R.; Theorell, T. *Healthy Work: Stress, Productivity, and the Reconstruction of Working Life*; Basic Books: New York, NY, USA, 1990.
23. Kivimäki, M.; Jokela, M.; Nyberg, S.T.; Singh-Manoux, A.; Fransson, E.; Alfredsson, L.; Bjorner, J.B.; Borritz, M.; Burr, H.; Casini, A.; et al. Long working hours and risk of coronary heart disease and stroke: A systematic review and meta-analysis of published and unpublished data for 603,838 individuals. *Lancet* **2015**, *386*, 1739–1746. [CrossRef]
24. Kraatz, S.; Lang, J.; Kraus, T.; Münster, E.; Ochsmann, E. The incremental effect of psychosocial workplace factors on the development of neck and shoulder disorders: A systematic review of longitudinal studies. *Int. Arch. Occup. Envir. Health* **2013**, *86*, 375–395. [CrossRef] [PubMed]
25. Madsen, I.E.; Nyberg, S.T.; Hanson, L.M.; Ferrie, J.E.; Ahola, K.; Alfredsson, L.; Batty, G.D.; Bjorner, B.; Borritz, M.; Burr, H.; et al. Job strain as a risk factor for clinical depression: Systematic review and meta-analysis with additional individual participant data. *Psychol. Med.* **2017**, *47*, 1342–1356. [CrossRef] [PubMed]
26. Falk, A.; Hanson, B.S.; Isacsson, S.-O.; Ostergren, P.-O. Job strain and mortality in elderly men: Social network, support, and influence as buffers. *Amer. J. Public Health* **1992**, *82*, 1136–1139. [CrossRef]
27. Lindström, M. Psychosocial work conditions, social participation and social capital: A causal pathway investigated in a longitunal study. *Soc. Sci. Med.* **2006**, *62*, 280–291. [CrossRef]
28. Nilsen, C.; Agahi, N.; Kåreholt, I. Work stressors in late midlife and physical functioning in old age. *J. Aging Health* **2017**, *29*, 893–911. [CrossRef] [PubMed]
29. James, B.; Wilson, R.; Barnes, L.; Bennet, D. Late-life social activity and cognitive decline in old age. *J. Int. Neuropsychol. Soc.* **2011**, *17*, 998–1005. [CrossRef] [PubMed]
30. Carlsson, F.; Merlo, J.; Lindström, M.; Östergren, P.-O.; Lithman, T. Representativity of a postal public health questionnaire survey in Sweden, with special reference to ethnic differences in participation. *Scand. J. Public Health* **2006**, *34*, 132–139. [CrossRef]
31. Lindström, M.; Merlo, J.; Ostergren, P.-O. Individual and neighbourhood determinants of social participation and social capital: A multilevel analysis of the city of Malmö, Sweden. *Soc. Sci. Med.* **2002**, *54*, 1779–1791. [CrossRef]
32. Hanson, B.S.; Östergren, P.-O.; Elmståhl, S.; Isacsson, S.-O.; Ranstam, J. Reliability and validity assessments of measures of social networks, social support and control—Results from the Malmö Shoulder and Neck Study. *Scand. J. Soc. Med.* **1997**, *25*, 249–257. [CrossRef]
33. Karasek, R.; Brisson, C.; Kawakami, N.; Houtman, I.; Bongers, P.; Amick, B. The Job Content Questionnaire (JCQ): An instrument for internationally comparative assessments of psychosocial job characteristics. *J. Occup Health Psychol.* **1998**, *3*, 322. [CrossRef]
34. Karasek, R. Job demands, job decision latitude, and mental strain: Implication for job redesign. *Admin. Sci. Quart.* **1979**, *24*, 285–308. [CrossRef]
35. Kaplan, G.A.; Camacho, T. Perceived health and mortality: A nine-year follow-up of the human population laboratory cohort. *Amer. J. Epidemiol.* **1983**, *117*, 292–304. [CrossRef]
36. Schnittker, J.; Baćak, V. The Increasing Predictive Validity of Self-Rated Health. *PLoS ONE* **2014**, *9*, e84933. [CrossRef]
37. Ware, J.E.; Kosinski, M.; Keller, S.D. A 12-Item Short-Form Health Survey: Construction of Scales and Preliminary Tests of Reliability and Validity. *Med. Care* **1996**, *34*, 220–233. [CrossRef] [PubMed]
38. Björner, J.; Sondergaard, K.T.; Orth-Gomér, K.; Tibblin, G.; Sullivan, M.; Westerholm, P. *Self-Rated Health: A Useful Concept in Research, Prevention and Clinical Medicine*; Swedish Council for Planning and Coordonation of Research: Stockholm, Sweden, 1996.
39. Rothman, J. *Modern Epidemiology*; Little, Brown and Company: Boston, MD, USA, 1986.
40. Marmot, M. Social determinants of health inequalities. *Lancet* **2005**, *365*, 1099–1104. [CrossRef]
41. Fransson, E.I.; Heikkilä, K.; Nyberg, S.T.; Zins, M.; Westerlund, H.; Westerholm, P.; Väänänen, A.; Virtanen, M.; Vahtera, J.; Theorell, T.; et al. Job strain as a risk factor for leisure-time physical inactivity: An individual-participant meta-analysis of up to 170,000 men and women: The IPD-Work Consortium. *Amer. J. Epidemiol.* **2012**, *176*, 1078–1089. [CrossRef]

42. Heikkilä, K.; Fransson, E.I.; Nyberg, S.T.; Zins, M.; Westerlund, H.; Westerholm, P.; Virtanen, M.; Vahtera, J.; Suominen, S.; Steptoe, A.; et al. Job strain and health-related lifestyle: Findings from an individual-participant meta-analysis of 118,000 working adults. *Amer. J. Public Health* **2013**, *103*, 2090–2097. [CrossRef]
43. Breheny, M.; Griffiths, Z. "I had a good time when I was young": Interpreting descriptions of continuity among older people. *J. Aging Stud.* **2017**, *41*, 36–43. [CrossRef]
44. Utz, R.L.; Carr, D.; Nesse, R.; Wortman, C.B. The effect of widowhood on older adults' social participation: An evaluation of activity, disengagement, and continuity theories. *Gerontologist* **2002**, *42*, 522–533. [CrossRef]
45. Kulmala, J.; von Bonsdorff, M.B.; Stenholm, S.; Törmäkangas, T.; von Bonsdorff, M.E.; Nygård, C.H.; Klockars, M.; Seitsamo, J.; Ilmarinen, J.; Rantanen, R. Perceived stress symptoms in midlife predict disability in old age: A 28-year prospective cohort study. *J. Gerontol. Ser. A* **2013**, *68*, 984–991. [CrossRef]
46. Kulmala, J.; Hinrichs, T.; Törmäkangas, T.; von Bonsdorff, M.; von Bonsdorff, M.; Nygård, C.-H.; Klockars, M.; Seitsamo, J.; Ilmarinen, J.; Rantanen, T. Work-related stress in midlife is associated with higher number of mobility limitation in older age—Results from the FLAME study. *AGE* **2014**, *36*, 9722. [CrossRef]
47. Nilsen, C.; Andel, R.; Fors, S.; Meinow, B.; Mattsson, A.D.; Kåreholt, I. Associations between work-related stress in late midlife, educational attainment, and serious health problems in old age: A longitudinal study with over 20 years of follow-up. *BMC Public Health* **2014**, *14*, 1–12. [CrossRef]
48. Parker, V.; Andel, R.; Nilsen, C.; Kåreholt, I. The association between mid-life socioeconomic position and health after retirement—Exploring the role of working conditions. *J. Aging Health* **2013**, *25*, 863–881. [CrossRef]
49. Sindi, S.; Hagman, G.; Håkansson, K.; Kulmala, J.; Nilsen, C.; Kåreholt, I.; Soininen, H.; Solomon, A.; Kivipelto, M. Midlife Work-Related Stress Increases Dementia Risk in Later Life: The CAIDE 30-Year Study. *J. Gerontol. Ser. B* **2016**, *72*, 1044–1053. [CrossRef] [PubMed]
50. Howrey, B.T.; Hand, C. Measuring social participation in the and retirement study. *Gerontologist* **2019**, *59*, e415–e423. [CrossRef]
51. Wilcock, A.; Hocking, C. *An Occupational Perspective of Health*, 3rd ed.; Slack Incorporated: Thorofare, NJ, USA, 2015.
52. Sirven, N.; Debrand, T. Social participation and healthy ageing: An international comparison using SHARE data. *Soc. Sci. Med.* **2008**, *67*, 2017–2026. [CrossRef] [PubMed]
53. Sirven, N.; Debrand, T. Social Participation of Elderly People in Europe. *Retraite Soc.* **2013**, *2*, 59–80. [CrossRef]
54. European Union Information Agency for Occupational Safety and Health; European Centre for the Development of Vocational Trainong; European Foundation for the Improvement of Living and Working Conditions; European Institute for Gender Equality; Dubois, H.; Jungblut, J.-M.; Wilkens, M.; Vermeylen, G.; Vargas Llave, O. *Towards Age-Friendly Work in Europe: A Life Course Perspective on Work and Ageing from EU Agencies*; Publications Office of the European Union: Luxembourg, 2017.
55. Nilsson, K. Interventions to reduce injuries among older workers in agriculture: A review of evaluated intervention projects. *Work.* **2016**, *55*, 471–480. [CrossRef]
56. Nilsson, K. The influence of work environment and motivation factors on seniors' attitudes to an extended working life or retire. A cross sectional study with employees 55–74 years of age. *Open J. Soc. Sci.* **2017**, *5*, 30.
57. Anxo, D.; Ericson, T.; Herbert, A.; Rönnmar, M. *To Stay or not to Stay. That is the Question: Beyond Retirement: Stayers on the Labour Market*; Linnaeus University: Växjö, Sweden, 2017.
58. Prakash, K.; Neupane, S.; Leino-Arjas, P.; von Bonsdorff, M.B.; Rantanen, T.; von Bonsdorff, M.E.; Seitsamo, J.; Ilmarinen, J.; Nygard, C.-H. Work-related biomechanical exposure and job strain as separate and joint predictors of musculoskeletal diseases: A 28-year prospective follow-up study. *Amer. J. Epidemiol.* **2017**, *186*, 1256–1267. [CrossRef]
59. von Bonsdorff, M.E.; Rantanen, T.; Törmäkangas, T.; Kulmala, J.; Hinrichs, T.; Seitsamo, J.; Nygård, C.-H.; Ilmarinen, J.; von Bonsdorff, M.B. Midlife work ability and mobility limitation in old age among non-disability and disability retirees—A prospective study. *BMC Public Health* **2016**, *16*, 1–8. [CrossRef]
60. Oakman, J.; Neupane, S.; Prakash, K.; Nygård, C.H. What are the key workplace influences on pathways of workability? A six-year follow up. *Int. J. Environ. Res. Public Health* **2019**, *16*, 2363. [CrossRef]
61. Carr, E.; Hagger-Johnson, G.; Head, J.; Shelton, N.; Stafford, M.; Stansfeld, S.; Zaninotti, P. Working conditions as predictors of retirement intentions and exit from paid employment: A 10-year follow-up of the English Longitudinal Study of Ageing. *Eur. J. Ageing* **2016**, *13*, 39–48. [CrossRef]
62. Hofacker, D.; Naumann, E. The emerging trend of work beyond retirement age in Germany. *Z. Gerontol. Geriatr.* **2015**, *48*, 473–479. [CrossRef] [PubMed]
63. Nilsson, K.; Hydbom, A.R.; Rylander, L. How are self-rated health and diagnosed disease related to early or deferred retirement? A cross-sectional study of employees aged 55–64. *BMC Public Health* **2016**, *16*, 886. [CrossRef] [PubMed]
64. Sousa-Ribeiro, M.; Bernhard-Oettel, C.; Sverke, M.; Westerlund, H. Health and age-related workplace factors as predictors of preffered, ecpected, and actual retirement timing: Findings from a Swedish cohort study. *Int. J. Environ. Res. Public Health* **2021**, *18*, 1–23. [CrossRef] [PubMed]
65. Nilsson, K. A sustainable working life for all ages—The swAge-model. *Appl. Ergon.* **2020**, *86*, 103082. [CrossRef]

66. Nilsson, K. Conceptualisation of ageing in relation to factors of importance for extending working life—A review. *Scand. J. Public Health* **2016**, *44*, 490–505. [CrossRef]
67. Nilsson, K.; Nilsson, E. Organisational measures and strategies for healthy and sustainable extended working life and employability—A deductive content analysis with data including employees, first line managers, trade union representatives and HR-practioners. *Int. J. Environ. Res. Public Health* **2021**, *18*, 5226. [CrossRef]

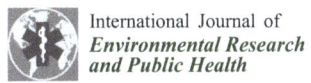

Article

Sustainable Working Life in Intensive Care: A Qualitative Study of Older Nurses

Marta Sousa-Ribeiro *, Petra Lindfors and Katinka Knudsen

Department of Psychology, Stockholm University, 11 419 Stockholm, Sweden; pls@psychology.su.se (P.L.); katinkaknudsen@hotmail.com (K.K.)
* Correspondence: marta.s.ribeiro@psychology.su.se

Abstract: To counteract the shortage of nurses in the workforce, healthcare organizations must encourage experienced nurses to extend their working lives. Intensive care (IC) has higher nurse-to-patient ratios than other settings, which includes a particular susceptibility to staff shortage. This qualitative study investigated how older IC nurses experienced their working life and their reflections on the late-career and retirement. Semi-structured interviews with 12 IC nurses in Sweden (aged 55–65 years) were analyzed using an interpretative phenomenological analysis approach. The results showed that nurses planned to continue working until the age of 65 and beyond. When reflecting on their late-career decisions, nurses considered nine areas covering individual, work, and organizational factors as being central to their ability and willingness to stay. Overall, the nurses had good health and were very satisfied and committed to their job and to the organization. They mentioned having both the job and personal resources required to cope with the physical and mental job demands, which were perceived as motivational challenges, rather than hinders. They also reflected on various human resource management practices that may promote aging-in-workplace. These findings may inform organizations aiming at providing adequate conditions for enabling healthy and sustainable working lives for IC nurses.

Keywords: retirement decisions; extended working lives; older nurses; intensive care; SwAge model; interpretative phenomenological analysis; qualitative

1. Introduction

During the last decades, many industrialized countries have seen the number and proportion of the population aged 65 years or older increase rapidly [1]. In Sweden, women and men aged 65 in 2018 would expect to live an additional average of respectively 22 and 19 years (for both women and men, 16 of these years were to involve no severe or moderate health problems) [2]. Moreover, in Sweden, the number of people aged 80 years or older is expected to increase by 50 percent by 2029 [3]. These changes in the age structures and demographic aging have profound implications at various levels and threaten the sustainability of healthcare, long-term care, and pension systems [1,2].

To respond to the challenges associated with the aging of the population, several European Union member states have implemented substantial reforms to their pension systems. Mainly, these reforms have focused on increasing the age of effective retirement and on tightening the eligibility requirements to qualify for retirement, with stronger disincentives to early retirement and advantages for postponed retirement [4]. These reforms have had an effect on the labor market participation of older workers (aged 55–64 years) in the European Union, with employment rates increasing from 38% in 2000 to 62% in 2019 [4].

The Swedish pension system is flexible and allows employees to work until a later age. In Sweden, there is no statutory retirement age, and employees have the possibility to retire between ages 62 and 68 (with financial benefits for later retirement), and most have a possibility to work beyond age 68 if the employer agrees [5]. For an increasing

Citation: Sousa-Ribeiro, M.; Lindfors, P.; Knudsen, K. Sustainable Working Life in Intensive Care: A Qualitative Study of Older Nurses. *IJERPH* **2022**, *19*, 6130. https://doi.org/10.3390/ijerph19106130

Academic Editors: Kerstin Nilsson, Tove Midtsundstad, Peter Lundqvist, Joanne Crawford, Clas-Håkan Nygård and Paul B. Tchounwou

Received: 29 April 2022
Accepted: 14 May 2022
Published: 18 May 2022

Publisher's Note: MDPI stays neutral with regard to jurisdictional claims in published maps and institutional affiliations.

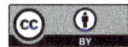

Copyright: © 2022 by the authors. Licensee MDPI, Basel, Switzerland. This article is an open access article distributed under the terms and conditions of the Creative Commons Attribution (CC BY) license (https://creativecommons.org/licenses/by/4.0/).

number of people, retirement decisions now mostly relate to decisions about when to start drawing a pension. Instead of an abrupt transition out of the workforce, retirement may involve a gradual process of labor market withdrawal. The pension can be drawn as 25–100 percent of the whole, and besides being allowed to suspend and subsequently restart the payment of the pension at any time, the retirees may continue to work and earn new pension entitlements after having started to draw their pensions [6]. Sweden has a relatively high employment rate of workers aged 60–64 (70%), but this rate decreases to 24% among workers aged 65–69 [7]. In 2019, the average age of starting to take up the retirement pension was 64.6 years. Although there is a relatively late-exit culture in Sweden, as compared with other countries [8], preferences for early retirement seem common. In a survey conducted in 2015 [2], the average age until which employees thought that they would be able to work in their current job or a similar one was 68.0 years for men and 67.1 years for women, whereas the average ages people wanted to work to were 63.3 years (men) and 62.8 years (women), respectively. Thus, many still prefer to retire much earlier than they probably can and will [9].

An aging workforce adds challenges to organizations which face shortages of qualified workers. Healthcare is a key sector that is particularly pressured by the increase in life expectancy and the number of older people, with associated increases in chronic diseases as well as healthcare needs and demands [1]. Nurses are key in healthcare organizations and are the largest group of health and social care workers in many OECD (Organisation for Economic Co-operation and Development) countries, corresponding to approximately 20–25% of all workers [1]. The age composition of nurses follows that of the general population [1] and is aging as well. In Sweden, the age distribution of nurses is relatively even, but the 50–54-year-olds constitute the largest group [10]. In 2020, the average retirement age was 63.8 years, with 5.8% of the nurses being aged 65 and older including those who postponed retirement and those who worked on an hourly basis after having started to receive their pension benefits [11].

In Sweden, as elsewhere, there is an enormous lack of qualified nurses [1,10,12]. In 2018, Swedish healthcare providers reported facing shortages of general and specialist registered nurses in all areas, including anesthesia, intensive care, and surgical care, which are key areas where 80 percent of the organizations reported a lack of staff [10]. This obviously challenges the capability to provide efficient and high-quality healthcare, with staff shortage also adding stress [13]. To address the shortage of nurses in an ever-increasing competitive labor market searching for registered nurses, healthcare organizations need to attract new staff and motivate their experienced nurses to postpone the point of fully retiring from the nursing profession [12]. For example, a report from the Swedish Association of Local Authorities and Regions in 2017 [14] stated that the recruitment needs of the Swedish welfare, including healthcare, until 2026, would decrease by 50,000 individuals by postponing the average retirement age by two years. Besides alleviating the staff shortage, older nurses who extend their working lives contribute to the organization with the experience, proficiency, and wisdom that they have acquired over the years [13,15,16]. This is important for the quality of the care provided as well as for the guidance of entry-level nurses [17]. In view of this, it is both timely and important to investigate how older nurses experience their working life and describe the factors that are important when considering a late career and whether to retire or not [18]. Such knowledge may be important for organizations and policymakers to design policies and practices enabling and motivating nursing staff to remain in the workforce [19].

An aging workforce is a global phenomenon, and retirement has turned into an important research topic. An increasing number of research literature has investigated older workers' late-career and retirement decisions (for meta-analyses and literature reviews, see [20–23]). Wang and Shi [24] systematized the factors that influence the retirement process into four categories: (1) individual attributes (e.g., demographic characteristics, health, and financial circumstances), (2) family factors (e.g., marital and dependent care status, and spouse's working status), (3) job and organizational factors (e.g., job characteristics, job attitudes, and age stereotypes at work), and (4) socioeconomic factors (e.g., social norms about retirement, and the social security system). Moreover, Browne et al. [25] focused their systematic review on the relationships between workplace psychosocial environments, retirement intentions, and actual retirement, and found that high job satisfaction and high job control were associated with later retirement intentions and actual retirement. However, occupations within human services, such as nursing, involve direct contact with people and are characterized by fewer opportunities for control and planning than occupations in other sectors [26].

A number of studies have investigated factors associated with nurses' retention [19,27], intention to remain [28–30], intention to leave [31–36], turnover [19,37,38], retirement planning [39,40], retirement preferences [16,18,41–49], and post-retirement work [50]. Although turnover and retirement constitute distinct types of organizational withdrawal, there are similarities [51], and all these outcomes are of interest when investigating older nurses' late-career decisions.

Research has found that there are several individual-related factors involved in older nurses' decisions regarding whether or not to remain in the workforce, including health status and work ability [16,43,46,48,49], financial motives [27,43,46,48,49], social motives [27,45,49], and family situation and leisure time [16,43,46,48]. The psychosocial work environment has also been found to impact significantly on older nurses' late-career plans [16,18], and a number of work-related factors have been found to be important, such as workload [46,48], work pace [46], autonomy and control [46], role clarity [30], flexible working conditions, flexible working schedules and work-time control [27,30,48], shift work [48], recovery opportunities [46], opportunities for competencies development [41,45,48], recognition [28,48], leadership style and supervisor support [16,30,48], challenging, varied, and interesting work [27,45], meaningful work [45], and job satisfaction [16,45].

Nursing work is often experienced as physically and mentally demanding [19,43,48], and has consistently been associated with poor health including musculoskeletal disorders, high levels of work-related stress, and burnout, as well as with job dissatisfaction [17,48,52]. Due to the particularly fast-paced work, excessive workload, limited decision authority, long work shifts, demands of continuous and close monitoring of severely ill and unstable patients, the need of handling sophisticated life support equipment, the frequent exposure to critical and traumatic events, and confrontation with ethical dilemmas, nursing work in intensive care (IC) units is associated with higher levels of physical and emotional demands, work stress, burnout, and depression as compared with other healthcare environments [36,53–55]. Furthermore, IC units require a higher nurse-to-patient ratio than other healthcare settings— in Sweden, this is normally 1:1–2 [56]. This means that IC units are particularly vulnerable to the shortage of nursing staff [36], something that has been aggravated during the COVID-19 pandemic [56]. However, despite the increasing importance of IC nurses to the sustainability of the healthcare sector, the characteristics of older IC nurses' late-career decisions seem understudied.

The Present Study

This study investigated how older IC nurses experienced working life and reflected on their late-careers and retirement. Using a qualitative interpretative phenomenological approach (IPA, [57,58]), we aimed to add to previous research findings and to provide a fine-grained perspective and new insights into IC nurses' sensemaking of their experiences of working and approaching retirement in IC, and their thoughts concerning what may influence their late-career decisions. The study findings may be important for organizations and policymakers in the design of policies and practices targeted at enabling healthy and sustainable working lives, and motivating experienced IC nursing staff to remain in the workforce longer.

2. Materials and Methods

2.1. Participants and Procedure

The study was part of a research project investigating older workers' retirement decision making and was approved by the Swedish Ethical Review Authority (ref no. 2017/1720-31/5). The recruitment of interviewees involved purposeful sampling of nurses in an IC unit in a general hospital in a large city in Sweden, which employed approximately 85 nurses, 26 of those aged 55 years or older, and followed three criteria: (1) working as a specialized nurse in the IC unit; (2) aged 55 years or older; and (3) not yet retired.

The third author contacted the head of the IC unit and the operational manager and presented the study aim and the sampling criteria. The managers granted permission for the implementation of the study at the unit, and a leaflet with information about the research project and contact details to the research team was distributed to the nurses. Those interested in participating contacted the team, received a brief description of the study again, and then provided written informed consent.

The participants included 12 IC nurses aged between 55 to 65 years who specialized in either IC or anesthesia. Four participants worked full time, while the others were working part time (ranging between 50% and 90% of a full-time schedule). Besides their clinical work within the IC unit, five nurses had other roles in the hospital, such as work in the emergency room, training and supervision of students, and IT and technical support of clinical devices. Organizational tenure ranged between 2 and 36 years; the nurses with the shortest tenures had long experiences of working as nurses elsewhere. All but four interviewees were women, which to some extent reflects the gender distribution of the nursing occupation in Sweden [26]. The relatively small and homogeneous sample of 12 IC nurses aligns with the IPA approach adopted in this study, which typically includes smaller samples ranging from 5 to 10 participants [58]. This allowed for a detailed and nuanced analysis, as well as for some variation in the subjective experiences while keeping with the ideographic focus characterizing the IPA approach.

2.2. Interviews

The semi-structured interviews took place in May–June 2019, in a private room at the hospital during working time, and lasted around 40–65 min. All interviews were audio-recorded and conducted in Swedish by the third author. The interviews were transcribed verbatim by the third author, with all names and other details that would somehow identify interviewees being masked during the process, to maintain interviewee integrity and to follow research ethics. The transcripts' length ranged between 4865 and 10,364 words (median 7363 words).

The interview guide covered the following main topics: (1) experience of working as an IC nurse at the organization; (2) perceptions of aging in the workplace, (3) attitudes toward work and retirement, and (4) thoughts and preferences regarding the retirement transition. The questions were open-ended and the interviewees were encouraged to expand freely on the topic. Example questions were as follows: "How do you experience your work as an IC nurse at this unit?", "What place has work in your life?", and "What are your thoughts on retirement?". Potential prompts were prepared to facilitate the flow of the interview. The interview guide was first pilot tested with two older nurses, which resulted in minor language adjustments in order to improve the clarity of the questions and ensure the validity of the interview guide.

2.3. Analytic Approach

The methodological approach used in this study was primarily the IPA [57]. The IPA was chosen due to us being interested in exploring the nurses' sensemaking of their experiences of working in IC, and of approaching retirement. Specifically, the use of IPA allows for an in-depth exploration of subjective experiences in a particular context [57]. It involves a so-called double hermeneutic, as the researcher aims at interpreting and making sense of the participants' sensemaking of their own lived experiences [57]. The use of IPA follows an inductive approach to interpret interview data, departing from the participants' narratives and then forming theoretically driven interpretations of the meanings identified in the transcripts.

The analyses of the transcripts were conducted separately by the first and third authors. This was followed by a discussion around the possible interpretations of the extracts and a construction of a thematic structure that increased the validity of the study findings. At first, the analytical process followed the heuristic framework proposed by Smith [57] for analyzing qualitative data using the IPA approach. In brief, each transcript was carefully read and re-read a few times, with initial notes being made on the extracts that were to be considered of interest for the study. Some of these notes were purely descriptive, while others were more conceptual and interpretative. Then, the analyses involved establishing associations and patterns of meaning across the initial notes within each transcript. This allowed for the identification of emergent themes, which reflect both the interviewee's narrative and the researcher's interpretations while keeping an ideographic focus on the individual voices. This process was followed by the development of an initial structure, built on the relationships across the emergent themes that were considered relevant for the study aim. This, in turn, resulted in the development of higher-level "superordinate themes", which clustered together a number of related "subordinate themes", and represented a higher concept of meaning. Finally, the analyses focused on identifying commonalities and convergences, as well as nuances and divergences across the different transcripts, and the themes were retained on the basis of their meaningfulness in representing the subjective meanings of the experiences of the interviewees and the relevance of the theme for the study aim. In the final phase, this inductive and data-driven analytic approach, which identified themes emerging from the narratives, was combined with a more deductive approach, which was informed by the SwAge model (sustainable working life for all ages) [59], a theoretical model for sustainable working life for all ages that proposes nine areas to be determinant to the individual decisions of whether to extend the working life or to retire. This combination of the inductive and deductive approaches contributed to refining the thematic structure and guided the final labeling of the superordinate or higher-order themes.

3. Results

The analysis generated ten superordinate themes, the first centering on the nurses' retirement decision making, and nine themes that reflect the nine determinant areas proposed by the SwAge model [59] to be involved in the individual's decision of whether to extend the working life or to retire: (1) self-rated health, diagnoses, and functional diversity; (2) physical work environment; (3) mental work environment; (4) work schedule, work pace, and recovery time; (5) personal finances; (6) personal social environment and private life; (7) social work environment, discrimination, leadership style, and age management; (8) motivation, satisfaction, and stimulation in the execution of work tasks; and (9) competence, use of skills, knowledge, and opportunities for development at work (see Table 1 for an overview).

Table 1. Thematic structure.

Superordinate Themes	Subordinate Themes
1. Retirement decision making	1.1. Ambivalent attitudes towards retirement 1.2. Retirement preferences 1.3. The transition to retirement
2. Self-rated health, diagnoses, and functional diversity	2.1. Being healthy as a condition to continue working 2.2. Being healthy as a condition to enjoy retirement
3. Physical work environment	3.1. Continuous noise causes stress 3.2. A physically demanding job

Table 1. *Cont.*

Superordinate Themes	Subordinate Themes
4. Mental work environment	4.1. Being in control despite the unpredictable context 4.2. Job demands—the "ethical stress" and the "nursing dilemma" 4.3. Job demands also perceived as positive challenges
5. Work schedule, work pace, and recovery time	5.1. Irregular working time may be a hinder for a sustainable and healthy working life 5.2. Recovery strategies 5.3. Post-retirement work as a way to work in a flexible schedule
6. Personal finances	6.1. Financial considerations
7. Personal social environment and private life	7.1. Attitudes towards leisure 7.2. Family situation plays a role in the work centrality and retirement plans
8. Social work environment, discrimination, leadership style, and age management	8.1. Organization-based self-esteem 8.2. The importance of a supportive working team 8.3. A supportive leadership is central for job retention 8.4. Age-friendly work environment 8.5. Age management practices that may promote a more sustainable working life
9. Motivation, satisfaction, and stimulation in the execution of work tasks	9.1. A rewarding and meaningful job 9.2. Variety at work 9.3. Job satisfaction
10. Competence, use of skills, knowledge, and opportunities for development at work	10.1. Opportunities for use of accumulated knowledge and competences 10.2. Occupational self-efficacy and the positive side of being an older worker—"the clinical eye" and "the tacit knowledge" 10.3. Importance of keeping skills up-to-date 10.4. Internal and external employability

3.1. Retirement Decision Making

3.1.1. Ambivalent Attitudes towards Retirement

The interviewees reflected on their transition to retirement and held both positive and negative attitudes towards retiring and the retiree role. The prospect of ending the working life was perceived as pleasant, as they would be freed from the obligations of work and have control of how to use their time; however, simultaneously, they were apprehensive that ending an important facet of their lives would feel strange, and they feared to miss having a job that added meaning to their daily lives and to become restless and empty. Conversely, those who considered themselves being further away from retirement had avoided thinking about it.

> *First of all, it feels very unreal, ahem, I've not really taken it in yet. (. . .) No, but it brings, well it brings joy, that you will have time off, and be free and maybe do things that you yourself think are nice, to travel and such, but then again, it is a big part of your life that somehow comes to an end. (. . .) Yes* [laughs] *I think it will be weird* [the day she stops working]*. Then again, it might probably be nice too.* [Celine]

3.1.2. Retirement Preferences

In general, the age of 65 was the preferred and most likely age at which the interviewees would start receiving their pensions. However, this was not necessarily perceived as the time to fully exit working life, and to continue working after 65 (but not full time) was in some of the nurses' plans. Post-retirement work may take various forms, such as part-time employment, or hourly paid work, which was considered more flexible. Yngve expressed the flexibility of the Swedish pension system, which allows the employee to decide the time to begin receiving pension benefits within a certain age range and combine retirement with paid work.

> *I will most likely retire when I turn 65, then I will stop working full time. And as a start, then I will use my pension benefits and work in some way, but I have not decided in what way. I have no idea whether I will continue to work on an hourly basis, or just work now and then, or continue to work part-time or something. But I will continue working in one way or another, I will.*

3.1.3. The Transition to Retirement

Interviewees emphasized the importance of retirement planning and the voluntariness of the timing of the retirement. When asked about how he would feel the day he would stop working, Sten stated:

> Then I think I would have picked that day carefully; I would have decided for myself and be happy with it. (...) When I retire, I would have planned for it. (...) I know when to do it and I would have tied up all the loose ends ahem, and I would have nothing hanging over me and I won't feel cast away. Because I think it's important that you get to retire when you want to, not because your age stops you or that you become ill or something. (...) I think this difference is essential to feel that you're done. It wasn't working life that was done with me, but it was I who were done with working life. I think this is important.

There was a clear preference for a gradual transition to retirement, as expressed by Daniella, who returned to work part time after regretting having fully retired.

> For me retirement isn't ... no, I've felt it has been quite difficult (...) 'was it just this, eh? To make a cut?' (...) I wanted to practice a bit [the retirement life]. (...) I've felt that it has been quite difficult to retire, the age, it's not that fun to grow old (...). And then I felt a bit like well (...), this is probably good, to work part-time for six months and then I'll cut [completely]. And here you can work on an hourly basis.

Post-retirement work was seen as an intermediate state and a means to adapt smoothly to the retiree role.

> I think you need to have some place to go, and that's the dilemma when you retire, that you have nowhere to go. Then perhaps you could work a bit as a nurse somewhere, on an hourly basis. [Alice]

3.2. Self-Rated Health, Diagnoses, and Functional Diversity

3.2.1. Being Healthy as a Condition to Continue Working

Despite not having the same energy as in the past, and needing longer to recover, interviewees were in relatively good health and did not feel that their age physically limited their work. Being healthy was seen as the most important requirement in considering working until age 65 and beyond.

> So, I don't know how many years after my retirement I can work part-time, I don't know, but if I'm healthy and feel that this is fun, then I can probably see myself working in the healthcare. [Nina]

> I think it is most likely that I'll continue working after 65, perhaps part-time, but I don't know how my body will feel, but if I feel good and got the strength, then I think I'll cut down to part-time. [Petter]

3.2.2. Being Healthy as a Condition to Enjoy Retirement

Besides being central for work ability, good health was also considered necessary to enjoy the retirement years. Fredrik, who planned to retire at 63, was worried about not having the health and time to do everything he would want to do after his retirement.

> But we also know that, especially we who work in this sector know that, it's not a question of whether the diseases will come, it's rather the question of when they will come. And then you also want to enjoy your retirement, I've worked well beyond 30 years. (...) It would be awful, really, if you were to come back as a patient instead. No, I wouldn't want that. And not to get to experience all this that I want to do, go on all these fantastic cruises, there are a lot of retired people there, and that's nice.

3.3. Physical Work Environment

3.3.1. Continuous Noise Causes Stress

The IC room was placed in a temporary building, and the room was very warm and considered small for the number of patients. The continuous noise from the equipment and the alarms was considered disturbing and stressful, and affected both the nurses and the patients.

> *It is noisy and very warm. And then you must constantly be careful to avoid tripping on any cable hanging five centimeters above the floor (…) so that constantly, to be responsible for the patient's life and at the same time be so* [aware of your surroundings] *(…) that you don't hurt yourself or unplug a cable from any advanced equipment. (…) Eh, yes, I think it affects me and increases stress. (…) I don't think anyone works well under pressure when it is noisy (…) and then you have to think about, it's difficult for the staff but … what how about the patient? That is, patients who are lying down, who cannot turn over by themselves and staring at the ceiling or looking into a wall, and hear all these alarms, knowing that these alarms concern themselves, but don't understand what they mean. (…) We know that we have patients who have nightmares about alarms after they recover from intensive care.* [Sten]

3.3.2. A Physically Demanding Job

Working in an IC unit was considered to involve a comprehensive task list experienced as more physically demanding with aging.

> *We care for* [patients], *we have to wash, care for, make their beds, turn, eh. Patients who are anesthetized, it's very heavy, sometimes they weigh a lot too. They have to be moved in beds and sometimes, uh, we need to go for X-rays, tomographies (…). I probably do the same amount* [as when I was younger], *but it's a bit heavier, I cannot cope in the same way (…) it takes its toll on my body, I think. I think back when I was the same age as the younger nurses.* [Marie]

3.4. Mental Work Environment

3.4.1. Being in Control despite the Unpredictable Context

Work was to a large extent perceived as unpredictable, as there were often unforeseeable events that interviewees needed to deal with when taking care of seriously ill patients. However, this apparent lack of control was not experienced as too stressful and was seen as an inherent quality of the job.

> [I feel control over work] *to a fairly large extent, so you live in a chaotic world, because we live with people whose bodies have gone into chaos. We try, what we do is that we try to control this chaos, eh. Of course, it's not possible, if we could, they wouldn't have been in the intensive care unit (…), but I strive for it* [control] *and I try to avoid thinking of the things that can go wrong, and if needed, to be prepared, materially and mentally. This is what an intensive care nurse quickly learns to do, to think about what might happen. (…) And once I have it in place, then I feel I have control, even if it* [something serious] *happens.* [Petter]

The IC unit stood out among others in the clear routines and guidelines, and this was felt as providing some sense of control when dealing with emergencies.

> *I like working here, that's why I came back too. (…) I feel that in this unit, things are in order, (…) there is a lot of routines that need to be followed. (…) I was away a few years and came back, I have been around and seen how it works in other places, I felt then that it worked much better when I was here, with the routines and everything like that.* [Helen]

> *That is, when the environment becomes stressful, when we are pushed to our limits, then we need have a working communication system and stick to it. Avoid running, stay in the box, and know your function.* [Sten]

3.4.2. Job Demands—The "Ethical Stress" and the "Nursing Dilemma"

Work was seen as mentally demanding. There was a heavy workload in which critical moments were felt as difficult to handle. In these situations, it caused what Marie called "ethical stress".

> *Sometimes the workload becomes so high that you don't have the control that you need to fulfil patient safety. (...) It's difficult, so difficult, it's the most difficult thing about this, it is the most difficult part of the job, the ethical stress, not being able to meet adequate needs in an adequate way.*

Petter, in turn, talked about the "nursing dilemma", that is the need to make priorities in the care that is to be provided and to delegate some tasks to nursing assistants.

> *There is a constant frustration in not having time for the basic nursing, I don't have time to carry out the core of the nursing profession, you have to hand it over to assistant nurses, and this is far from good. (...) We have far too much, we have more to do than we squeeze in on a working day, that is the nurse's dilemma.*

Work was sometimes experienced as emotionally demanding. Interviewees also mentioned the conflicting demands and described the stresses of such demands.

> *Because, you can stand there and mix a very important infusion that will soon run out in a seriously ill patient, and then something else happens to the other* [patient], *which needs to be taken care of immediately. It gets extremely stressful, ahem, if you're lucky, the colleague in the room next door may help you, but sometimes you can end up in almost impossible situations.* [Marie]

Furthermore, nurses felt they were responsible for their patients' lives. In this, having to handle the relatives of the patients, while being perceived as an important task, still involved an additional strain.

> *'Too many irons in the fire' and you work with human life, yes. So, my evaluations affect patient health, or what happens to the patient, we handle very advanced drugs, and very advanced technological equipment. If we do anything wrong, the result can be bad, so it is always important to focus.* [Ida]

Ultimately, the demands of the job can be a motive for stopping to work in IC after the age of 65. Marie was especially critical of the recent changes in the Swedish pension system not taking into consideration the type of occupation, as some occupations including those in healthcare, seem more demanding than others.

> *But I really think they should differentiate that because ahem, assistant nurses for example who work hard, it's not okay, ahem ... you sit in the office, I don't say that you don't work, but it doesn't add wear and tear to your body. (...) Like lifting a lot, because they are the ones who do all the heavy lifting.*

She added that in the nursing occupation, the lack of energy and work ability may have different and more serious consequences than other occupations.

> *When we don't really keep up with everything as we should, then it's people who are affected, and it's a huge difference between having to wait a long time for pain relief or having to wait a long time for a newly bought car to be delivered.*

3.4.3. Job Demands Also Perceived as Positive Challenges

Notwithstanding experiences of stress at work, interviewees generally considered this to be manageable to a certain extent, as expressed by Ida, who felt that she could rapidly recover from stress.

> *Eh, yes it* [stress] *is about not always having time to do what you have to do. It's an issue of having too many ill patients, it is too demanding to deal with. It can be stressful but it is not something that affects me long-term, only the moment when it happens.*

Similarly, Marie, even if she perceived her job to involve various types of demands, felt she could cope well with them, *"Ehm, it's going well. I'm tired in my body after a day, but I'm fine. I do exercise, I'm careful to keep myself physically active in my free time too!"*.

Furthermore, job demands were also positively perceived as providing the nurses with some challenges, which were appreciated and a job characteristic nurses would miss when fully retiring.

> *This is a bit of an intellectual challenge, so it's not just a job that you go to and* [plodding along] *like this. You have to be alert and attentive all the time. (. . .) above all* [what I would miss the most are] *these challenges at work and solving the problems.* [Helen]

3.5. Work Schedule, Work Pace, and Recovery Time

3.5.1. Irregular Working Time May Be a Hinder for a Sustainable and Healthy Working Life

An IC unit functions 24/7 and requires healthcare staff to work days, evenings, nights, and weekends. In this particular unit, all nurses were required to work in two shifts and some weekend days every month. However, there was some flexibility and, whenever possible, the work time would be scheduled according to the employees' preferences, which was very appreciated by the nurses, even if it was not always possible.

> *Maybe that you would work less during the weekends* [would facilitate extended working lives]. *Above all, one thing, and it works here, is that you don't have to work three shifts, but there can be a choice. There are many units where you have to work three shifts, which many find very tiring. And not having to work nights when you're older, (. . .) then you just work days and evenings. But this, well it already works here, for everyone.* [Helen]

Cecilia felt that shift work was particularly demanding, and was happy to be able to work only the day shift two weeks a month, which allowed for some stability.

> *It's difficult to have irregular working hours, I think it wears more on the body ahem.* [Working more days and having more weekends off] *means a lot, I think, I have longed for it a bit, to be able to do this, and it is great (. . .) it makes wonders for the routine, I sleep much better.*

Working nights was considered demanding and a health risk, as mentioned by Helena, who no longer did night shifts.

> *Working nights, I felt that, no, it wasn't for me. My body and mind simply could not cope; it didn't work at all. I couldn't sleep, neither during the days nor nights, I slept very badly, and now I have, I just feel like this, that now* [after stopping working night shifts], *I go home and just go to bed, and then I fall asleep.*

However, the nurses did see advantages of working nights and weekends, as it provided an extra income, reduced the number of weekly work hours, and provided some free days during the week. Moreover, it allowed some variation and work in a calmer environment.

> *I* [like] *working weekends, I like having weekdays off. (. . .) There are less people* [at the unit] *and the fewer you are the less messy it becomes, it's a bit quitter in that way.* [Nina]

In the long term, irregular working hours were nevertheless seen as a potential hindrance for extended working lives.

> *I don't know how I will feel in ten years, but it may be the working hours that are tiring in the long run. (. . .) You get more tired in the future (. . .), so it's quite tiring to work late evenings and get up early in the morning, and work night shifts maybe, and you may not have the energy.* [Ida]

3.5.2. Recovery Strategies

To work with seriously ill patients did not allow taking breaks at regular times of the day, as the breaks were dependent on the tasks that needed to be performed, and it was not always possible to predict the duration of such tasks. The nurses had no possibilities to take longer breaks as they were needed at the unit: *there is a person there, a seriously ill person, and I need to be there.* [Marie]

Sometimes, the nurses experienced difficulties recovering from critical events at work: *Sometimes, sometimes, it depends on how tough [it is] but, it can take weeks to handle events at work [such as] patients who have had bad experiences. (. . .) I'm tired for days.* [Petter]

Furthermore, nurses felt a greater need for recovery as they were aging.

I have a greater need to rest and recover, I do. (. . .) Sleeping, that's what I need to do. I feel that, I didn't need that before, then I could stay up much longer, but over the years I feel more tired. [Alice]

To decrease one's working time was seen as an important strategy to increase the time for recovery and to protect long-term health: *It takes many, many hours before I unwind. I'm tired the next day. I work part-time (. . .) To have a little more recovery.* [Marie]

However, this impacted on income and future pensions.

I don't work full-time [works 90%], I'm absolutely sure that I won't work full-time [until retiring], very few nurses above 30 years of age want to work full-time. (. . .) [I work] 90 [%], which is too much. (. . .) I would like to cut down my working hours. But then, well, it affects my income and pension, so this is what holds me back. [Petter]

While the nurses welcomed the possibility to work part time, there was concern that this would lead to a loss of competence.

And at the same time, I think that (. . .) you shouldn't work too few hours. Not in healthcare, if you are to continue working (. . .) because then you might not be able to keep up, then it will be too burdensome. So, there may be a limit to how few hours you can work if you are to stay. [Lotte]

To perform other tasks outside the unit was also a strategy to recover from the particularly demanding job as an IC nurse and to facilitate a longer working life in the nursing profession.

Getting a break, if I worked here full-time maybe I would not be as happy, maybe I would consider it to be more tiring. But I get a break by doing two different things and that's satisfying, yes. [Ida]

3.5.3. Post-Retirement Work as a Way to Work in a Flexible Schedule

Post-retirement work was seen as a way to gain control over one's work time and to have a more flexible schedule. This freedom, along with the possibility to remove undesired tasks and responsibilities, seemed very attractive to nurses when they thought about their late career options.

Because I'm really tired of working weekends, I'm really, really tired of it, so it would be nice [to be able to decide when to work or not]. (. . .) When working on an hourly basis, you can have a lot of influence [regarding decisions when to work]. (. . .) Now I cannot influence this that much [the working hours]. We put in, we have a wish list. So, we can influence it to a certain extent, but, when working on an hourly basis, you can influence this a lot. [Daniella]

3.6. Personal Finances

3.6.1. Financial Considerations

Although the nurses thought that they would have a relatively comfortable economic situation when retiring, one of the attractive factors in working until the age 65 and beyond was to guarantee a higher pension-related income after retirement.

I like money (laughs), to get a little more, increase the pay desk actually (. . .). Not because I have a huge need, I'm fine. I can manage, absolutely. (. . .) But I still think

that this feeling of getting some money and feeling that you have done something would be good, would be good, at least in the beginning [of the retirement life]. [Alice]

3.7. Personal Social Environment and Private Life

3.7.1. Attitudes towards Leisure

Notwithstanding the diversity regarding the relative importance that work and leisure had in their lives, the nurses' overall experience was that work did not prevent them from enjoying their time off nor from engaging in family and leisure activities, and they felt they had a relatively good work/personal life balance. To decrease the working time was nevertheless seen as attractive and a possibility for more leisure time, if they were economically independent. The interviewees reflected on their aging and were increasingly aware of the fact that life is limited in time. Their future time perspectives, and the importance of having a fulfilling private life in their remaining time, while still keeping up their health, played a role in the attitudes towards leisure.

And, I have a limited time left, statistically I'll only have about 23 years left to live, and out of those 23 years, maybe I have 15, what do I know, with a body that works, when I still think it's nice to do things, (...) so I don't have so many years. (...) Then I need to use the years I have left and spend my time on nice things. (...) Most [of the dying people] *regretted what they didn't do. Knowing this, then I think that I may well try to do nice things (...) in the years I have left.* [Yngve]

Despite this awareness of a limited life time to engage in meaningful activities, Yngve acknowledged that work continued to play an important role, in having a relevant social function, as was the case, to some extent, for the other nurses too.

I think I value my work more today. I took it more for granted earlier eh, also, (...) it means more. But it can also be me being in a different social situation than I was before. (...) Yes, so I have fewer social contacts, that's why I agree that I have to create a social life outside work and I do that gradually as well.

3.7.2. Family Situation Plays a Role in Work Centrality and Retirement Plans

The family context played a role when reflecting on the importance of work, the timing of retirement, and engaging or not in post-retirement work.

It [work] *has a big place in my life, I think what I do is fun, and since I don't have a family of my own, then work takes up more space. (...) If I had my own family and grandchildren and all this, then I don't know what it would have been like. But since I don't have it, work adds a dimension, yes, it gets a bigger space.* [Marie]

There was a wish to coordinate retirement plans with the partner, as recognized by Celine:

Yes, my husband of course [will affect my retirement decision]. *He's six years younger than me, so we have talked a lot about, how we should handle it, because it is perhaps not so fun to go home and wait for someone for six years, it has to be some kind of compromise.* [Laughs] *Yes, but it makes me think that maybe I should work ahem, a bit on an hourly basis, so, I've started to think, or we've discussed it a bit, and that he might also do that, so that we can get more time off together.*

The existence of (grand)children or parents to care for was also referred to as an important factor to take into account in the retirement decisions.

I want (...) to try to spend more time with grandchildren, so perhaps you can pick them up from preschool, (...) if you retire, you can then set aside one day a week when you do these things, well that's it. (...) My parents are still alive ahem, yes, you talk about it [retirement] *a bit, and so. (...) Yes, my parents think I should leave earlier* [laughs]. [Celine]

3.8. Social Work Environment, Discrimination, Leadership Style, and Age Management

3.8.1. Organization-Based Self-Esteem

The nurses felt very respected and appreciated, both by their colleagues and managers. Their long experience and knowledge were recognized, and they thought they had a valuable and important role at the unit.

> I'm a very experienced nurse ahem, and I also get recognition for that, both from colleagues, but also from managers. (. . .) Colleagues, both nurses and assistant nurses, come and ask, 'What do you think?' 'Would you, can you have a look?' 'What would you do in this situation?' [Managers say] that I'm capable, that I'm being helpful, that I don't snap back at them and that I (. . .) 'you do a good, a very good job' and that I'm one of the most competent, they say. (. . .) And that, I have that with me, and then I feel that I can be happy that the colleagues I work with encourage me and say that we have . . . we work well together. [Lotte]

3.8.2. The Importance of a Supportive Working Team

The social work environment was perceived as very supportive, which was considered to play an important role in balancing the impact of job demands as well as for the satisfaction the nurses mentioned having at work, which in turn contributed to the motivation to continue working. Colleagues were a strong asset and a vital resource, particularly when handling critical events involving patients, which were common at the unit.

> I always feel secure when I work together with other people, (. . .) we always work in a team, we do it together, and it works incredibly well at this hospital, I think, this unit where I work, that we work together. So, I'm confident that if it's not me, there's always someone else who can do it. And we help each other, and then it works well. [Yngve]

3.8.3. A Supportive Leadership Is Central for Job Retention

The nurses were very satisfied with the leadership at the unit, which they described as having the ability to motivate the group.

> I've never been at a workplace where so many are so positive regarding their manager as here, it's fascinating, because I've worked for a long time and been at many different places, so he is very good, he is here and he sees us and he is there for us. (. . .) I feel this all the time. (. . .) And I also know other hospitals have concerns regarding the salaries and work time models, and stuff like that, we don't have to think about it that much. We know that this will be sorted, and so do they, so they [managers] do that. So, I'm very happy. [Yngve]

Managers, both those at the front line and at a higher hierarchical level in the unit, were perceived as being present, accessible, open, fair, and close to the employees. To give honest and timely feedback was also mentioned as an important quality that they recognized in their leaders.

> I think that it is [a fairly open climate], they also deal with things. They [the managers] work, they are a bit different, but everyone tries to provide feedback (. . .) [a good manager] should be able to see me. (. . .) She should be able to provide feedback. [Lotte]

The feeling of having a supportive leadership played a central role in job satisfaction and their willingness to stay at the unit and continue working.

> I think he is understanding and he, if you have something, you can go and talk to him and he will listen, and he takes his time and so on, he does. (. . .) He is extremely popular among the employees in the unit. (. . .) We have many employees who have worked here for many years, and I still think that part of it, why you stay, is because you know you can reach your manager and meet them. [Alice]

3.8.4. Age-Friendly Work Environment

The working team was age diverse and age neutral, and the nurses did not feel that they were discriminated against due to their age. They welcomed the opportunity to use their accumulated knowledge and experience to help their younger colleagues and simultaneously felt that they could learn from the younger ones.

I think it's great [to collaborate with younger employees], *ahem that you feel much younger and then it's they who know about the latest findings. It's been a number of years since I went to school. (. . .) I learn from them and they learn from me, so that, yes, I think it's a lot of fun. (. . .) They know that you've been through a lot more and have a lot to teach. (. . .) They ask, ask questions, come and ask for help, want to know 'that I'm doing the right thing', that is it.* [Nina]

3.8.5. Age Management Practices That May Promote a More Sustainable Working Life

The nurses did not find many possibilities to adapt some of their responsibilities and working tasks to their age, potential changes in work ability and interests, and thought that work would become more manageable in a long-term perspective if such adaptations were possible.

But it's still like that you have the same expectations on yourself, as when you started working as a 23-year-old, as when you leave as a 65-year-old with 45 years of experience. You should do as much on your first day as you should do on your last day, that's absurd. [Petter]

As Marie noted, increasing the staff would allow for a decrease in the workload and facilitate extended working lives: *Increased staffing. (. . .) That you didn't have to stress around so much, and hurry through the whole workday. We often drive at full speed the entire work shift, and it is not healthy.*

Nina, in turn, welcomed the possibility for lateral job movements.

If you could combine not only working on the floor, but maybe get some administrative (. . .) administrative tasks or something else on the side. (. . .) That is, if you get older you won't have as much strength, it will be heavy to run around here, and stand, lift. So that, making use of the knowledge that the older nurses have.

The nurses said that they sometimes assumed a mentoring role. However, this was perceived as rather informal and not organized. To formalize such a role and promote the systematic transfer and knowledge exchange with the younger colleagues was seen as a practice that would benefit the unit and facilitate extended working lives.

That you are some kind of senior nurse and walk around and support those who don't ahem, these newcomers who have just arrived, and be a support, but then, maybe not have so many patients of your own, but to work more, like a mentor maybe. And support the [younger nurses], *to help them out in these situations that turn out to be more demanding, and in the daily, well the regular work as well.* [Helen]

To retire and engage in post-retirement work was considered as an attractive strategy to skip some of the responsibilities at work while continuing to work with more suitable and interesting tasks within nursing: *As it is now, it's the case that when you turn 65, then you get rid of these other tasks, as you no longer have a permanent position.* [Lotte]

There is a responsibility that you let go of. A responsibility in a broader perspective, which I think I should have, and I have, for the workplace. It doesn't continue, I'll then [after retirement] *come in and solve specific issues, and then I don't have to solve the problems with the storing of the medication, or stand in the sorting room, and things like that.* [Marie]

3.9. Motivation, Satisfaction, and Stimulation in the Execution of Work Tasks

3.9.1. A Rewarding and Meaningful Job

When asked the "lottery question", the nurses reflected on motives for work. While the income was a strong motive, they would continue to work to some extent even if they would receive a large amount of money.

I would probably like to work less, yes, I would probably like to do that, but I wouldn't want to stop working, no. (. . .) Because I think it's fun to work, it's a satisfaction, it's as I say, all the people you meet enrich your life. [Ida]

I don't think [money] *is a driver of whether I should work or not, I think I would like to continue working in any case, even if I would end up in a financial situation where I wouldn't have to work another day in my life, but I don't work for the money. I actually work for the feeling of being in a context where I've something to contribute and where I feel good about it, so that I actually don't think that . . . it's not for the sake of my own profit that I do things.* [Sten]

The interviewees thought that their work as nurses in an IC unit, where their daily focus was saving the lives of patients with extremely delicate health conditions, was very rewarding and meaningful: *It* [the job] *gives incredibly much back, a job in healthcare, it gives a lot back, at the human and social levels, so that is perhaps what I value most, yes* [in having a job]. [Ida]

The meaningfulness of work was considered as a strong motive to continue working beyond the age of 65.

I don't think I could quit the job [if I won the lottery], *I don't think so (. . .) it's the incredible need for acknowledgment, I think. But to feel that I mean something (. . .) to me is an important part. (. . .) Because I know what drives me somewhere and what I think is important. (. . .) I'm a bit scared when I quit. Just this feeling of being needed and being able to really give things and get the acknowledgment. (. . .) Because a day, it ends, when I don't work then. Then I just hope I've found myself in that 'now it's enough, now I have other things I want to do'.* [Yngve]

3.9.2. Variety at Work

The nurses very much appreciated the variation they found in their work. They enjoyed the unpredictability and working in a place "where things happen". Moreover, feeling that their job was interesting and stimulating influenced their willingness to continue working beyond retirement.

It [willingness to work beyond 65] *is probably partly because I think it's fun, partly because I think I can do it, and it's stimulating, intellectually stimulating, socially stimulating, and financially stimulating.* [Petter]

3.9.3. Job Satisfaction

The interviewees mentioned being very satisfied with their jobs as IC nurses and with the organization, and reflected on this in different ways during the interviews. Job satisfaction was central for staff retention, and for the openness to extended working lives.

As long as it feels like this and I've a good workplace to go to, I'll continue [to work full time until retirement]. *(. . .) Because I enjoy my job. (. . .) The organization works well (. . .) it is good on so many levels. (. . .) I don't think I would have this elsewhere.* [Yngve]

3.10. Competence, Use of Skills, Knowledge, and Opportunities for Development at Work

3.10.1. Opportunities for Use of Accumulated Knowledge and Competences

The nurses very much valued the opportunity to use the specialized knowledge and range of competencies that they developed throughout their academic and working life.

Mm, I think (...) that my knowledge is used in a good way. (...) [what you appreciate most about having a job] is, ahem, it's simple, it's to be able to work with what I've been trained for, that's right. [Celine]

3.10.2. Occupational Self-Efficacy and the Positive Side of Being an Older Worker—"the Clinical Eye" and "the Tacit Knowledge"

The nurses were very confident of being competent to perform their job well, as well as when dealing with critical events: *I can see, immediately take things in* [I have to do this, I have to do that]. *It's a clinical eye, yes, it's a clinical eye.* [Sten]

The "clinical eye", resulting from the experience accumulated during the years, provided nurses some calm, and to some extent buffered the impact of both job demands and lack of control, which were seen as inherent characteristics of the IC job.

Ahem, it's because I've been here so long, and been through so much, I think. Then it feels like I, I can handle most situations, then I perhaps think that things can be more or less difficult, but I can usually handle it. [Celine]

Fredrik referred to it as "tacit knowledge", which is the way his experience is being expressed at work.

This tacit knowledge. So, you've been involved in and through a number of things, then you get a feeling for the situation, and you also get a feeling for the course of events. And it's very, very difficult sometimes to teach, but it's something that you learn when you've experienced it a number of times and I think it, it's actually really invaluable. (...) You have, you develop some kind of emotional antennae, "what are things going to be like for this patient?" Although you don't see any signals yet, older nurses have already their heads wrapped around it, yes.

The long work experience also helped to recover emotionally from tragic work-related events.

But before, I would probably turn in my bed for quite a long time [after a tragic event at work]*, but I have no problem with this anymore, I can go home and go to bed and sleep. (...) It* [what helps a faster recovery] *is the experience, absolutely, and then the more you see and the more you come across, so yes, you gain a lot of knowledge from different experiences, you use it too, I'd say.* [Helen]

3.10.3. Importance of Keeping Skills Up-to-Date

The organization provided opportunities for training and development, and overall, the interviewees considered themselves to have had their skills updated: *Good* [opportunities for skills development]*, I think. (...) A lot of courses (...) we have a continuous training at work, we have a lot.* [Petter]

This was highly valued and recognized by the nurses, who considered it important to follow the development in their area of expertise, despite not feeling any need for extensive training, given their seniority and being near retirement.

I want to develop my competencies very much, I want that (...) because you can always learn something new, and there will be new findings as I said before, so all who work at the unit need to take part, I'd say. [Celine]

3.10.4. Internal and External Employability

The interviewees mentioned that as senior, competent, and experienced nurses, they had good opportunities to continue working after retirement, at the same, or at some other, hospital.

Oops, the [current job market in healthcare] *is huge. There are many job opportunities, both in Sweden and Norway. (...) There is no age discrimination, instead they appreciate that you are experienced and stuff like that, I'm still very much in demand on the labour market.* [Yngve]

The high perceived internal and external employability seemed to have a strong impact on the motivation to continue working.

> Yes, but we have several of those who retired recently, they are back, working. There's no difference. So, most who retire return (. . .) and work on an hourly basis. (. . .) I think I have the prerequisites [to continue working after retirement]. I have a job that I'm happy with, (. . .) I have endless opportunities to continue working with things that I know. And then, I mean, I can do it until that day I that say 'no, now I'm happy, now this is enough'. [Sten]

4. Discussion

This interview study investigated older IC nurses' experiences of working life and their reflections about the late career and retirement. The interviewees provided rich accounts of their experiences, and the interpretative phenomenological analysis resulted in ten superordinate themes, with the first centering on the nurses' retirement decision making and nine themes reflecting the nine determinant areas proposed by the SwAge model [59] involved in individuals' decisions on whether to extend their working lives or to retire. The discussion of the results will follow the thematic structure identified in the study.

4.1. Retirement Decision Making

Retirement is a major life transition [60] that may have a deep impact on individual lifestyles and social networks. About 10–25 percent of older workers have difficulties in adjusting to retirement [61]. Thus, retirement is a transition that can generate an ambivalence, as the individual, in the moment of choosing whether or not to retire, often considers both positive and negative outcomes of work and retirement [62]. Indeed, the nurses participating in this study expressed ambivalent attitudes towards the retirement transition and the role as retiree; this included both positive and negative valence. Moreover, some of their retirement plans included continuing working after the age of 65, which reflects the flexibility of the Swedish pension system and its facilitation of a steady transition to full retirement and extended working life. Importantly, retirement was perceived as a new career stage [24,63], with post-retirement work being considered an opportunity to engage in new roles in a more attractive employment form, while simultaneously allowing for a gradual disengagement of the working role and adaptation to life as a retiree. Post-retirement work may help individuals to maintain their identity of a work role [20], to avoid an abrupt discontinuity of their life structure after retirement [64–66], and to achieve a balance between the gradual distancing from work and continuity in life [67].

The importance of planning for retirement and the voluntariness of retirement were mentioned by the nurses. Indeed, Shultz and colleagues [68] found that the extent to which a retirement decision was perceived as voluntary or not impacted on retirement wellbeing. Importantly, individuals who retire due to different factors forcing them out of the workforce (so-called "push factors", such as poor health or skills obsolescence), report poorer retirement wellbeing [68,69]. Although retirement planning and preparation is considered beneficial to the quality of adjusting to retirement [70,71], it is not frequent among older nurses [40,72].

4.2. Self-Rated Health, Diagnoses, and Functional Diversity

The nurses reported having relatively good health, without any significant physical ailments. In an occupation frequently associated with back pain, musculoskeletal disorders, psychological distress [48], and high turnover rates [38], they can be considered "survivors". Consistent with the literature, the nurses in this study considered health as a major requirement for continuing to work. While good health has been associated with preferences for late retirement [73,74], poor health is indeed one of the strongest predictors of early retirement [20,23]. De Wind et al. [75] identified four pathways through which poor health leads to retirement: (1) the employee's total incapacity to work due to health problems;

(2) the employee being pushed out from work by the employer due to health problems; (3) the employee's perceived decline in the (future) work ability caused by poor health; and (4) the employee's fear of further health declines. The latter two pathways have also been found by Pond et al. [76] (p. 527) and were named "the health protection pathway". Moreover, the current study findings showed that health was considered a pre-condition for enjoying the retirement years as well, and the nurses expressed that they wanted to retire while still having a good health, which aligns with findings reported by De Wind et al. [75] and in Pond et al. [76], where this pathway was referred to as the "maximization of life" exit pathway (p. 527).

4.3. Physical Work Environment

The physical work environment includes features such as noise, air quality, cleanness of the space, total area of the premises, temperature, and lighting [77,78]. The quality of the physical healthcare environment influences the quality of healthcare provision [78] and older nurses' retirement timing [16]. The nurses in the present study complained with regard to their physical work environment, in particular the small rooms, with its implications for their and patients' safety, and the constant noises coming from the life support equipment. The noise level is a particularly relevant work stressor with a negative impact for the nurses' performance [77]. As older nurses are more prone to physical injuries, a good physical work environment that is well-equipped and has a reasonable sound level is an important factor that adds to their job satisfaction to a larger extent than it does for younger nurses [45]. Importantly, the nurses perceived nursing work as more physically demanding as the nurses became older. Research has found that working in more physically challenging environments is perceived by older nurses as tiring and a challenge to their continuity in the nursing profession [79]. Handling patients, including the repeated bending, lifting, and twisting may result in musculoskeletal injuries. Such injuries may accumulate over time and add to other physical problems that can occur with aging and thus make older nurses more vulnerable to the occupational risks that are commonly found in healthcare [13,15,80]. This means that organizations need to consider these issues, and make efforts to promote the use of ergonomic aids and design functional, comfortable, and safe workplaces, which provide a healthy and sustainable working life for all ages [15,59].

4.4. Mental Work Environment

The lack of control experienced by the nurses was seen as an inherent characteristic of their work with severely ill patients at the IC unit. However, the nurses considered the clear guidelines and routines at the unit as adding some control, even in the case of unforeseen events. The nurses experienced stress and pressure that came from a heavy workload, which led to time pressure and feelings of insufficiency, guilt, and frustration, and fears of risking the quality of patient care. Overall, they felt being capable to meet the demands of the job, but excessive job demands would still be a reason for not continuing IC work after retirement. Yet, the job demands were to some extent perceived as positive challenges and motivating job characteristics that the nurses would miss when leaving the profession. This follows Furunes and colleagues [73] finding that older workers appreciated high job demands, due to this making their work more interesting and challenging. Furthermore, a decrease in such demands was a reason to retire and not continue working. Importantly, these findings align with distinguishing between "job hindrances", that is, the demands that elicit negative emotions, and "job challenges", which refer to demands that, despite depleting energy, have stimulating characteristics [81]. Similarly, LePine et al. [82] in a two-dimensional model of stressors and performance, distinguished between "bad stress" and "good stress", with the first resulting from hindrance stressors, including the inadequacy of resources, role ambiguity, interpersonal conflicts, and the latter resulting from challenge stressors (such as job demands and workloads) that may be associated with high performance. Providing the access to resources and practices to manage stress and reduce the levels of strain (such as support, time for social and physical activities, and training to prioritize tasks) may protect against any costs of challenge stressors for the long-term health of nurses [82].

4.5. Work Schedule, Work Pace, and Recovery Time

The opportunity to control work time is considered important to older nurses' job satisfaction [45]. The nurses taking part in this study reported that the unit had a two-shift working schedule. However, older nurses were not required to work night shifts, which has been identified as a type of work schedule that is associated with nurses' intentions to leave the organization [32]. Moreover, managers tried to consider the nurses' preferences for shift schedules, something that was much appreciated by the nurses. Indeed, the results of a large longitudinal European study [83] has shown that fulfilling nurses' wishes regarding shift work patterns may sustain nurses' work ability and health, which in turn facilitates extended working lives. Moreover, Leineweber et al. [35] found that satisfaction with schedule flexibility was associated with a lower intention to leave the nursing profession or the organization.

Irregular working hours or rotating shifts are typical stressors of nursing work that become more difficult to handle with aging [13,48]. In the present study, this emerged as an occupational hazard that, in the long term, would potentially hinder the nurses' ability to extend their working lives. Yet, this can be balanced by flexible schedules and freedom in choosing when and how to work. These were characteristics of post-retirement work that the nurses considered as very attractive—a finding which follows previous studies of older nurses [42,50,84,85]. The majority of the nurses that were interviewed worked part time. This was a strategy to increase recovery time. Importantly, recovery was perceived as key for health, wellbeing, and the ability to perform at work, and consequently, for remaining longer in the nursing profession. Another recovery strategy was to distance oneself from the IC work, and to carry out other types of activities considered less emotionally laden outside the unit.

4.6. Personal Finances

Financial resources available for retirement is one of the most frequently recurring factors in older employees' conceptualizations of extended working lives [20,23]. However, the role of financial factors for extended working lives is not straightforward [86,87]. While some studies show that higher pay and pension incomes are negatively associated with the likelihood of post-retirement work [88], other studies find that wealth does not predict the decision to continue working after retirement [89]. Some findings suggest a U-shaped relationship, according to which post-retirement work participation is higher among individuals with lower and higher retirement incomes, as compared with those in the middle [90]. The nurses interviewed in the present study considered finances to play a role in their retirement plans. However, this was not the core motivational driver for continuing to work, which is something that has been found in other qualitative studies with more heterogeneous samples [47,91,92]. The nurses thought they would continue working to some extent even if they would win a large amount of money in the lottery. Rather than financial needs in its strictest sense, the main finances-related motives for working until the age 65 and beyond seemed to involve a guarantee of a higher pension income, to maintain a certain living standard, and to afford some extras, such as traveling.

4.7. Personal Social Environment and Private Life

The nurses mentioned that being engaged in several activities during their leisure time, including having a relatively good work/private life balance, was important for their wellbeing. However, there was an increasing awareness of the fact that a human's lifetime is limited, which created an urgency to make the best of one's remaining time. This finding can be related to the socioemotional selectivity theory [93], which argues that perceptions of the amount of time left in life impact profoundly on individual motivation and priorities. Importantly, when perceiving that time is limited, individuals seem to become more motivated to prioritize their emotional satisfaction, and focus on deepening their relationships, and on enjoying life.

The mentioning of work having a continued and important role in providing opportunities for socialization, particularly for those not living with a partner, has been found in other studies of older nurses [27,45,49,50]. For instance, continuing to work due to social reasons seems particularly common among older women [94]. Yet, the importance of having time for family life and sharing leisure activities has been reported in previous research as well [16,43,46,48]. Specifically, nurses with a partner expressed a wish to coordinate their retirement and the potential engagement in post-retirement work with those of their partner. These findings suggest that healthcare organizations that facilitate work–life balance, through flexible work arrangements, may delay full retirement of older nurses who may wish to retire at the same time as their partners, who may be older and entitled to retire earlier.

4.8. Social Work Environment, Discrimination, Leadership Style, and Age Management

The extent to which employees perceive themselves as capable, meaningful, and valuable to the organization employing them has been referred to as "organization-based self-esteem" (OBSE) [95]. OBSE has been linked to employee motivation, job satisfaction, organizational commitment, performance, and mentoring behaviors, as well as to lower levels of both turnover intention and actual turnover [95]. The nurses participating in the present study mentioned being respected and appreciated both by their colleagues and managers at the IC unit. Importantly, both colleagues and managers recognized the value of the expertise and the quality of the care that the nurses provided. Similar to previous studies of older nurses [28,45,48,84,85], the esteem and appreciation reported by the IC nurses seemed to play an important role for their satisfaction, but also for their commitment and sense of belonging to the workplace. This has been underscored as important to consider for organizations, for instance by implementing a "culture of appreciation" to attract "silver workers", or active retirees, in order to recognize the older employees' accumulated experience and expertise [96] (p. 152).

According to the job demands–resources (JD-R) model [97,98], social support is a job resource that promotes work engagement, and buffers the impact of high demands, particularly in highly demanding jobs [97,99], such as IC nursing. Here, the nurses mentioned getting much support from their colleagues, which they considered an important resource that helped to counterbalance the negative impact of work stressors. Moreover, the support seemed to increased their job satisfaction, commitment to work, and health. This aligns with a systematic review [100], which reports linkages between social support and lower risks for burnout among emergency care nurses.

The leadership was also perceived as very supportive, in contributing to a good work environment, which in turn seemed to have a positive impact on the nurses' job satisfaction as well as on their willingness to stay with the organization. This finding follows those of a systematic review of the effects of leadership styles for nurses [101]. Specifically, leaders who make use of their emotional skills and are empathetic and responsive to work concerns and emotional needs of the staff, and promote the best use of staff competencies and expertise, seem to empower nurses while also adding to their job satisfaction, satisfaction with the leader, productivity and effectiveness, and organizational commitment, as well as to reduced retention. Importantly, such leaders, in making use of their skills, contribute to a variety of positive outcomes for the nurses, for the work environment, and the organization [101].

The nurses who were interviewed did not feel being discriminated against by their age, and were very committed in passing on their knowledge and expertise to younger nurses, thus showing high levels of generativity [102]. In a recent meta-analysis [103], this has been found to have several positive consequences, including job satisfaction, work motivation, occupational self-efficacy and a motivation to continue working. Here, the nurses mentioned that their mentoring of entry-level nurses was rather informal and not systematic. Thus, the interviewees suggested that creating formal mentoring programs including senior and more experienced nursing staff would be a practice that would encourage employees to extend their working life in the organization, something that has been suggested in the literature as well [13,17,42]. Moreover, the nurses thought that their work would be more sustainable in the long term if they would have the possibility to reduce their workload and reassign some responsibilities and working tasks as a way to address their interests and potential limitations related to aging. This means that they suggested the organization to offer older workers opportunities to engage in job crafting behaviors in order to promote person–job fit and foster successful aging at work [104], to extend their working lives.

4.9. Motivation, Satisfaction, and Stimulation in the Execution of Work Tasks

The nurses mentioned being very committed to their work and satisfied with their jobs and considered this to be important for prolonging their working lives—a finding that has been reported in previous studies as well [16,45]. For instance, previous research has found a U-shaped relationship between nurses' age, seniority, and job satisfaction with higher levels of job satisfaction at the entry level and after the age of 50 [105]. For the older nurses, this may be explained by an increased expertise, better working schedules, and salaries, and better work–family balance. However, for older nurses, the increasing job satisfaction may reflect a selection effect, that is, the less satisfied and the dissatisfied nurses may have left the job. Such a selection may also apply to the present study findings.

The IC nurses felt intrinsically motivated to work, that is, were driven by the work content and the inner joy of the work itself cf. [106]. As has been suggested [80,107], the intrinsic rewards of healthcare may promote work ability as well as work engagement. In particular, work engagement may counteract burnout [107], which is common in healthcare occupations. Here, the nurses described their nursing work at the IC unit as varied, interesting, and stimulating, as well as very rewarding and meaningful. Importantly, this was a strong motive for continuing to work beyond the age of 65. This finding is in line with previous research [74,108], showing that individuals who extend their work careers typically feel important to other people and that they have meaningful tasks.

4.10. Knowledge, Skills, and Competence

In the present study, the opportunity to use skills and knowledge acquired over the years of work seemed a key factor linked to the nurses' job satisfaction, which has been reported in previous studies as well [45]. Importantly, they felt very confident regarding their competencies to perform and to be efficient when caring for patients, which in turn, contributed to a sense of control in critical and high-stress situations that characterize much of the IC work. The sense of accomplishment and performance success, in turn, provided the nurses with feelings of being capable (i.e., self-efficacy) [109]. Self-efficacy has been found to be relevant both for older workers' motivation at work, for their motivation to work [110], as well as for nurses' willingness to work longer [44]. Self-efficacy and self-esteem are considered personal resources [111] that may protect and buffer the negative effects of heavy workload on nurses' burnout. Thus, to promote aging-in-workplace and encourage extended working lives, healthcare organizations would need to develop practices that promote the development of nurses' personal resources, including their occupational self-efficacy. Here, the possibilities for continuous learning and development that the IC unit provided, something that the nurses valued, may play a key role in developing personal resources, as this gave them opportunities to prevent skills obsolescence and to keep up with the rapid technological advances in the highly specialized environment of the IC unit.

4.11. Methodological Considerations and Suggestions for Future Research

The present study used a relatively small and homogenous sample of 12 nurses working in the same IC unit, which restricts generalizability to other organizations and nursing occupations while also restricting representativity. Yet, IPA studies often include smaller samples (between 5 and 10 participants) [58], which allow for keeping with the ideographic focus characterizing this approach [57]. The use of the IPA in this study involved a detailed and systematic analysis of the subjective experiences of working as an IC nurse, the perceptions of aging in the workplace, and thoughts regarding extended working lives in a particular healthcare setting in Sweden. The nurses that were interviewed had a good health and were very satisfied with their job and the organization, which means that there is a risk of sample selection issues resulting from a potential "healthy worker effect" [112]. This means that nurses with poorer health or those dissatisfied with their job or the workplace may have already left nursing or decided to not participate in this study. Moreover, the data were collected before the COVID-19 pandemic. Although most of the findings would stand in the present, the pandemic put an enormous pressure on IC healthcare workers who had to deal with an unknown, life-threatening disease, while the units also had to accommodate new and less experienced nursing staff in a very short time in order to respond to the higher IC needs [56]. Future research should thus investigate how the COVID-19 pandemic affected older IC nurses' experiences of work and their late-career decisions. Additionally, interview studies with IC nurses in less supportive organizational contexts and in settings with more rigid pension systems, including nurses at different stages of their careers and specializing in different nursing occupations, may broaden the overall understanding of the topic of sustainable working lives in nursing.

5. Conclusions

The COVID-19 pandemic has put an enormous strain on the already pressured healthcare services all over the world [1]. Specifically, the health crisis brought about by the pandemic increased the demand for qualified healthcare staff and underscored the central role of nurses [1]. The characteristics of IC work have specifics that turn it into a particularly demanding environment—one with the highest staffing shortages in healthcare. Using a phenomenological approach, this study sought to add a fine-grained analysis to the research literature but also to provide policymakers and healthcare organizations with insights regarding IC nurses' ways of conceptualizing and making sense of their experiences of work as well as their late-career decisions when approaching retirement, topics which seem understudied.

The IC nurses participating in this study planned to remain in the nursing profession and in the organization, and considered working until 65 and beyond. To work after retirement on an hourly basis was considered an attractive employment form in that it allows for flexibility in working time and more control over the type of tasks to be performed while simultaneously including a gradual disengagement from the working role, which in turn, can facilitate adapting to life as a retiree. The flexibility of the Swedish pension system, the labor demand for qualified nurses, and the openness of the organization to employ retired nurses were considered important contextual facilitators. While some of the emerging themes that resulted from the analysis follow existing findings from large quantitative studies with heterogeneous samples of older employees, the access to detailed and rich first-person accounts collected through the interviews with IC nurses served as a means to add the "lived experiences" of a specific profession and to provide a constellation of other individual, work, and organizational factors that seem central for ability and willingness to remain. Moreover, by combining an inductive and data-driven approach to identify themes emerging from the narratives with a deductive approach, informed by the SwAge model [59], to refine the thematic structure, this study also contributed to empirical validation of this model and to the research literature regarding sustainable working lives.

In terms of implications of the study, an improved focus on ergonomics, possibilities to adjust some tasks to age-related physical limitations and interests, a possibility for lateral job movement, and a formal mentoring program taking advantage of older nurses' expertise while at the same time freeing them from some of the heavier tasks, were considered as examples of human resources management practices that would contribute to aging-in-workplace and increase the motivation to postpone the moment of fully exiting the nursing profession. Importantly, the findings from this study show that raising statutory retirement ages and establishing financial benefits for late retirement may constitute incentives for extended working lives; however, such incentives seem far from enough in order to encourage older nurses to postpone the timing of their exit from the labor market. Notably, it is important to ensure that older nurses want to, and will be able to, work longer, which is something that may be facilitated by providing adequate working conditions that enable a healthy and sustainable working life throughout the life-span.

Author Contributions: Analysis, M.S.-R. and K.K.; writing—original draft preparation, M.S.-R. and P.L.; writing—review and editing, M.S.-R., P.L. and K.K.; funding acquisition, M.S.-R. All authors have read and agreed to the published version of the manuscript.

Funding: This research was funded by a grant from FORTE: Swedish Research Council for Health, Working Life and Welfare (grant number 2014–1662) to the first author.

Institutional Review Board Statement: The study was conducted according to the guidelines of the Declaration of Helsinki and approved by the Swedish Ethical Review Authority (ref no. 2017/1720-31/5).

Informed Consent Statement: Informed consent was obtained from all subjects involved in the study.

Data Availability Statement: The data are not publicly available due to legal restrictions that protect the integrity of research participants. Detailed analyses of the masked transcripts are available on request from the corresponding author [M.S.-R.].

Conflicts of Interest: The authors declare no conflict of interest.

References

1. OECD. *Health at a Glance 2021: OECD Indicators*; OECD Publishing: Paris, France, 2021.
2. European Union. Ageing Europe. Looking at the Lives of Older People in the EU. Luxembourg: Publications Office of the European Union. 2020. Available online: https://ec.europa.eu/eurostat/statistics-explained/index.php?title=Ageing_Europe_-_looking_at_the_lives_of_older_people_in_the_EU (accessed on 28 February 2022).
3. Statistics Sweden. Sveriges framtida befolkning 2020–2070. In *The Future Population of Sweden 2020–2070*; Statistikmyndigheten SCB: Örebro, Sweden, 2020; Available online: https://www.scb.se/contentassets/9c8e50dfe0484fda8fed2be33e374f46/be0401_2020i70_sm_be18sm2001.pdf (accessed on 25 January 2021).
4. European Commission. The Ageing Report. European Economy Institutional, Paper 148. May 2021. Available online: https://ec.europa.eu/info/publications/economic-and-financial-affairs-publications_en (accessed on 28 February 2022).
5. Swedish Pensions Agency. Pensionsåldrar och arbetslivets längd–Svar på regleringsbrevsuppdrag 2020. In *Retirement Ages and Length of Working Life*; Report No. PID176578; Pensionsmyndigheten: Stockholm, Sweden, 2020.
6. Government Offices of Sweden. The Swedish Old-Age Pension System. In *How the Income Pension, Premium Pension and Guarantee Pension Work*; Article No: S2017.001; Ministry of Health and Social Affairs: Stockholm, Sweden, 2016. Available online: https://www.government.se/49aff8/contentassets/f48ac850ff0f4ed4be065ac3b0bcab15/the-swedish-old-age-pension-system_webb.pdf (accessed on 16 December 2021).
7. OECD. *Pensions at a Glance 2019: OECD and G20 Indicators*; OECD Publishing: Paris, France, 2019.
8. Poulsen, O.M.; Fridriksson, J.F.; Tómasson, K.; Midtsundstad, T.; Mehlum, I.S.; Nilsson, K.; Albin, M. *Working Environment and Work Retention*; Nordic Council of Ministers: Copenhagen, Denmark, 2017; p. 559.
9. Sousa-Ribeiro, M.; Bernhard-Oettel, C.; Sverke, M.; Westerlund, H. Health- and age-related workplace factors as predictors of preferred, expected, and actual retirement timing: Findings from a Swedish cohort study. *Int. J. Environ. Res. Public Health* **2021**, *18*, 2746. [CrossRef] [PubMed]
10. Swedish National Board of Health and Welfare. *Bedömning av Tillgång och Efterfrågan på Legitimerad Personal i Hälso- och Sjukvård Samt Tandvård [Assessment of Supply and Demand for Licensed Personnel in Healthcare and Dentalcare]*; Socialstyrelsen: Stockholm, Sweden, 2019.
11. Swedish Association of Local Authorities and Regions. *Personalen i Välfärden [Welfare Staff]*; Sveriges Kommuner och Regioner: Stockholm, Sweden, 2021.
12. Swedish Association of Local Authorities and Regions. *Hälso-och Sjukvårdsrapporten [Healthcare Sector Report]*; Sveriges Kommuner och Regioner: Stockholm, Sweden, 2020.
13. Fitzgerald, D.C. Aging, experienced nurses: Their value and needs. *Contemp. Nurse* **2007**, *24*, 237–243. [CrossRef] [PubMed]

14. Swedish Association of Local Authorities and Regions. Sveriges viktigaste jobb finns inom välfärden. In *Rekryteringsrapport 2018 [Sweden's Most Important Jobs Are in Welfare. Recruitment Report]*; Sveriges Kommuner och Landsting: Stockholm, Sweden, 2017.
15. Hatcher, B.J.; Bleich, M.R.; Connolly, C.H.; O'Neilly, H.P.; Stokley, H.K. *Wisdom at Work: The Importance of the Older and Experienced Nurse in the Workplace*; Robert Wood Johnson Foundation: Princeton, NJ, USA, 2006.
16. Markowski, M.; Cleaver, K.; Weldon, S.M. An integrative review of the factors influencing older nurses' timing of retirement. *J. Adv. Nurs.* **2020**, *76*, 2266–2285. [CrossRef]
17. Leners, D.W.; Wilson, W.D.; Connor, P.; Fenton, J. Mentorship: Increasing retention probabilities. *J. Nurs. Manag.* **2006**, *14*, 652–654. [CrossRef]
18. Wargo-Sugleris, M.; Robbins, W.; Lane, C.J.; Phillips, L.R. Job satisfaction, work environment and successful ageing: Determinants of delaying retirement among acute care nurses. *J. Adv. Nurs.* **2018**, *74*, 900–913. [CrossRef] [PubMed]
19. Moseley, A.; Jeffers, L.; Paterson, J. The retention of the older nursing workforce: A literature review exploring factors that influence the retention and turnover of older nurses. *Contemp. Nurse* **2008**, *30*, 46–56. [CrossRef]
20. Fisher, G.G.; Chaffee, D.S.; Sonnega, A. Retirement Timing: A Review and Recommendations for Future Research. *Work. Aging Retire.* **2016**, *2*, 230–261. [CrossRef]
21. Scharn, M.; Sewdas, R.; Boot, C.R.L.; Huisman, M.; Lindeboom, M.; van der Beek, A.J. Domains and determinants of retirement timing: A systematic review of longitudinal studies. *BMC Public Health* **2018**, *18*, 1083. [CrossRef]
22. Topa, G.; Moriano, J.A.; Depolo, M.; Alcover, C.-M.; Morales, J.F. Antecedents and consequences of retirement planning and decision-making: A meta-analysis and model. *J. Vocat. Behav.* **2009**, *75*, 38–55. [CrossRef]
23. Topa, G.; Depolo, M.; Alcover, C.M. Early retirement: A meta-analysis of its antecedent and subsequent correlates. *Front. Psychol.* **2018**, *8*, 2157. [CrossRef]
24. Wang, M.; Shi, J. Psychological Research on Retirement. *Annu. Rev. Psychol.* **2014**, *65*, 209–233. [CrossRef] [PubMed]
25. Browne, P.; Carr, E.; Fleischmann, M.; Xue, B.; Stansfeld, S.A. The relationship between workplace psychosocial environment and retirement intentions and actual retirement: A systematic review. *Eur. J. Ageing* **2019**, *16*, 73–82. [CrossRef] [PubMed]
26. Sverke, M.; Falkenberg, H.; Kecklund, G.; Magnusson Hanson, L.; Lindfors, P. *Women and Men and Their Working Conditions: The Importance of Organizational and Psychosocial Factors for Work-Related and Health-Related Outcomes*; Swedish Work Environment Authority: Stockholm, Sweden, 2017.
27. Graham, E.; Donoghue, J.; Duffield, C.; Griffiths, R.; Bichel-Findlay, J.; Demitireis, S. Why do older RNs keep working? *J. Nurs. Adm.* **2014**, *44*, 591–597. [CrossRef] [PubMed]
28. Armstrong-Stassen, M.; Schlosser, F. Perceived organizational membership and the retention of older workers. *J. Organ. Behav.* **2011**, *32*, 319–344. [CrossRef]
29. Armstrong-Stassen, M.; Stassen, K. Professional development, target-specific satisfaction, and older nurse retention. *Career Dev. Int.* **2013**, *18*, 673–693. [CrossRef]
30. Liebermann, S.C.; Müller, A.; Weigl, M.; Wegge, J. Antecedents of the expectation of remaining in nursing until retirement age. *J. Adv. Nurs.* **2015**, *71*, 1624–1638. [CrossRef]
31. Camerino, D.; Conway, P.M.; Van Der Heijden, B.I.J.M.; Estryn-Behar, M.; Consonni, D.; Gould, D.; Hasselhorn, H.-M. the NEXT-Study Group Low-perceived work ability, ageing and intention to leave nursing: A comparison among 10 European countries. *J. Adv. Nurs.* **2006**, *56*, 542–552. [CrossRef]
32. Chan, Z.C.; Tam, W.S.; Lung, M.K.; Wong, W.Y.; Chau, C.W. A systematic literature review of nurse shortage and the intention to leave. *J. Nurs. Manag.* **2013**, *21*, 605–613. [CrossRef]
33. De Oliveira, D.R.; Griep, R.H.; Portela, L.F.; Rotenberg, L. Intention to leave profession, psychosocial environment and self-rated health among registered nurses from large hospitals in Brazil: A cross-sectional study. *BMC Health Serv. Res.* **2017**, *17*, 21. [CrossRef]
34. Hasselhorn, H.M.; Tackenberg, P.; Kuemmerling, A.; Wittenberg, J.; Simon, M.; Conway, P.M.; Bertazzi, P.A.; Beermann, B.; Büscher, A.; Mueller, B.H.; et al. Nurses' health, age and the wish to leave the profession–findings from the European NEXT-Study. *La Med. Del Lav.* **2006**, *97*, 207–214.
35. Leineweber, C.; Chungkham, H.S.; Lindqvist, R.; Westerlund, H.; Runesdotter, S.; Alenius, L.S.; Tishelman, C. Nurses' practice environment and satisfaction with schedule flexibility is related to intention to leave due to dissatisfaction: A multi-country, multilevel study. *Int. J. Nurs. Stud.* **2016**, *58*, 47–58. [CrossRef] [PubMed]
36. Salehi, T.; Barzegar, M.; Yekaninejad, M.; Ranjbar, H. Relationship between healthy work environment, job satisfaction and anticipated turnover among nurses in intensive care unit (ICUs). *Ann. Med. Health Sci. Res.* **2020**, *10*, 825–826.
37. Daouk-Öyry, L.; Anouze, A.-L.; Otaki, F.; Dumit, N.Y.; Osman, I. The JOINT model of nurse absenteeism and turnover: A systematic review. *Int. J. Nurs. Stud.* **2014**, *51*, 93–110. [CrossRef] [PubMed]
38. Nei, D.; Snyder, L.A.; Litwiller, B.J. Promoting retention of nurses: A meta-analytic examination of causes of nurse turnover. *Health Care Manag. Rev.* **2015**, *40*, 237–253. [CrossRef]
39. Li, H.; Xing, Z.; Li, Y.; Wan, Z.; Sun, D.; Zhao, M.; Sun, J. Retirement planning: The perceptions of pre-retirement nurses within different hospitals in China. *Int. Nurs. Rev.* **2020**, *67*, 173–182. [CrossRef]
40. Liu, P.-C.; Zhang, H.-H.; Zhang, M.-L.; Ying, J.; Shi, Y.; Wang, S.-Q.; Sun, J.; Rn, P.L.; Rn, H.Z.; Rn, M.Z. Retirement planning and work-related variables in Chinese older nurses: A cross-sectional study. *J. Nurs. Manag.* **2018**, *26*, 180–191. [CrossRef]

41. Boumans, N.P.; De Jong, A.H.; Vanderlinden, L. Determinants of early retirement intentions among Belgian nurses. *J. Adv. Nurs.* **2008**, *63*, 64–74. [CrossRef]
42. Cleaver, K.; Markowski, M.; Wels, J. Factors influencing older nurses' decision making around the timing of retirement: An explorative mixed-method study. *J. Nurs. Manag.* **2022**, *30*, 169–178. [CrossRef]
43. Duffield, C.; Graham, E.; Donoghue, J.; Griffiths, R.; Bichel-Findlay, J.; Dimitrelis, S. Why older nurses leave the workforce and the implications of them staying. *J. Clin. Nurs.* **2015**, *24*, 824–831. [CrossRef]
44. Molero, M.d.M.; Pérez-Fuentes, M.d.C.; Gázquez, J.J. Analysis of the mediating role of self-efficacy and self-esteem on the effect of workload on burnout's influence on nurses' plans to work longer. *Front. Psychol.* **2018**, *9*, 2605. [CrossRef] [PubMed]
45. Nilsson, K. Arbetstillfredsställelse hos äldre läkare och sjuksköterskor. In *Work Satisfaction among Older Physician and Nurses*; Swedish National Institute of Working Life: Malmö, Sweden, 2003.
46. Nilsson, K. *Äldre Medarbetares Attityder till ett Långt Arbetsliv. Skillnader Mellan Olika Yrkesgrupper inom Hälso- och Sjukvården [Older Employees' Attitudes to a Long Working Life. Differences between Different Occupational Groups in Healthcare]*; Arbetsliv i Omvandling, 10; Arbetslivsinstitutet: Stockholm, Sweden, 2006.
47. Stattin, M.; Bengs, C. Leaving early or staying on? Retirement preferences and motives among older healthcare professionals. *Ageing Soc.* **2021**, 1–27. [CrossRef]
48. Uthaman, T.; Chua, T.L.; Ang, S.Y. Older nurses: A literature review on challenges, factors in early retirement and workforce retention. *Proc. Singap. Healthc.* **2016**, *25*, 50–55. [CrossRef]
49. Valencia, D.; Raingruber, B. Registered Nurses' Views about Work and Retirement. *Clin. Nurs. Res.* **2010**, *19*, 266–288. [CrossRef] [PubMed]
50. MacLeod, M.L.P.; Zimmer, L.V.; Kosteniuk, J.G.; Penz, K.L.; Stewart, N.J. The meaning of nursing practice for nurses who are retired yet continue to work in a rural or remote community. *BMC Nurs.* **2021**, *20*, 220. [CrossRef]
51. Adams, G.A.; Beehr, T.A. Turnover and retirement: A comparison of their similarities and differences. *Pers. Psychol.* **1998**, *51*, 643–665. [CrossRef]
52. Van Bogaert, P.; Peremans, L.; Van Heusden, D.; Verspuy, M.; Kureckova, V.; Van de Cruys, Z.; Franck, E. Predictors of burnout, work engagement and nurse reported job outcomes and quality of care: A mixed method study. *BMC Nurs.* **2017**, *16*, 5. [CrossRef]
53. Bae, S. Intensive care nurse staffing and nurse outcomes: A systematic review. *Nurs. Crit. Care* **2021**, *26*, 457–466. [CrossRef]
54. Bakker, A.B.; Le Blanc, P.M.; Schaufeli, W. Burnout contagion among intensive care nurses. *J. Adv. Nurs.* **2005**, *51*, 276–287. [CrossRef]
55. Huang, H.; Xia, Y.; Zeng, X.; Lü, A. Prevalence of depression and depressive symptoms among intensive care nurses: A meta-analysis. *Nurs. Crit. Care* **2022**. [CrossRef]
56. Bergman, L.; Falk, A.; Wolf, A.; Larsson, I. Registered nurses' experiences of working in the intensive care unit during the COVID-19 pandemic. *Nurs. Crit. Care* **2021**, *26*, 467–475. [CrossRef]
57. Smith, J.A.; Flowers, P.; Larkin, M. *Interpretative Phenomenological Analysis: Theory, Method and Research*; Sage: London, UK, 2009.
58. Smith, J.A. Reflecting on the development of interpretative phenomenological analysis and its contribution to qualitative re-search in psychology. *Qual. Res. Psychol.* **2004**, *1*, 39–54. [CrossRef]
59. Nilsson, K. A sustainable working life for all ages—The swAge-model. *Appl. Ergon.* **2020**, *86*, 103082. [CrossRef] [PubMed]
60. Zhan, Y.; Wang, M.; Daniel, V. Lifespan perspectives on the work-to-retirement transition. In *Work Across the Lifespan*; Baltes, B.B., Rudolph, C.W., Zacher, H., Eds.; Elsevier: New York, NY, USA, 2019; pp. 581–604.
61. Van Solinge, H. Adjustment to Retirement. In *The Oxford Handbook of Retirement*; Wang, M., Ed.; Oxford University Press: Oxford, UK, 2012; pp. 313–324.
62. Newman, D.A.; Jeon, G.; Hulin, C.L. Retirement attitudes: Considering etiology, measurement, attitude-behavior relationships, and attitudinal ambivalence. In *The Oxford Handbook of Retirement*; Wang, M., Ed.; Oxford University Press: Oxford, UK, 2012; pp. 228–248.
63. Platts, L.G.; Ignatowicz, A.; Westerlund, H.; Rasoal, D. The nature of paid work in the retirement years. *Ageing Soc.* **2021**, 1–23. [CrossRef]
64. Kim, S.; Feldman, D.C. Working in retirement: The antecedents of bridge employment and its consequences for quality of life in retirement. *Acad. Manag. J.* **2000**, *43*, 1105–1210.
65. Zhan, Y.; Wang, M. Bridge Employment: Conceptualizations and New Directions for Future Research. In *Aging Workers and the Employee-Employer Relationship*; Bal, P.M., Kooij, D.T.A.M., Rousseau, D.M., Eds.; Springer International Publishing: New York, NY, USA, 2015; pp. 203–220. [CrossRef]
66. Burkert, C.; Hochfellner, D. Employment Trajectories beyond Retirement. *J. Aging Soc. Policy* **2017**, *29*, 143–167. [CrossRef]
67. Schalk, R.; Desmette, D. Intentions to continue working and its predictors. In *Aging Workers and the Employee-Employer Relationship*; Bal, P.M., Kooij, D.T.A.M., Rousseau, D.M., Eds.; Springer International Publishing: New York, NY, USA, 2015; pp. 187–201.
68. Shultz, K.S.; Morton, K.R.; Weckerle, J.R. The influence of push and pull factors on voluntary and involuntary early retirees' retirement decision and adjustment. *J. Vocat. Behav.* **1998**, *53*, 45–57. [CrossRef]
69. Nordenmark, M.; Stattin, M. Psychosocial wellbeing and reasons for retirement in Sweden. *Ageing Soc.* **2009**, *29*, 413–430. [CrossRef]
70. Reitzes, D.C.; Mutran, E.J. The transition into retirement: Stages and factors that influence retirement adjustment. *Int. J. Aging Hum. Dev.* **2004**, *59*, 63–84. [CrossRef]

71. Yeung, D.Y.; Zhou, X. Planning for Retirement: Longitudinal Effect on Retirement Resources and Post-retirement Well-being. *Front. Psychol.* **2017**, *8*, 1300. [CrossRef]
72. Blakeley, J.; Ribeiro, V. Are nurses prepared for retirement? *J. Nurs. Manag.* **2008**, *16*, 744–752. [CrossRef]
73. Furunes, T.; Mykletun, R.J.; Solem, P.E.; De Lange, A.H.; Syse, A.; Schaufeli, W.; Ilmarinen, J. Late Career Decision-Making: A Qualitative Panel Study. *Work. Aging Retire.* **2015**, *1*, 284–295. [CrossRef]
74. Nilsson, K. Why work beyond 65? Discourse on the Decision to Continue Working or Retire Early. *Nord. J. Work. Life Stud.* **2012**, *2*, 7–28. [CrossRef]
75. De Wind, A.; Geuskens, G.A.; Reeuwijk, K.G.; Westerman, M.J.; Ybema, J.F.; Burdorf, A.; Bongers, P.M.; Van Der Beek, A.J. Pathways through which health influences early retirement: A qualitative study. *BMC Public Health* **2013**, *13*, 292. [CrossRef]
76. Pond, R.; Stephens, C.; Alpass, F. How health affects retirement decisions: Three pathways taken by middle-older aged New Zealanders. *Ageing Soc.* **2010**, *30*, 527–545. [CrossRef]
77. Björn, C.; Lindberg, M.; Rissén, D. Significant factors for work attractiveness and how these differ from the current work situation among operating department nurses. *J. Clin. Nurs.* **2015**, *25*, 109–116. [CrossRef] [PubMed]
78. Elf, M.; Nordin, S.; Wijk, H.; McKee, K.J. A systematic review of the psychometric properties of instruments for assessing the quality of the physical environment in healthcare. *J. Adv. Nurs.* **2017**, *73*, 2796–2816. [CrossRef]
79. Clendon, J.; Walker, L. The juxtaposition of ageing and nursing: The challenges and enablers of continuing to work in the latter stages of a nursing career. *J. Adv. Nurs.* **2016**, *72*, 1065–1074. [CrossRef]
80. Stimpfel, A.W.; Arabadjian, M.; Liang, E.; Sheikhzadeh, A.; Weiner, S.S.; Dickson, V.V. Organization of Work Factors Associated with Work Ability among Aging Nurses. *West. J. Nurs. Res.* **2020**, *42*, 397–404. [CrossRef]
81. Van den Broeck, A.; De Cuyper, N.; De Witte, H.; Vansteenkiste, M. Not all job demands are equal: Differentiating job hindrances and job challenges in the Job Demands–Resources model. *Eur. J. Work Organ. Psychol.* **2010**, *19*, 735–759. [CrossRef]
82. Lepine, J.A.; Podsakoff, N.P.; Lepine, M.A. A Meta-Analytic Test of the Challenge Stressor–Hindrance Stressor Framework: An Explanation for Inconsistent Relationships among Stressors and Performance. *Acad. Manag. J.* **2005**, *48*, 764–775. [CrossRef]
83. Galatsch, M.; Li, J.; DeRycke, H.; Müller, B.H.; Hasselhorn, H.M. Effects of requested, forced and denied shift schedule change on work ability and health of nurses in Europe -Results from the European NEXT-Study. *BMC Public Health* **2013**, *13*, 1137. [CrossRef] [PubMed]
84. Armstrong-Stassen, M. Human resource management strategies and the retention of older RNs. *Nurs. Leadersh.* **2005**, *18*, 50–64. [CrossRef] [PubMed]
85. Clendon, J.; Walker, L. Nurses aged over 50 and their perceptions of flexible working. *J. Nurs. Manag.* **2015**, *24*, 336–346. [CrossRef] [PubMed]
86. Beehr, T.A.; Bennett, M.M. Working after Retirement: Features of Bridge Employment and Research Directions. *Work. Aging Retire.* **2015**, *1*, 112–128. [CrossRef]
87. Rudolph, C.W.; De Lange, A.H.; Van der Heijden, B. Adjustment processes in bridge employment: Where we are and where we need to go. In *Aging Workers and the Employee-Employer Relationship*; Bal, P.M., Kooij, D.T.A.M., Rousseau, D.M., Eds.; Springer International Publishing: New York, NY, USA, 2015; pp. 221–242.
88. Dingemans, E.; Henkens, K.; Van Solinge, H. Working retirees in Europe: Individual and societal determinants. *Work. Employ. Soc.* **2017**, *31*, 972–991. [CrossRef]
89. Wang, M.; Zhan, Y.; Liu, S.; Shultz, K.S. Antecedents of bridge employment: A longitudinal investigation. *J. Appl. Psychol.* **2008**, *93*, 818–830. [CrossRef]
90. Cahill, K.E.; Giandrea, M.D.; Quinn, J.F. To What Extent is Gradual Retirement a Product of Financial Necessity? *Work. Aging Retire.* **2017**, *3*, 25–54. [CrossRef]
91. Loretto, W.; Vickerstaff, S. The domestic and gendered context for retirement. *Hum. Relat.* **2013**, *66*, 65–86. [CrossRef]
92. Sewdas, R.; De Wind, A.; Van Der Zwaan, L.G.; Van Der Borg, W.E.; Steenbeek, R.; Van Der Beek, A.J.; Boot, C.R. Why older workers work beyond the retirement age: A qualitative study. *BMC Public Health* **2017**, *17*, 672. [CrossRef]
93. Carstensen, L.L.; Mikels, J.A.; Mather, M. Aging and the intersection of cognition, motivation, and emotion. In *Handbook of the Psychology of Aging*; Birren, J.E., Schaire, K.W., Eds.; Elsevier Academic Press: Amsterdam, The Netherlands, 2006; pp. 343–362.
94. Loretto, W.; White, P. Work, More Work and Retirement: Older Workers' Perspectives. *Soc. Policy Soc.* **2006**, *5*, 495–506. [CrossRef]
95. Pierce, J.L.; Gardner, D. Self-Esteem within the Work and Organizational Context: A Review of the Organization-Based Self-Esteem Literature. *J. Manag.* **2004**, *30*, 591–622. [CrossRef]
96. Deller, J.; Liedtke, P.; Maxin, L. Old-Age Security and Silver Workers: An Empirical Survey Identifies Challenges for Compa-nies, Insurers and Society. *Geneva Pap. Risk Insur.–Issues Pract.* **2009**, *34*, 137–157. [CrossRef]
97. Bakker, A.B.; Demerouti, E. Job demands–resources theory: Taking stock and looking forward. *J. Occup. Health Psychol.* **2017**, *22*, 273–285. [CrossRef] [PubMed]
98. Demerouti, E.; Bakker, A.B.; Nachreiner, F.; Schaufeli, W.B. The job demands-resources model of burnout. *J. Appl. Psychol.* **2001**, *86*, 499–512. [CrossRef] [PubMed]
99. Bakker, A.B.; van Wingerden, J. Do personal resources and strengths use increase work engagement? The effects of a training intervention. *J. Occup. Health Psychol.* **2021**, *26*, 20–30. [CrossRef]
100. Adriaenssens, J.; De Gucht, V.; Maes, S. Determinants and prevalence of burnout in emergency nurses: A systematic review of 25 years of research. *Int. J. Nurs. Stud.* **2015**, *52*, 649–661. [CrossRef]

101. Cummings, G.G.; MacGregor, T.; Davey, M.; Lee, H.; Wong, C.A.; Lo, E.; Muise, M.; Stafford, E. Leadership styles and outcome patterns for the nursing workforce and work environment: A systematic review. *Int. J. Nurs. Stud.* **2010**, *47*, 363–385. [CrossRef]
102. Erikson, E.H. *The Life Cycle Completed: A Review*; Norton: New York, NY, USA, 1982.
103. Doerwald, F.; Zacher, H.; Van Yperen, N.W.; Scheibe, S. Generativity at work: A meta-analysis. *J. Vocat. Behav.* **2021**, *125*, 103521. [CrossRef]
104. Kooij, D.T.A.M.; van Woerkom, M.; Wilkenloh, J.; Dorenbosch, L.; Denissen, J.J.A. Job crafting towards strengths and interests: The effects of a job crafting intervention person–job fit and the role of age. *J. Appl. Psychol.* **2017**, *102*, 971–981. [CrossRef]
105. Stordeur, S.; D'hoore, W.; Heijden, B.; Dibisceglie, M.; Laine, M.; van der Schoot, E. Leadership, job satisfaction and nurses' commitment. In *Working Conditions and Intention to Leave Profession among Nursing Staff in Europe*; Nurses Early Exit Study Report; National Institute for Working Life: Stockholm, Sweden, 2003; pp. 28–45.
106. Gagné, M.; Deci, E.L. Self-determination theory and work motivation. *J. Organ. Behav.* **2005**, *26*, 331–362. [CrossRef]
107. Fragoso, Z.L.; Holcombe, K.J.; McCluney, C.L.; Fisher, G.G.; McGonagle, A.K.; Friebe, S.J. Burnout and Engagement. *Work. Health Saf.* **2016**, *64*, 479–487. [CrossRef] [PubMed]
108. Hansson, I.; Zulka, L.E.; Kivi, M.; Hassing, L.B.; Johansson, B. *Att Arbeta Vidare efter 65—vem gör det och Varför? [To Continue Working after 65—Who Does it and Why?]*; Rapport 14; Delegationen för Senior Arbetskraft: Stockholm, Sweden, 2019.
109. Bandura, A. *Self-Efficacy: The Exercise of Control*; Freeman: New York, NY, USA, 1997.
110. Kooij, D.T.A.M.; Kanfer, R. Lifespan perspectives on work motivation. In *Work across the Lifespan*; Baltes, B.B., Rudolph, C.W., Zacher, H., Eds.; Elsevier Academic Press: Cambridge, MA, USA, 2019; pp. 475–493.
111. Xanthopoulou, D.; Bakker, A.B.; Demerouti, E.; Schaufeli, W.B. The role of personal resources in the job demands-resources model. *Int. J. Stress Manag.* **2007**, *14*, 121–141. [CrossRef]
112. McMichael, A.J. Standardized Mortality Ratios and the "Healthy Worker Effect": Scratching Beneath the Surface. *J. Occup. Environ. Med.* **1976**, *18*, 165–168. [CrossRef] [PubMed]

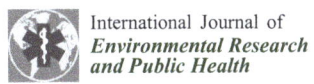

International Journal of
Environmental Research and Public Health

Article

Factors Influencing Retirement Decisions among Blue-Collar Workers in a Global Manufacturing Company—Implications for Age Management from A System Perspective

Ellen Jaldestad [1,*], Andrea Eriksson [1], Philip Blom [2] and Britt Östlund [1]

1 Department of Biomedical Engineering and Health Systems, KTH Royal Institute of Technology, SE-141 57 Huddinge, Sweden; andrea4@kth.se (A.E.); brittost@kth.se (B.Ö.)
2 Scania CV AB, Health & Work Environment, 8000 AP Zwolle, The Netherlands; philip.blom@scania.com
* Correspondence: ellkar@kth.se

Citation: Jaldestad, E.; Eriksson, A.; Blom, P.; Östlund, B. Factors Influencing Retirement Decisions among Blue-Collar Workers in a Global Manufacturing Company—Implications for Age Management from A System Perspective. *IJERPH* **2021**, *18*, 10945. https://doi.org/10.3390/ijerph182010945

Academic Editors: Kerstin Nilsson, Tove Midtsundstad, Peter Lundqvist, Joanne Crawford and Nygård Clas-Håkan

Received: 2 September 2021
Accepted: 12 October 2021
Published: 18 October 2021

Publisher's Note: MDPI stays neutral with regard to jurisdictional claims in published maps and institutional affiliations.

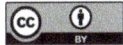

Copyright: © 2021 by the authors. Licensee MDPI, Basel, Switzerland. This article is an open access article distributed under the terms and conditions of the Creative Commons Attribution (CC BY) license (https://creativecommons.org/licenses/by/4.0/).

Abstract: The maintenance of older workers and determining the appropriate age for retirement are growing issues related to the fact that fewer people, still active in working life, have to provide for more non-working people due to increased life expectancy. As a result, retirement age has started to rise in many countries, and employers need to find ways to maintain an older and healthy work force, not least to avoid the loss of important experience. The aim of the current study was to increase the knowledge of factors influencing the retirement decisions among blue-collar workers in different national settings. A survey and semi-structured interviews were conducted with a sample of 100 blue-collar workers in Sweden, the Netherlands, and France, aged 55 years and older, within a global manufacturing company. Based on the results, implications for companies' age management strategies were discussed from a system perspective. Factors contributing to both retirement and to a prolonged work life were found on individual, organisational, and societal levels. This indicates the importance of a system perspective when planning for age management interventions.

Keywords: international study; job crafting; older workers; prolonged work life; sustainable work

1. Introduction

As the average life expectancy in the western world continues to increase, the possibility of continuing to work also increases for those who have health and motivation. Socioeconomic factors and work conditions such as physical and psychological strain impact aging employees' possibilities and/or individual motivation to retain more years at work. Today, we know quite well what is influencing retirement [1], but the problem is the lack of knowledge and age management strategies on how to influence decisions to postpone retirement. Age management can be defined as taking the employee's age and age-related factors into account in daily work management, work planning, and work organisation, thus enabling everyone, regardless of age, to achieve personal and organisational targets healthily and safely [2,3].

The decision to leave the labour force is a complex one including a range of factors that need to be considered in a company's age management. A poor physical work environment tends to influence employees' motivation to retire early. So do psychosocial factors, the organisation of work, and the content of job tasks, especially the degree of influence at work and the opportunity to pass experiences on to younger generations [1,4–11], as well as ill health and disabilities due to musculoskeletal disorders [12–14]. Other considerations that affect retirement decisions concern financial incentives for retirement, e.g., uncertainty regarding being able to provide for the household without a full income [14–17], as well as family and social life outside work. Family members' retirement also increases the risk of early retirement [6,14,18]. Opportunities for development and influence at work, responsibility for others, and satisfaction with working hours and meaningful tasks reduce that risk [6,8,14,17,19].

There are indications that continuing working has a positive relation to health [20] and early retirement has negative health effects [21]. Good health has also been shown to be an important factor for positive attitudes towards job retainment [8]. The duration of working life varies between company branches and between men and women. Research points out that some groups are overrepresented in terms of working longer in old age, especially farmers, while knowledge about retirement age for other businesses and for employees in technology companies is lacking [2]. Manufacturing is one of the strongly overrepresented industries in the labour market in terms of reported occupational accidents and diseases, physical disorders, and fatigue [22,23].

There is also limited research on how organisations can support and motivate older employees to continue to work beyond retirement age, but existing results point to the fact that employability and productivity can be maintained much further than we would normally expect [5,24]. To implement, and focus, age management is beneficial, regardless of sector and size of the organisation [25]. Bottom-up employee-driven job crafting interventions for older employees have in this context been advocated, because they have been shown to increase motivation for prolonged working life [20] as well as increase production and decrease absenteeism [26]. The concept of job crafting can encourage employees to reshape and improve the fit between the characteristics of the work and their own needs, abilities, and preferences [27,28]. Three types of crafting related to age management were published in Pit, Shrestha, Schofield, and Passey [13]; new skills to prevent jobs becoming monotonous, interpersonal relationships, and employees' cognitive stance toward their work by positively reframing the manner in which they think about aspects of the job. Other studies confirm that job crafting interventions in general working populations may increase individuals' well-being and health [29,30] with an even bigger effect on older workers [31].

However, there is also a need for organisational structures and management support for implementation of age management interventions. To educate managers to be 'age aware' and to establish an environment that enhance the workability and effort of older employees, e.g., developing strategies for mentoring and age management education for managers, can in this context be seen as important [32]. An environment supporting and encouraging older employees to keep on developing and to actively counteract age discrimination was shown to be especially important for work engagement and affective commitment to work and the employer [33].

Overall, research reviews have shown that age management interventions yielded better results if they included more than one organisational dimension than if they focused on one aspect [34]. It is therefore suggested that combined measurements on different organisational levels can support consistent results rather than interventions merely directed towards individuals [24,35]. System perspectives have in decades been advocated for workplace health interventions [36] and have recently also been suggested for considering the inter-relationships between different factors impacting a prolonged working life [1]. However, this kind of system approach has rarely been adopted in age management interventions. Nilsson [24] presents the swAge-model, which argues the importance of an age awareness in working life. The model holds a system perspective on sustainable age management in which different forms of ageing (i.e., biological, chronological, social, and cognitive ageing) are related to areas important to older employees' ability and willingness to continue working. Strategies to enable individuals to retain in work are, according to the model, formed by structures in both the organisational (meso) level and in the societal (macro) level. A system approach like the swAge-model allows for a holistic approach to different factors in interlinked subsystems, affecting the health and motivation of older workers to continue working. System models commonly contain structures on different levels, and the interaction between these subsystems are highlighted [35,37,38]. This study was based on a system model including a time perspective (chrono), a societal level (macro), two different organisational levels (meso and micro), and one individual level [37], as presented below and in Figure 1. According to the swAge-model [24] employers need to take into account that their older employees age differently. They are, for example, differently affected by biological changes. Thus biological ageing interacts with aspects on the individual level; one employee might need more variation in work than another to be able to stay healthy at work. On the meso-level chronological ageing is, following the swAge-model [24], connected to personal economics through, for example, statutory retirement age; employees in one country may have to work longer than their colleagues in other countries. On the macro- and micro-levels, organisational and manager attitudes towards older workers are related to social ageing in the swAge-model [24], and can influence willingness to stay in work. Examples of aspects that, according to the swAge-model, are connected to a person's cognitive ageing include opportunities to participate in professional development and work satisfaction [24]. These aspects are found on the micro-level and on the individual level, respectively. Thus, many aspects interrelate on different levels, as well as with the individual's ageing process. This indicates the need for adjusting work to the individual worker, from their current state of health.

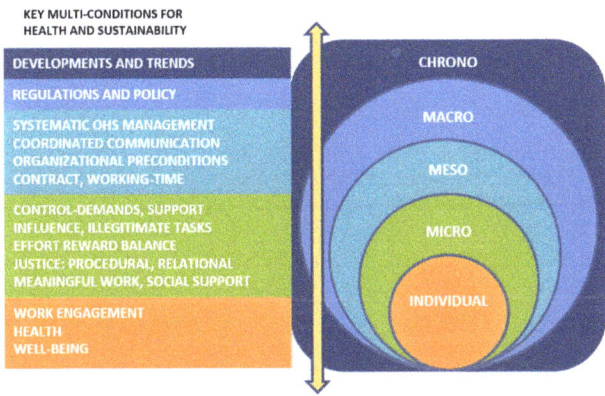

Figure 1. Examples of aspects on the different system levels included in the study. The arrow indicates the interplay between the levels (modified from [35]).

The chrono-system level is a time factor and is here described as, for example, trends in society that may have importance for workers' health and wellbeing, such as political decisions and changing pension regulations [35]. A rising life expectancy is also included in the chrono-level, as well as the different forms of ageing presented above [24]. The macro-system level includes policies and legislation and can in this context be the national retirement legislation that companies need to consider and follow. The meso-system level is manifested by organisational structures and organisational culture and includes health and safety management systems, company policies related to age management, and organisational preconditions for age management. The micro-system level is directly experienced by the employees and is where interactions between colleagues, and between managers and subordinates, occur. Work demands, resources, control, and social support are manifested at the micro-system level. The individual level includes individuals' handling strategies related to work and identity, motivation, health, and wellbeing. The individual level also holds a person's knowledge, capability, attitudes, values, lifestyle, and behaviour [35].

In conclusion, an integrated system model for how employee wellbeing could be crafted through managerial work and managerial strategies can be applied to analyse preconditions for more holistic age management interventions and implementing those [24,35]. The application of this kind of system approach may facilitate a work organisation's understanding of the complex and interrelated factors influencing a worker's retirement decision [1]. To our knowledge, there is no previous study investigating factors contributing to blue-collar workers' retirement decisions from a system perspective, conducted in a global manufacturing organisation. The aim of the study was, thus, to increase the knowledge of factors influencing the retirement decisions among blue-collar workers in different national settings. This was done from a system perspective, and implications for companies' age management strategies was discussed accordingly.

2. Method

2.1. Company Presentation and Pension Systems

Scania CV AB, with its head office in Sweden, was founded in 1891 and is now a worldwide provider of transport solutions, including trucks and buses for heavy transport applications. In 2017, the company had around 49,300 employees in about 100 countries. Production takes place in Europe, Latin America, and Asia.

The company is working actively with age management with the aim to enable blue-collar workers to continue working longer, with retained health and work capacity. The company has an internal occupational health service, which aims to work proactively; developing a safe, healthy, inspiring and productive workplace that rewards good performance. Representatives of occupational health service connect the work with age management to one of the company's core values 'respect for the individual'; meaning the individual stands at the centre in all aspects.

The blue-collar workers in this study worked on different kinds of workshop tasks. Most of them worked on the assembly line, putting different parts of a truck in place on a fixed time cycle. They worked in teams and rotated regularly between different workstations during the day. Some respondents worked in stations outside of the assembly line, for example in painting and in engine testing, or assembled the final parts of the vehicle. Those stations were not on a fixed time cycle. Some respondents worked in logistics within the production plants. They were able to plan their day largely than the other groups of respondents. Among the tasks was also quality control, which was considered as a 'calmer' work task, where, for example, assembled parts on a vehicle were controlled. Other 'calmer' tasks, such as cleaning, had earlier been available for older workers or people on rehabilitation. However, those tasks were now outsourced or included in other work tasks, reducing the opportunities for older employees to work at a slower pace and with a less heavy physical workload and more autonomy.

Acting on a global arena, the company is affected by national and local pension schemes in the different countries (see Table 1).

Table 1. Pension systems and local agreements in the different countries.

	Sweden	The Netherlands	France
Statutory retirement age	61–67 In 2017, state pension was available from age 61, and guarantee pension was available from age 65. Age for state pension will rise from 62 in 2020, to 63 in 2023 and 64 in 2026.	65 in 2017, 66 in 2018 and 67 in 2021. From 2022, the state pension will be calculated according to year of birth and life expectancy.	62 Full state pension available from 62 years of age or more, if one has worked for 167 quarters for people born between 1958 to 1960; 168 quarters for people born between 1961 to 1963 and so on.
Effective (average) retirement age (men/women)	65/64 [39]	63/62 [39]	59/60 [39]
Local agreements at the company	Blue-collar workers aged 62 who has been employed for at least 30 years, or aged 63 and employed for at least 25 years, can retire with full occupational pension (compared to age 65). When turning 60, employees are entitled to part-time retirement.	When approaching retirement age, workers can use saved holidays to take one or more days off each week. When retiring before the calculated pension age, the occupational pension will pay out less accordingly.	Normal working time is 35 h per week. Blue-collar workers at the company work 37 h per week. Extra hours can currently be used as reduction of working time to start retirement earlier.

2.2. Data Collection

Data was collected during 2016 and 2017 and included a sample of 100 blue-collar workers aged 55 and older in Sweden ($n = 29$), the Netherlands ($n = 37$), and France ($n = 34$). Respondents were selected within five production plants; three in Sweden, one in the Netherlands, and one in France. The data collection was mainly conducted using a survey, including factors previously shown as contributing to retirement, distributed to all blue-collar workers in the sample, and semi-structured interviews with all blue-collar workers in the sample with the aim to provide a deeper understanding of the survey data.

The respondents included full-time workers, part-time workers, and full-time retired workers. All respondents had been employed as blue-collar workers at the company for at least the latest four years (currently employed or before retirement). The retired respondents had all retired within the last 12 months. Respondents were asked to participate voluntarily by selection from the oldest person available and downward in age (see Table 2).

Table 2. Sample characteristics.

		SE	NL	FR	Total
Respondents	Men	24	36	34	94
	Women	5	1	0	6
	Total	29	37	34	100
Age	Range	59–69	57–67	56–62	56–69
	Average	63 (62.9)	65 (64.62)	58 (58.29)	62 (61.87)
	Std	2.41	2.06	1.96	3.46
Years of employment at Scania	Range	5–44	4–51	4–25	4–51
	Average	30 (29.6)	37 (36.92)	20 (20.47)	29 (29.2)
	Std	12.4	9.46	6.57	11.78
Work/retirement	Full-time working	20 (89%)	29 (78.4%)	30 (88.2%)	79 (79%)
	Part-time working	1 (3.4%)	2 (5.4%)	4 (11.8%)	7 (7%)
	Full-time retirement	8 (27.6%)	6 (16.2%)	0	14 (14%)

(SE = Sweden. NL = the Netherlands. FR = France).

A computerized survey, based on previous research in the area (see Table 3), was conducted individually guided by either an internal or an external interviewer. The internal interviewers worked either in HR or in the occupational health and safety department. The external interviewers were the first author of this article, one HR-student, and one HR-trainee. In Sweden and in the Netherlands there were both internal and external interviewers. In France, one external interviewer conducted the interviews. The first author of this article trained all interviewers. The survey was open for comments and followed by the semi-structured interview with open-ended questions. All interviews were held in the first language of each country (Swedish, Dutch, and French) by a native-born interviewer.

A pilot study was initially conducted with respondents in Sweden and in the Netherlands, to test and adapt the survey questions and the interview guide to the study settings. During this phase, interviews were also held with trade union and workers council representatives, as well as HR partners in all countries, which resulted in some adding of interview questions. All questions were professionally translated from Swedish into Dutch and French and thereafter discussed within the project group of each country to ensure that the questions were perceived in the same manner in the different cultural contexts. This was a process that included many steps back and forth between the researcher team and project teams, to ensure a proper translation and mutual understanding of the questions included in the survey and in the interviews with the blue-collar workers. In this process, some aspects were removed from the French version of the survey, e.g., "sense of coherence", and "experience of ageism". The reason for this was that the French project group was not able to find a suitable formulation of the aspect, or considered the aspect too personal to ask in a work setting.

Table 3. Factors and examples of items included in the survey.

Factors	Examples of Items ("Which of the Following Aspects are Crucial When You Consider Retirement?")	References
Physical work environment	Heavy workload; Repetitive tasks; Disturbing noise	[1,4–10]
Psychosocial work environment	Demand and control of the work; Experienced work-related stress (e.g., due to lack of time or insufficient resources); Cooperation and possibility to get help when needed	[1,4–7,9,10,17]
Work organisation	Working hours and pauses; Setup of working shift and job rotation	[1,6,8,9,11,19,32]
Job task characteristics	Interesting job assignments; Having meaningful work tasks	[1,6,8,14,17,19]
Personal effort	To be content with your own effort; Commitment and attachment to the job and the company	[1,6,8,9,14,17,19]
Economic situation	Need to keep working to provide for your basic needs; How you consider national and local pension systems (e.g., generous or tough)	[1,9,14,16,17]
Health	Self-experienced physical and mental health; How you think your health will change during the following years	[1,8,9,12–14,17]
Attitude towards an older work force	How you experience the attitude towards an older workforce at your job; -among your family and friends	[1]
Personal factors	Having a spouse who is already retired; Wanting to spend more time with family and friends, or on leisure activities	[1,6,8,9,14,18]

During the study, the first author of the article, to gain an understanding of the work environment and work settings for the older workers, visited all five production plants. Notes were taken during an integrative walk through with company representatives. To complete the data collection the first author of the article was provided with some internal personnel information, such as age and gender distribution in the different production plants and countries. This data, and the observations of the plants, were not analysed.

The Ethical Review Board in Stockholm approved the study and informed consent was applied; all respondents were informed verbally and in written text about the study before accepting participation. The respondents were also informed that the interview could be stopped at any time, with no further questions asked and that no data would be kept. All material was handled confidentially within the company and coded when reported back to the first author of the article, to ensure anonymity.

In the survey, the respondents were asked to take a stand on different aspects of given factors shown by previous research to influence retirement decisions (see Table 3 for item examples). The respondents were asked to state whether the aspects contributed to retirement or motivated them to prolong work life, with the stem questions "Which of the following aspects are crucial when you consider retirement?", and "In what way are the chosen aspect(s) crucial—Do they contribute to retirement or to a prolonged work life?" The term "retirement" included both "early retirement" (retirement before statutory retirement age), and "retirement on statutory retirement age'. All questions were open for comments. In the semi-structured interview, the respondents were, for example, asked about how to improve the work environment for older employees, and if they considered other aspects than the ones in the survey to be crucial for their decision about retirement; e.g., "What changes would you like to see at your job that can contribute to a better work environment for older workers?" and "Beyond the aspects you previously took a stand on, are/were there any other aspects important to your decision regarding retirement?".

2.3. Analysis

The results from the survey were first descriptively organized into percentages of respondents in the different countries who stated the aspects of the different factors either as contributing to retirement or to a prolonged work life, or if the aspect had no impact on the decision. If the respondent had stated that the aspect was important, but not commented in what direction, the interview answers were used to understand in what way the aspect was considered as important. Secondly, the semi-structured interviews, as well as the comments in the survey, were used in order to gain understanding and give substance to the individual answers from the survey. In all, the analysis of the empirical data was conducted in three steps;

1. The survey data indicated if the aspect was crucial or not to the decision about retirement.
2. The comments in the survey were used to code in what direction the aspect was considered as crucial; to retirement or to a prolonged work life.
3. The individual answers from the interviews were used to understand in what way the aspect was considered as crucial in the present context, e.g., "shift work is hard, especially night shifts, and has been so for at least ten years" (blue-collar worker in Sweden), and "the opportunity to work daytime is the main reason for me to be able to continue working" (blue-collar worker in the Netherlands).

The qualitative data were further analysed from the themes in the survey. This meant that how similarities and differences in between different individuals (e.g., the individuals' current health status), different workplace contexts (e.g., support from colleagues and superiors), and different national contexts (e.g., local pension systems) influenced the perceived importance of an aspect was analysed. The qualitative data thus deepened the understanding of why and in what ways a specific aspect was important to the respondents. It also showed how aspects on different system levels interacted in the respondents' decision about retirement. The qualitative data were therefor used in the development of the proposed system model and intervention activities discussed below. To summarize and visualize the results, we used the system model presented in the introduction. There were aspects considered crucial to the blue-collar workers' decision about retirement in all system levels except the chrono-level. The chrono-level was not used in the survey, nor in the analysis. The chrono-level was, however, used when discussing the results.

3. Results

In this section, results that represent differences between the countries, as well as the interplay between different system levels, are presented. This is done in order to lay the foundation for the intervention actions discussed below. In Table 4, we summarize what we consider the most important findings on the different system levels, as well as the main differences between the countries. All of the descriptive results from the survey are presented in Table 5. The table holds the percentages of aspects considered as crucial to either retirement or to a prolonged work life, or as having no effect on the decision. This is presented for each country and in total.

Table 4. Most important findings and main differences between the countries.

System Level	Most Important Findings	Main Differences between the Countries
Macro	On the macro-level national pension systems were considered tough.	This was mainly found in Sweden and the Netherlands. In Sweden the local pension system still enabled workers to retire earlier, whereas workers in both France and the Netherlands said they needed to keep working to provide for their basic needs.
Meso	Setup of working shifts, and work distribution were the most prominent aspects on the meso-level.	Shift work, especially over night shifts, were considered tough by respondents in Sweden and the Netherlands. French respondents were more positive to shift work in general. Swedish respondents were more negatively affected by the work distribution than respondents in the other countries, where comments were that work enabled variation and recovery during the day.

Table 4. Cont.

System Level	Most Important Findings	Main Differences between the Countries
Micro	The most positive aspects to prolong work life on the micro-level were social support from colleagues and superiors, and the atmosphere at work. Most negative aspects were physical work load, repetitive work tasks, and work related stress.	French respondents said the support from closest superior was lacking, and that the positive atmosphere at work had decreased. Thus, both aspects had a negative impact on their retirement decision, in contrast to the respondents in Sweden and the Netherlands.
Individual	Self-experienced physical and mental health, expected future health, and to spend more time with family and friends, were the most important aspects to retirement in all countries. The economic situation was the most prominent factor to prolong work life.	The local pension system, as mentioned above, was the only thing that differed between the countries on this level, which enabled Swedish respondents to retire earlier.

Table 5. Result of the survey; percentages of respondents considering the aspects as either contributing to retirement or to a prolonged work life, or as having no effect on the decision. Percentages is presented within each country and in total.

	Sweden			The Netherlands			France			Total		
	No Effect	To Retirement	To A Prolonged Work Life	No Effect	To Retirement	To A Prolonged Work Life	No Effect	To Retirement	To A Prolonged Work Life	No Effect	To Retirement	To A Prolonged Work Life
Physical Work Environment												
ASPECT												
Physical workload	58.6	34.5	6.9	56.8	35.1	8.1	79.4	20.6	0	65	30	5
Ergonomic tools and adequate safety equipment	86.2	10.3	3.4	83.8	0	16.2	79.4	2.9	17.6	83	4	13
Repetitive work	75.9	20.7	3.4	83.8	10.8	5.4	70.6	29.4	0	77	20	3
Working position/posture	82.8	17.2	0	100	0	0	79.4	20.6	0	88	12	0
Variation and recovery	72.4	20.7	6.9	48.6	18.9	32.4	73.5	8.8	17.6	64	16	20
Lightning	96.6	3.4	0	97.3	2.7	0	91.2	8.8	0	95	5	0
Disturbing noise	86.2	13.8	0	100	0	0	88.2	11.8	0	92	8	0
Vibrations	89.7	10.3	0	97.3	2.7	0	88.2	11.8	0	92	8	0
Temperature	93.1	6.9	0	97.3	2.7	0	94.1	5.9	0	95	5	0
High risk of work-related injuries	89.7	10.3	0	100	0	0	79.4	20.6	0	90	10	0
Exposed to chemicals	93.1	6.9	0	100	0	0	94.1	5.9	0	96	4	0
Psychosocial work environment												
ASPECT												
Demands and control in work	89.7	10.3	0	51.4	27	21.6	67.6	26.5	5.9	68	22	10
Work-related stress	51.7	48.3	0	81.1	18.9	0	61.8	38.2	0	66	34	0

Table 5. *Cont.*

	Sweden			The Netherlands			France			Total		
	No Effect	To Retirement	To A Prolonged Work Life	No Effect	To Retirement	To A Prolonged Work Life	No Effect	To Retirement	To A Prolonged Work Life	No Effect	To Retirement	To A Prolonged Work Life
Clear organisational goals	96.6	3.4	0	97.3	2.7	0	88.2	8.8	2.9	94	5	1
Social support from colleagues	89.7	3.4	6.9	40.5	2.7	56.8	67.6	17.6	14.7	64	8	28
Support from closest superior	79.3	6.9	13.8	43.2	10.8	45.9	64.7	26.5	8.8	61	15	24
The atmosphere and comfort at work	72.4	6.9	20.7	29.7	5.4	64.9	47.1	38.2	14.7	48	17	35
Cooperation and possibility of getting help when needed	82.8	3.4	13.8	64.9	2.7	32.4	70.6	26.5	2.9	72	11	17
Relationship with co-workers and superior(s)	75.9	10.3	13.8	51.4	2.7	45.9	70.6	23.5	5.9	65	12	23
Work organisation												
ASPECT												
Work distribution during the day	89.7	10.3	0	48.6	13.5	37.8	67.6	11.8	20.6	67	12	21
Working hours and pauses	82.8	10.3	6.9	81.1	8.1	10.8	70.6	14.7	14.7	78	11	11
Setup of working shifts	69	20.7	10.3	37.8	48.6	13.5	79.4	11.8	8.8	61	28	11
Setup of job rotation	82.8	13.8	3.4	86.5	2.7	10.8	67.6	8.8	23.5	79	8	13
Work station in order	96.6	3.4	0	97.3	2.7	0	76.5	17.6	5.9	90	8	2
Clear job description	93.1	3.4	3.4	97.3	2.7	0	79.4	5.9	14.7	90	4	6
Knowing who to ask if needed	100	0	0	97.3	2.7	0	Question was not used in France			98.5 †	1.5 †	0 †
Correct and functioning information flow	89.7	10.3	0	97.3	2.7	0	88.2	5.9	5.9	92	6	2
Management approach	82.8	13.8	3.4	67.6	18.9	13.5	67.6	26.5	5.9	72	20	8
Experienced development opportunities	86.2	6.9	6.9	97.3	2.7	0	88.2	8.8	2.9	91	6	3
Job task characteristics												
ASPECT												

Table 5. Cont.

	Sweden			The Netherlands			France			Total		
	No Effect	To Retirement	To A Prolonged Work Life	No Effect	To Retirement	To A Prolonged Work Life	No Effect	To Retirement	To A Prolonged Work Life	No Effect	To Retirement	To A Prolonged Work Life
Interesting and meaningful job assignments	65.5	3.4	31	86.5	2.7	10.8	52.9	23.5	23.5	69	10	21
Influence and responsibility for others as well as for the work procedures	72.4	3.4	24.1	89.2	2.7	8.1	Question was not used in France			81.8 †	3 †	15.2 †
Suitable competence to conduct job assignments	86.2	0	13.8	94.6	2.7	2.7	67.6	11.8	20.6	83	5	12
Personal effort												
ASPECT												
One's professional identity	75.9	6.9	17.2	89.2	2.7	8.1	73.5	5.9	20.6	80	5	15
To be content with one's own effort	62.1	3.4	34.5	91.9	2.7	5.4	52.9	14.7	32.4	70	7	23
Appreciation from others on work conducted	65.5	6.9	27.6	83.8	0	16.2	73.5	8.8	17.6	75	5	20
Meaningful job assignments and mission	65.5	3.4	31	81.1	2.7	16.2	85.3	2.9	11.8	78	3	19
Being able to use one's competence, education, and experience in a relevant way	72.4	6.9	20.7	91.9	2.7	5.4	73.5	14.7	11.8	80	8	12
Commitment and attachment to the job and the company	72.4	3.4	24.1	89.2	2.7	8.1	67.6	11.8	20.6	77	6	17
Economic situation												
ASPECT												
Need to keep working to provide for one's basic needs	89.7	3.4	6.9	29.7	2.7	67.6	50	2.9	47.1	54	3	43
Choose to work some extra years to raise one's future pension	75.9	0	24.1	94.6	0	5.4	67.6	2.9	29.4	80	1	19
Pension is not enough to provide the life-style one is used to	82.8	6.9	10.3	78.4	2.7	18.9	82.4	2.9	14.7	81	4	15

Table 5. Cont.

	Sweden			The Netherlands			France			Total		
	No Effect	To Retirement	To A Prolonged Work Life	No Effect	To Retirement	To A Prolonged Work Life	No Effect	To Retirement	To A Prolonged Work Life	No Effect	To Retirement	To A Prolonged Work Life
Providing for others in household	93.1	0	6.9	89.2	2.7	8.1	91.2	2.9	5.9	91	2	7
Pension enough to provide without income	58.6	41.4	0	91.9	8.1	0	85.3	0	14.7	80	15	5
Having another income	100	0	0	97.3	2.7	0	100	0	0	99	1	0
National and local pension systems considered tough or generous	72.4	6.9	20.7	78.4	8.1	13.5	97.1	0	2.9	83	5	12
Health												
ASPECT												
Self-experienced physical and mental health	37.9	41.4	20.7	45.9	40.5	13.5	41.2	52.9	5.9	42	45	13
Feeling good or feeling bad in general	62.1	27.6	10.3	75.7	16.2	8.1	Question was not used in France			69.7 †	21.2 †	9.1 †
Sense of coherence	82.8	17.2	0	100	0	0	Question was not used in France			92.4 †	7.6 †	0
In control of matters that affect one's life	82.8	17.2	0	100	0	0	67.6	26.5	5.9	84	14	2
Confronted with life crisis	86.2	13.8	0	83.8	10.8	5.4	79.4	17.6	2.9	83	14	3
Expected future health	48.3	44.8	6.9	43.2	56.8	0	85.3	14.7	0	59	39	2
Attitude towards an older work force												
ASPECT												
Attitude at one's work place	79.3	6.9	13.8	91.9	5.4	2.7	91.2	8.8	0	88	7	5
Attitude among family and friends	93.1	0	6.9	100	0	0	97.1	0	2.9	97	0	3
Attitude in the society	86.2	6.9	6.9	97.3	2.7	0	97.1	2.9	0	94	4	2
Attitude in the culture	100	0	0	97.3	2.7	0	Question was not used in France			98.5 †	1.5 †	0
Affected by stereotyping	96.6	3.4	0	100	0	0	97.1	2.9	0	98	2	0
Experience of ageism	93.1	6.9	0	97.3	2.7	0	Question was not used in France			95.5 †	4.5 †	0 †
Personal factors												
ASPECT												
Partner's retirement	82.8	3.4	13.8	86.5	13.5	0	85.3	11.8	2.9	85	10	5

Table 5. Cont.

	Sweden			The Netherlands			France			Total		
	No Effect	To Retirement	To A Prolonged Work Life	No Effect	To Retirement	To A Prolonged Work Life	No Effect	To Retirement	To A Prolonged Work Life	No Effect	To Retirement	To A Prolonged Work Life
Social life connected to work	100	0	0	100	0	0	100	0	0	100	0	0
More time for family, friends, and leisure activities	41.4	58.6	0	59.5	40.5	0	73.5	26.5	0	59	41	0
More time for a spare-time job or volunteer work	79.3	17.2	3.4	100	0	0	79.4	20.6	0	87	12	1

† French respondents excluded from the total.

3.1. Macro Level

(Laws and regulations; e.g., national retirement legislation, culture and values, and attitude towards an older workforce)

In both Sweden and the Netherlands, the national pension system was considered tough. According to the comments, the respondents tried to 'adapt the size of the wallet' and use personal savings to handle the upcoming changes in their personal economy. The respondents also talked about a general view that older people should 'leave room for the younger ones', indicating a negative perception of the attitude towards an older work force in the society.

3.2. Meso Level

(Policies and company culture, attitude towards an older work force, local pension agreements, strategic management and communication, and working hours)

On the meso-level, within the factor work organisation, the setup of working shifts (28%) was the most crucial aspect to retirement, whilst work distribution (21%) and setup of job rotation (13%) were important to prolonging work life.

The aspect setup of working shifts as contributing to retirement was most prominent in the Netherlands (48.6%) compared to Sweden (20.7%) and France (11.8%). Shift work in general, and night shift in particular, were considered tough and were said to highly influence the decision regarding retirement. Working extra hours (e.g., 'flex-time') and on weekends had a negative impact, and some respondents requested to work daytime only. However, the work distribution and setup of the working hours and working shifts were also important aspects to consider for a prolonged work life, since shift work was mentioned as a positive aspect due to enhanced variation. Setup of work and breaks, and job rotation were also considered positive factors.

Regarding the local pension agreement, 41.4% of the Swedish respondents said they had, or would have, enough pension to provide an income without working past retirement age. The local pension agreement in Sweden was mentioned positively among several of them.

3.3. Micro Level

(Psychosocial work environment, responsibility and influence, management approach, attitude towards an older work force, and a physical work environment)

Within the factor of physical work environment, physical workload (30%), repetitive work (20%), and (lack of) variation and recovery (16%) were the most prominent aspects considered crucial to decisions about retirement. Heavy workload and repetitive tasks, as well as not being able to sit down during work, were said to be tiring and hard for the older workers. Some respondents said they had had injuries due to the physical work and some said that noise, worse lighting, vibrations, and working in uncomfortable positions could, or had, affected their decision about retirement. Variation and recovery (20%) was considered as an important aspect to prolong work life, especially in the Netherlands where 32.4% percent of the respondents had this opinion, as well as to have influence and responsibility for others (15.2%; France excluded), and to be appreciated by others (20%),

In total, 13% of the respondents considered the availability of ergonomic tools and safety equipment as important to prolonging work life. In Sweden the corresponding number was 3.4%, and comments were that ergonomic tools were not available. Workers on the assembly line said they were very tired after work and needed to rest to recover during evenings and weekends. They did not want their reduced energy levels to affect work, but it affected their spare time and their social life outside work more than ever. A gradual transition to retirement was therefore requested to reduce the physical workload.

Within the factor of psychosocial work environment, work-related stress (34%) and demands and control (22%) were the most prominent aspects crucial to retirement. These were followed by the atmosphere and comfort at work (17%) and support from closest superior (15%). Some respondents expressed that the stress had increased; '... more is to be produced with the same staff', and the older workers were not able to keep up with the pace on the assembly line. In France, the atmosphere (38.2%) and support from the closest superior (26.5%) were mentioned as factors contributing to retirement to a greater extent than to a prolonged work life (14.7% and 8.8%, respectively), with respondents commenting that they lacked support, recognition, and respect from their closest superior, and that the pressure had increased. Comments were that the closest superiors were 'too busy fulfilling their personal goals' instead of managing their group. Superiors were also said to have a lack of understanding of the challenges the older workers faces, as well as of how to make use of older workers' competence.

The atmosphere and comfort at work (35%) and support from closest superior (23%), along with social support from colleagues (28%), were also the most important aspects for a prolonged work life within the same factor. Social activities outside work, to talk to and get to know one's colleagues, as well as the possibility to plan their own work day, were said to have a positive effect on the amount of work-related stress and on the balance between work demands and control. Among the respondents who considered these aspects important to prolonging work life were those who said they actively tried to improve relations with both colleagues and supervisors, for example by socialising with colleagues during the day and developing a trusting relationship with their managers. The respondents in the Netherlands considered most of the aspects of the psychosocial work environment as important to prolong work life (e.g., social support from colleagues and superiors, cooperation, and the atmosphere at work) whereas the respondents in France mostly considered the same aspects as contributing to retirement.

There were different experiences of the attitude towards an older work force within the company among the respondents; some said they had not noticed anything regarding the attitude, whereas some had experienced only, or almost only, positive attitudes among colleagues and supervisors. Some said negative attitudes and comments at work due to age occurred. Even though most respondents thought it was positive to work in mixed groups with different ages, genders and cultures, some felt excluded by the working group due to their age.

3.4. Individual Level

(Economic situation, health and meaningfulness, competence and experience, engagement and belonging, and personal effort)

To experience work as interesting and meaningful (21%) and to have suitable competence to conduct work (12%) were important aspects for a prolonged work life within the factor 'job task characteristics'. However, in the Netherlands neither of these aspects were considered important in any direction by more than 11% of the respondents, and in

France the same amount of respondents (23.5% respectively) considered interesting and meaningful job assignments as important to retirement as to a prolonged work life.

The opinions in all countries also differed between those who said their work was interesting and meaningful and those who said they wished they had had more opportunity to develop within their work. Among the respondents who considered the job task characteristics meaningful and interesting, and also important to prolonging work life, there were those who said they had the opportunity to change and develop work to better suit their personal goals and needs, and to adjust work in discussions with colleagues and supervisors, for example in weekly quality meetings. Contrasting to this, those who considered the aspects contributing to retirement said work was too strict and standardised, leaving no room for individual changes. According to the comments, more development opportunities would have had contributed to a prolonged work life. In France some did not consider work as adding meaning to life; "work is work and not what gives life meaning".

In terms of personal effort, 14.7% of the French respondents said that being content with one's own effort influenced their decision about retirement. The same amount of respondents also said that being able to use one's competence was crucial, indicating in their comments that they used to be more content with work some years ago but that different aspects, such as more pressure and a different atmosphere, had changed that view. In total, to be content with one's own effort (23%) and to find the job meaningful (19%) were the most important aspects to a prolonged work life within the factor of "job task characteristics". Many respondents were proud of their jobs, and of the company. The personal mind-set and motivation were said to be important for being content with one's own work.

Many of the respondents said they had to keep working to retirement age or beyond in order to provide for basic needs (43%) and/or to maintain their current lifestyle (15%). This was largely seen in the Netherlands and in France, compared to Sweden. As mentioned above, personal savings were said to be a way to enable retirement, as well as to 'adapt to the size of the wallet' and to 'plan one's spending' more carefully. Even though the economic situation affected many respondents in their retirement decisions, some said 'there are more important factors,' such as health and spending time with family and friends.

Current health (45%) as well as future expected health (39%) were among the most crucial reasons contributing to retirement in the entire survey. Among the comments were: 'It is important to have a healthy life when retired', and 'I want to retire with my health left intact'. There were, however, also respondents who said they already had diseases and injuries to cope with, but that they would rather go to work than stay at home; 'It is better to work than to sit at home'.

Respondents who had experienced a life crisis or sickness themselves, or among family and friends, said this affected their decision to retire as early as possible. Having good health—current and expected—also influenced their decision to prolong work life; to work helped the respondents to feel well.

Among personal factors, to spend more time with family, friends, and on leisure activities was the most prominent aspect towards retirement (41%). There were also those who said they wanted to retire because of this aspect, but that they were not financially able to. According to open answers and comments, partners' retirement influenced the decision in different directions; there were those who said they wanted to keep working because their spouse was younger and those who wanted to stop working at the same time as their older spouse. However, there were also those who said they had to keep working because of their economic situation even though their partner was already retired. Overall, to enable a gradual transition to retirement was recurrently requested, in order to be more prepared for the upcoming changes in social life and in general life structure.

4. Discussion

The aim of the study was to increase the knowledge of factors influencing the retirement decisions among blue-collar workers in different national settings. This was done within a global manufacturing company. The results of the study found factors influencing the retirement decision on different system levels. In this particular study we chose to look at the results from the following levels; chrono- (time factor), macro- (societal level), meso- (organisational level), micro- (work group/department level), and individual level (see Figure 1). In the following section, the results are compared and contrasted to previous research from those system levels. Based on the results, age management intervention actions are also discussed from a system perspective (see Figure 2).

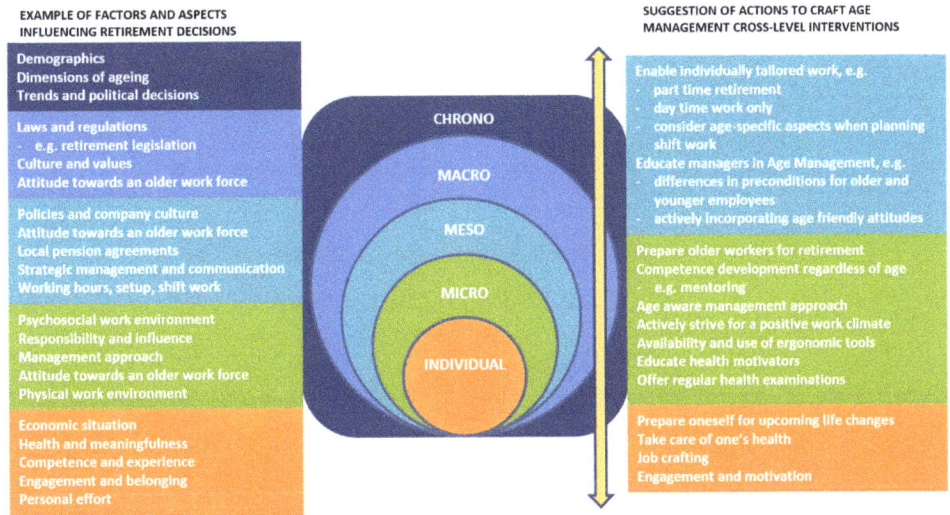

Figure 2. Examples of important aspects and age management actions suggestions based on the results. The arrow indicates the interplay between the levels (modified from [35]).

On the macro-level (e.g., policies and legislations on the national level), aspects said to be important to the respondents' decision about retirement included national retirement legislation. The statutory retirement age in the three countries in the study differed and global manufacturing companies thus need to consider that their blue-collar workers in some countries may have to work several years longer than in others. On the societal macro-level the culture and values in each country, as well as the attitude towards an older work force, might also differ. Among the respondents, there were those who said that the older workers should leave room for younger ones, even though most respondents considered the attitude towards older workers as positive. This aspect was not considered as influencing the decision about retirement largely; however, a global company should be aware of that when you are considered an older worker, a social aspect of ageing, might differ between countries [24].

An important aspect on the meso-level (i.e., organisational level) was access to the Swedish local retirement program. Several Swedish respondents in this study had access to the early retirement program, and most of them planned to take advantage of it, even though they said they felt healthy enough to continue working longer. Even though part-time retirement seem to have a positive outcome on keeping industrial employees in work beyond retirement age [40], agreements that enable people to stop working earlier may not encourage them to stay longer in the company [16,41]. However, such an agreement will likely be beneficial for the individuals' health as pensioners. Age management interventions that include individually tailored work, such as part-time retirement, could be strategic to keep older workers and their competence within the company [24,40]. Among the respondents were also people with immigrant backgrounds who had not been living in Sweden long enough to be able to benefit from the local retirement program. Similar to the respondents in the other countries, where no such retirement program existed, they had to keep working longer. In France, comments regarding pension legislation included 'I'll stop when I´ve reached my quartiles', indicating a possible social and cultural aspect of ageing, in not working longer than needed [24]. Age-specific aspects are also suggested to be considered in shift work planning [42], especially when non-senior older workers are involved. Due to, for example, multiple careers or emigration the older workers are not necessarily the most senior workers. Older shift workers who lack experience are probably the worst candidates working in non-traditional shift work [32].

The respondents had different ways to cope with work pressure and to gain and maintain energy, such as resting during evenings and weekends. They also talked about keeping healthy and having a positive attitude to work and life in general. Those are strategies on the individual level used by the blue-collar workers to handle challenges on other system levels. To reduce or eliminate the stressful work on the assembly line was suggested in all countries, as well as to work daytime only, to avoid flex work and over time, and to work shorter days. Even though shift work mostly was considered tiring, there were those who said shift work enabled variation, once again indicating the positive potential of more individualized work. In this study, the opinions of shift work differed the most between the Netherlands and France. In the Netherlands, where 48.6% of the respondents said shift work contributed to retirement, the average age of the respondents was 65 years. In France, the corresponding number was 11.8% and the average age of the respondents was 58 years. In France, the work shifts were also differently planned than in the Netherlands, and did not include overnight shifts. Both the age difference among the respondents and the fact that less respondents worked late shifts in France could explain why more respondents in the Netherlands than in France considered the aspect as contributing to retirement. To implement daytime work only may therefore not lead to the expected outcome in the different countries; the French workers may benefit less from such an implementation. These differences in the results also mirror the ambiguous findings of Blok and de Looze [42] who found differences between older and younger shift workers, but no evidence of more problems related to shift work among older workers. From the results of this study, a global company is also encouraged to strive for common values of older workers, and to consider how different aspects in the work environment affect those employees. This can be done by educating managers in age management and by developing strategies for internal communication to spread information within the organisation. Comments among the respondents regarding the attitude towards older workers in the company were overall positive, even though it was mentioned that the closest superior often lacked an understanding of the work situation for older workers. The attitudes towards older workers can differ on the different system levels, indicating the importance of having a common view on the meso-level to be spread through the organisation.

On the micro-level (i.e., workplace level) respondents in all countries asked for a gradual and smoother transition to retirement—to successively reduce the workload and to be more prepared for the upcoming changes in social life and in general life structure, which is also supported by the findings of, for example, Ilmarinen [5]. Mentoring younger and/or new colleagues can lead to learning and development as well as to more variation, skills transferring, and reduced workload for older workers, as well as to fully use the older workers' competence. The respondents also indicated that their closest managers (e.g., team leaders) often were young and more focused on making a career of their own than to understand the challenges faced by older workers, e.g., they were 'too busy fulfilling their own goals'. The understanding and interaction between managers and employees develop through time and attention, and are of importance in developing the company's age management strategies [43]. To organise for mentoring and an age-aware environment on both the micro- and meso-system levels are in line with the suggestions of Nilsson [24], Popkin, Morrow, Di Domenico, and Howarth [32], van Dam, van Vuuren, and Kemps [33], Widell Blomé, et al. [44], and BestAgers [45], who all indicated the importance of including the older workers, as well as providing training regardless of age, and to educate managers in age management. By letting, and encouraging, older workers to participate in training and education, relevant tacit knowledge can also be made available to managers and younger colleagues [43]. To actively seek a positive working climate that takes ageing and cultural aspects of work into account is also indicated on the micro-level. Overall, the general development of a positive work climate can be seen as a facilitator of a prolonged working life [33]. The respondents were keen to keep a positive atmosphere at work and to enjoy social activities outside work. To work in mixed groups, with people of different ages, genders, and cultures were considered positive for the psychosocial work environment. Most of the respondents also said they were proud to work for the company; its brand had high value. Intrinsic job value is positively related to employability, work engagement, and affective commitment [33]. There was, however, a national difference in the survey, in which the respondents in France had a more negative view of both the atmosphere at work, and of the social support from colleagues and supervisors compared to the other countries. A cultural difference in how work was interpreted may be the reason for this. Comments from the French respondents were that the attitude within the company had changed over the years, as well as that work was not considered as adding meaning to life; 'work is work, and not what gives life meaning'.

Availability of, and encouragement to use, ergonomic tools is an important aspect to reduce physical work load [24]. Some of the Swedish workers considered ergonomic tools and safety equipment to be an aspect contributing to retirement, whereas workers in the other countries considered this aspect as contributing to a prolonged work life. According to the Swedish respondents with this assumption, work was conducted with 'less resources than before' and featured 'heavy load and lifting without ergonomic tools'. Since older workers benefit more from ergonomic tools [32], and since the production plants in the study were more or less identical, it is assumed that the respondents who considered ergonomic tools as contributing to early retirement experienced a lack of them. To enable alteration between physically and mentally demanding tasks it is thus suggested to increase the variation in work load [24,46]. Based on these findings, and in line with Lichtenthaler and Fischbach [20] and Loch, Sting, Bauer, and Mauermann [26], we propose a bottom-up management approach to involve the employees in the intervention process.

Age management interventions, regardless of which level they are planned on, aim to enable individual workers to stay healthy at work [3,47]. The individual worker is the key to realizing this. However, the organisation must in this context be responsible for developing preconditions for individuals to make healthy choices [24]. On the individual level the economic situation was the most important reason for the respondents to keep working; thus, the need to prepare oneself for the upcoming changes in life, especially the economic situation, is supported. The respondents talked about 'adapting the size of the wallet', and personal savings, but many of them said they had to keep working because they were not able to provide for their basic needs. Self-experienced health was one of the most important aspect in the survey to retire as early as possible, both current (45%) and expected (39%) health. According to Nilsson, Hydbom and Rylander [47] self-experienced health is a better predictor of retirement decision than diagnosed health. This indicates the importance of keeping the health factor in focus on all levels whilst planning a company's age management strategies, as well as to encourage individual workers to take care of their own health e.g., by educating health motivators and providing regular health examinations with the occupational health care. The respondents also talked about being content with one's own effort, and being able to use one's competence and experiences in relevant ways. As mentioned previously, they wanted to be involved in organisational changes and to pass on their experience through mentoring. To enable more autonomy, influence, and freedom within work at individual level, which was requested in all countries, a bottom-up management approach is once more suggested. According to Widell Blomé, Borell, Nilsson, and Håkansson [44], organisational preconditions and attitudes need to be considered when planning age management interventions. These kinds of organisational conditions may promote individual job crafting; thus optimizing work to the employees' own abilities and energy [20,27]. Eaves, et al. [48] found that construction workers actively changed their work conditions to reduce challenging demands (e.g., safety risks), to make work easier, and to reduce musculoskeletal symptoms and increase overall health. This can be compared to Gaudart [49] who found that older assembly line workers developed strategies that enabled them to work at a steadier pace than their younger colleagues (e.g., by minimizing movements back and forth to collect gears) in order to protect them from physical strain. These examples of job crafting [28,50] can be compared to the respondents strategies found in this study, which included minor changes in the performance of tasks and to bring suggestions of improvements to the weekly quality meetings to reduce physical work load. Another job crafting activity found was to add meaning to one's job assignments. To reframe what to think of one's job in this way is one kind of cognitive crafting argued to be of particular value to older workers [51]. The perceived opportunities to job craft, however, differed among the respondents. Some said they had no opportunity to make any changes at all, whereas others were of a different opinion with a more positive mind set for making individual changes in work, in tasks, relations, and perception of work.

The survey did not include questions to cover the chrono-level. However, there are time-related aspects to consider when planning age management interventions in a global company. Firstly, the dimensions of ageing in the swAge-model interplay with the aspects found to be important to the blue-collar workers in this study. For example, the statutory retirement age differ between the three countries. This aspect is connected to chronological ageing and must be considered in a global company's age management. Secondly, it may not be possible for companies themselves to affect trends and political decisions, but it might be important to adapt to, or consider them in the companies' age management. One example is the statutory retirement age, currently rising in many European countries [52], as well as the fact that even though we live longer we do so with more chronic diseases, and not necessarily with a higher, or even maintained, work ability compared to previous generations. This is found especially among low-educated people [53]. Thirdly, the changing demographics with more older non-working people to provide for is perhaps one of the most obvious aspect to consider in age management strategies; ways to develop sustainable work settings that enable people to work longer with maintained health are needed. It is also important to consider the time factor when planning and implementing age management strategies within an organisation. For example, if a company chooses to educate their managers in age management, it will take time to educate all managers, as well as to implement the new knowledge in the company. There might also be a time difference in how fast the strategies can be adopted between the countries. In this study, the company already had a strategy for part time and early retirement through the local pension system in Sweden, which may offer better conditions for implementing certain age management strategies compared to the other countries.

To adapt the work to the individual workers, managerial decisions such as to enable part-time retirement, to customize work tasks, and to increase work autonomy can be effective ways to best make use of the competence of older workers [32,44].

Method Discussion and Limitations

It must be considered that the respondents may have interpreted the content of the questions differently, for example, if they considered themselves to be 'pushed' to retirement by some aspects in a negative sense or if they were positively 'pulled' towards their own decisions about working or retiring. There may also have been differences in how the concept 'prolonged work life' was interpreted; it did not necessarily mean to prolong work life beyond statutory retirement age, but to work as long as possible.

There may be differences in the degree of respondents' honesty and willingness to give information, depending on if the interviewer was someone from the company or an external person. In Sweden and the Netherlands there were also more than one interviewer, which may have had an effect on the data gathered, e.g., in terms of how comments were phrased. However, all the data was handled in the same manner when reported back to the first author of the article, and a close contact within the project teams during the entire study hopefully limited the effect on the results.

If the respondent had stated that the aspect was important, but not commented in what direction, the interview answers were used to understand in what way the aspect was considered as important. To be able to use both survey data and interview data is considered as a strength in the study design, although it is important to keep in mind that cultural differences may influence how appropriate the interview questions captured the essential opinions of the respondents. French blue-collar workers were not included in the pilot study, which can be seen as a weakness of the study design. If French respondents had been included in the pilot study, the survey and interview questions may have been more appropriate also to the French context and no aspects may have been removed from the French version of the survey.

The respondents were selected to provide us with the most genuine information; they were those who had retired most recently and those having the shortest amount of time left to retirement within the different production plants. In the planned study design, we hoped to include respondents that had left the company, or had been redeployed, due to sickness or physical issues. Those were however hard to track, and no respondent from that category was found. This may indicate 'the healthy worker effect'; that the interviewees represented a healthier sample than in the society on average [54]. We also had a small number of women among the respondents ($n = 6$). The low number of female respondents limits us in making any assumptions about gender differences. Even though the responses from the women in our study did not indicate any notable trends from the male respondents, there might be other aspects related to female blue-collar workers' situation than those appearing in this study.

The results of contributing aspects in this study are connected to the organisational context, and other known and unknown aspects in the area may not be covered. For example, an important health aspect in the physical work environment is vibrations. In our study, a rather low number of the respondents (8%) considered the aspect crucial to the decision about retirement, probably because most of the respondents did not consider themselves as exposed to vibrations. When asked about other possible aspects than the ones covered in the interview, comments were that there were none, and that work was not the most important factor to the decision. Instead health, family, and leisure time were said to be more important. Some said it was simply time to stop after a long work life.

5. Conclusions and Practical Implications

The results of this study contribute with a system perspective on age management, revealing aspects that a global company can affect, as well as some aspects on macro-, and chrono-levels that needs to be taken into account, when planning age management strategies. Both causes of early retirement and enablers of a prolonged work life were found on all levels; including individual-, organisational-, and societal levels.

The practical implications of this paper can contribute to the transition from work to retirement, from both employers' and employees' perspectives. For the employer this paper contributes with knowledge on what enables blue-collar workers to maintain in work, and how to facilitate this. From the employee perspective, the results can be used for raising their understanding and awareness of what factors might influence their willingness to prolong work life. As discussed above, this study found several factors influencing the retirement decisions among blue-collar workers, which cannot be solved separately. We also found differences among the respondents in the three different countries, but perhaps more importantly, there were differences between respondents within the same country and national settings. For example, in Sweden, some, but not all, respondents were able to retire early because of the local pension system. In all countries, there were also those who said they would like to retire with their health intact, but were not financially able to stop working. The results, above all, indicate that the different system levels interact and a system perspective is of great value when planning age management interventions in global organisations. Manufacturing companies that aim to enable blue-collar workers to work longer, and stay healthy whilst doing so, can thus benefit from using a system perspective, for example, the already established swAge-model [24], when planning and conducting age management interventions. Because of the individual differences among older workers, the possibility to craft their jobs, in a more autonomous setting, may be of particular importance. Further research, on how to conduct successful job crafting interventions for older blue-collar workers from a system perspective, is therefore suggested.

Author Contributions: Formal analysis, E.J., A.E. and B.Ö.; Methodology, E.J., P.B. and B.Ö.; Project administration, E.J., P.B. and B.Ö.; Resources, P.B. and B.Ö.; Supervision, A.E. and B.Ö.; Writing—original draft, E.J., A.E., P.B. and B.Ö.; Writing—review & editing, E.J., A.E. and B.Ö. All authors have read and agreed to the published version of the manuscript.

Funding: The study was partially funded by, and conducted in close collaboration with, the occupational health- and safety department in Scania CV AB.

Institutional Review Board Statement: The study was conducted according to the guidelines of the Declaration of Helsinki, and approved by the The Ethical Review Board in Stockholm (protocol code 2017/320-3. Date of approval 7 April 2017).

Informed Consent Statement: Informed consent was obtained from all subjects involved in the study.

Conflicts of Interest: The authors declare no conflict of interest.

References

1. Nilsson, K. Conceptualisation of ageing in relation to factors of importance for extending working life—A review. *Scand. J. Public Health* **2016**, *44*, 490–505. [CrossRef] [PubMed]
2. Nilsson, K.; Hydbom, A.R.; Rylander, L. Factors influencing the decision to extend working life or retire. *Scand. J. Work. Environ. Health* **2011**, *37*, 473–480. [CrossRef] [PubMed]
3. Walker, A. The emergence of age management in Europe. *Int. J. Organ. Behav.* **2005**, *10*, 685–697.
4. Von Bonsdorff, M.E.; Kokko, K.; Seitsamo, J.; von Bonsdorff, M.; Nygård, C.-H.; Ilmarinen, J.; Rantanen, T. Work strain in midlife and 28-year work ability trajectories. *Scand. J. Work. Environ. Health* **2011**, *37*, 455–463. [CrossRef]
5. Ilmarinen, J. *Towards a Longer Worklife: Ageing and the Quality of Worklife in the European Union*; Finnish Institute of Occupational Health, Ministry of Social Affairs and Health: Helsinki, Finland, 2005.
6. Seitsamo, J. Qualities of work, functioning and early retirement. A longitudinal study among Finnish ageing workers in 1981–1997. *Int. Congr. Ser.* **2005**, *1280*, 136–141. [CrossRef]
7. James, J.B.; McKechnie, S.; Swanberg, J. Predicting employee engagement in an age-diverse retail workforce. *J. Organ. Behav.* **2011**, *32*, 173–196. [CrossRef]
8. Jebens, E.; Medbø, J.I.; Knutsen, O.; Mamen, A.; Veiersted, K.B. Association between perceived present working conditions and demands versus attitude to early retirement among construction workers. *Work* **2014**, *48*, 217–228. [CrossRef]
9. Marcaletti, F. Age management and sustainable Careers for the Improvement of the Quality of Ageing at work. In *Active Ageing and Healthy Living. A Human Centered Approach in Research and Innovation as Source of Quality Life*; Riva, G., Marsan, P.A., Grassi, C., Eds.; IOS Press: Amsterdam, The Netherlands, 2014; Volume 13, pp. 134–144.
10. Kadefors, R. *Costs and Benefits of Best Agers Employment*; Department of Work Science University of Gothenburg: Gothenburg, Sweden, 2011.
11. Gommans, F.; Jansen, N.; Stynen, D.; De Grip, A.; Kant, I. The ageing shift worker: A prospective cohort study on need for recovery, disability, and retirement intentions. *Scand. J. Work. Environ. Health* **2015**, *41*, 356–367. [CrossRef]
12. Hult, C.; Stattin, M.; Janlert, U.; Järvholm, B. Timing of retirement and mortality—A cohort study of Swedish construction workers. *Soc. Sci. Med.* **2010**, *70*, 1480–1486. [CrossRef]
13. Pit, S.W.; Shrestha, R.; Schofield, D.; Passey, M. Health problems and retirement due to ill-health among Australian retirees aged 45–64 years. *Health Policy* **2010**, *94*, 175–181. [CrossRef] [PubMed]
14. de Wind, A.; Geuskens, G.A.; Ybema, J.F.; Blatter, B.M.; Burdorf, A.; Bongers, P.M.; van der Beek, A.J. Health, job characteristics, skills, and social and financial factors in relation to early retirement—Results from a longitudinal study in The Netherlands. *Scand. J. Work. Environ. Health* **2014**, *40*, 186–194. [CrossRef] [PubMed]
15. Henseke, G. Good jobs, good pay, better health? The effects of job quality on health among older European workers. *Eur. J. Health Econ.* **2018**, *19*, 59–73. [CrossRef] [PubMed]
16. Fischer, J.A.; Sousa-Poza, A. *The Institutional Determinants of Early Retirement in Europe*; Department of Economics, University of St. Gallen: Sent Gallen, Switzerland, 2006.

17. Proper, K.I.; Deeg, D.J.; Van Der Beek, A.J. Challenges at work and financial rewards to stimulate longer workforce participation. *Hum. Resour. Health* **2009**, *7*, 70–83. [CrossRef]
18. Cheung, F.; Wu, A.M.S. An investigation of predictors of successful aging in the workplace among Hong Kong Chinese older workers. *Int. Psychogeriat.* **2011**, *24*, 449–464. [CrossRef]
19. Vahidi, R.; Nekoui, M.; Sadeghi, V. Awareness of Aging Workers about Health Effects of Lifestyle. *Res. J. Biol. Sci.* **2008**, *3*, 35–38.
20. Lichtenthaler, P.W.; Fischbach, A. Job crafting and motivation to continue working beyond retirement age. *Career Dev. Int.* **2016**, *21*, 477–497. [CrossRef]
21. Kang, M.-Y.; Yoon, C.-G.; Yoon, J.-H. Influence of illness and unhealthy behavior on health-related early retirement in Korea: Results from a longitudinal study in Korea. *J. Occup. Health* **2015**, *57*, 28–38. [CrossRef]
22. Lind, C. Assessment and Design of Industrial Manual Handling to Reduce Physical Ergonomics Hazards: Use and Development of Assessment Tools. Ph.D. Thesis, KTH Royal Institute of Technology, Stockholm, Sweeden, 2017.
23. Schneider, E.; Copsey, S.; Irastorza, X. *OSH [Occupational Safety and Health] in Figures: Work-Related Musculoskeletal Disorders in the EU-Facts and Figures*; Office for Official Publications of the European Communities: Bruxelles, Belgium, 2010.
24. Nilsson, K. A sustainable working life for all ages–The swAge-model. *Appl. Ergon.* **2020**, *86*, 103082. [CrossRef]
25. Urbancová, H.; Vnoučková, L.; Linhart, Z.; Ježková Petrů, G.; Zuzák, R.; Holečková, L.; Prostějovská, Z. Impact of Age Management on Sustainability in Czech Organisations. *Sustainability* **2020**, *12*, 1064. [CrossRef]
26. Loch, C.H.; Sting, F.J.; Bauer, N.; Mauermann, H. How BMW is defusing the demographic time bomb. *Harv. Bus. Rev.* **2010**, *88*, 99–102.
27. Tuomi, K.; Huuhtanen, P.; Nykyri, E.; Ilmarinen, J. Promotion of work ability, the quality of work and retirement. *Occup. Med.* **2001**, *51*, 318–324. [CrossRef]
28. Wrzesniewski, A.; Dutton, J.E. Crafting a job: Revisioning employees as active crafters of their work. *Acad. Manag. Rev.* **2001**, *26*, 179–201. [CrossRef]
29. Van Wingerden, J.; Derks, D.; Bakker, A.B. The Impact of Personal Resources and Job Crafting Interventions on Work Engagement and Performance. *Hum. Resour. Manag.* **2017**, *56*, 51–67. [CrossRef]
30. Van den Heuvel, M.M.; Demerouti, E.; Peeters, M.C.W. The job crafting intervention: Effects on job resources, self-efficacy, and affective well-being. *J. Occup. Organ. Psychol.* **2015**, *88*, 511–532. [CrossRef]
31. Kooij, T.A.M.; van Woerkom, M.; Wilkenloh, J.; Dorenbosch, L.W.; Denissen, J.J.A. A job crafting intervention study. *Gerontologist* **2016**, *56*, 295. [CrossRef]
32. Popkin, S.M.; Morrow, S.L.; Di Domenico, T.E.; Howarth, H.D. Age is more than just a number: Implications for an aging workforce in the US transportation sector. *Appl. Ergon.* **2008**, *39*, 542–549. [CrossRef] [PubMed]
33. van Dam, K.; van Vuuren, T.; Kemps, S. Sustainable employment: The importance of intrinsically valuable work and an age-supportive climate. *Int. J. Hum. Resour. Manag.* **2016**, *28*, 2449–2472. [CrossRef]
34. Montano, D.; Hoven, H.; Siegrist, J. Effects of organisational-level interventions at work on employees' health: A systematic review. *BMC Public Health* **2014**, *14*, 135. [CrossRef] [PubMed]
35. Dellve, L.; Eriksson, A. Health-Promoting Managerial Work: A Theoretical Framework for a Leadership Program that Supports Knowledge and Capability to Craft Sustainable Work Practices in Daily Practice and During Organizational Change. *Societies* **2017**, *7*, 12. [CrossRef]
36. Eriksson, A.; Orvik, A.; Strandmark, M.; Nordsteien, A.; Torp, S. Management and Leadership Approaches to Health Promotion and Sustainable Workplaces: A Scoping Review. *Societies* **2017**, *7*, 14. [CrossRef]
37. Bone, K.D. The Bioecological Model: Applications in holistic workplace well-being management. *Int. J. Work. Health Manag.* **2015**, *8*, 256–271. [CrossRef]
38. Bronfenbrenner, U. Ecological systems theory. In *Encyclopedia of Psychology*; Kazdin, A., Ed.; Oxford University Press: New York, NY, USA, 2002; Volume 3, pp. 129–133.
39. Occupational Safety and Health Administration, Europa. 2020. Available online: https://visualisation.osha.europa.eu/ageing-and-osh#!/key-issue/early-exit-labour-market/AT/EU (accessed on 15 May 2020).
40. Principi, A.; Bauknecht, J.; Di Rosa, M.; Socci, M. Employees' Longer Working Lives in Europe: Drivers and Barriers in Companies. *Int. J. Environ. Res. Public Health* **2020**, *17*, 1658. [CrossRef]
41. Radl, J. Labour Market Exit and Social Stratification in Western Europe: The Effects of Social Class and Gender on the Timing of Retirement. *Eur. Sociol. Rev.* **2013**, *29*, 654–668. [CrossRef]
42. Blok, M.; De Looze, M. What is the evidence for less shift work tolerance in older workers? *Ergonomics* **2011**, *54*, 221–232. [CrossRef] [PubMed]
43. Liff, R.; Wikström, E. An interactional perspective on age management for prolonged working life. *Nord. Welf. Res.* **2020**, *5*, 137–139. [CrossRef]
44. Blomé, M.W.; Borell, J.; Håkansson, C.; Nilsson, K. Attitudes toward elderly workers and perceptions of integrated age management practices. *Int. J. Occup. Saf. Ergon.* **2018**, *26*, 112–120. [CrossRef]
45. BestAgers. The Labour Market and Demographic Change in the Baltic Sea Region Study Results and Recommendations of the Best Agers Project. 2012. Available online: http://eu.baltic.net/redaktion/General_Best%20Agers_October%202012.pdf (accessed on 11 October 2021).

46. Jahncke, H.; Hygge, S.; Mathiassen, S.E.; Hallman, D.; Mixter, S.; Lyskov, E. Variation at work: Alternations between physically and mentally demanding tasks in blue-collar occupations. *Ergonomics* **2017**, *60*, 1218–1227. [CrossRef]
47. Nilsson, K.; Hydbom, A.R.; Rylander, L. How are self-rated health and diagnosed disease related to early or deferred retirement? A cross-sectional study of employees aged 55–64. *BMC Public Health* **2016**, *16*, 886. [CrossRef]
48. Eaves, S.; Gyi, D.; Gibb, A. Building healthy construction workers: Their views on health, wellbeing and better workplace design. *Appl. Ergon.* **2016**, *54*, 10–18. [CrossRef]
49. Gaudart, C. Conditions for maintaining ageing operators at work—a case study conducted at an automobile manufacturing plant. *Appl. Ergon.* **2000**, *31*, 453–462. [CrossRef]
50. Tims, M.; Bakker, A.B. Job crafting: Towards a new model of individual job redesign. *SA J. Ind. Psychol.* **2010**, *36*, 9. [CrossRef]
51. Wong, C.M.; Tetrick, L.E. Job Crafting: Older Workers' Mechanism for Maintaining Person-Job Fit. *Front. Psychol.* **2017**, *8*. [CrossRef] [PubMed]
52. Occupational Safety and Health Administration, Europa. 2020. Available online: https://osha.europa.eu/sv/themes/osh-management-context-ageing-workforce (accessed on 15 May 2020).
53. Van Der Mark-Reeuwijk, K.G.; Weggemans, R.M.; Bültmann, U.; Burdorf, A.; Deeg, D.J.; Geuskens, G.A.; Henkens, K.C.; Kant, I.; De Lange, A.; Lindeboom, M.; et al. Health and prolonging working lives: An advisory report of the Health Council of The Netherlands. *Scand. J. Work. Environ. Health* **2019**, *45*, 514–519. [CrossRef] [PubMed]
54. Li, C.-Y.; Sung, F.-C. A review of the healthy worker effect in occupational epidemiology. *Occup. Med.* **1999**, *49*, 225–229. [CrossRef]

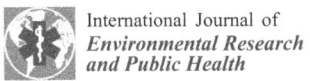

Article

School Principals' Work Participation in an Extended Working Life—Are They Able to, and Do They Want to? A Quantitative Study of the Work Situation

Kerstin Nilsson [1,2,*], Anna Oudin [1,3], Inger Arvidsson [1], Carita Håkansson [1], Kai Österberg [4], Ulf Leo [5] and Roger Persson [1,4]

1. Division of Occupational and Environmental Medicine, Lund University, SE-223 81 Lund, Sweden; anna.oudin@med.lu.se (A.O.); inger.arvidsson@med.lu.se (I.A.); carita.hakansson@med.lu.se (C.H.); roger.persson@psy.lu.se (R.P.)
2. Department of Public Health, Kristianstad University, SE-291 88 Kristianstad, Sweden
3. Department of Public Health and Clinical Medicine, Umeå University, SE-901 87 Umeå, Sweden
4. Department of Psychology, Lund University, SE-221 00 Lund, Sweden; kai.osterberg@psy.lu.se
5. Department of Centre for Principal Development, Umeå University, SE-901 87 Umeå, Sweden; ulf.leo@umu.se
* Correspondence: kerstin.nilsson@med.lu.se or kerstin.nilsson@hkr.se

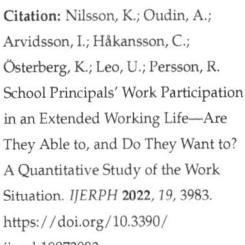

Citation: Nilsson, K.; Oudin, A.; Arvidsson, I.; Håkansson, C.; Österberg, K.; Leo, U.; Persson, R. School Principals' Work Participation in an Extended Working Life—Are They Able to, and Do They Want to? A Quantitative Study of the Work Situation. *IJERPH* **2022**, *19*, 3983. https://doi.org/10.3390/ijerph19073983

Academic Editor: Raphael M. Herr

Received: 6 January 2022
Accepted: 24 March 2022
Published: 27 March 2022

Publisher's Note: MDPI stays neutral with regard to jurisdictional claims in published maps and institutional affiliations.

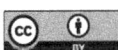

Copyright: © 2022 by the authors. Licensee MDPI, Basel, Switzerland. This article is an open access article distributed under the terms and conditions of the Creative Commons Attribution (CC BY) license (https://creativecommons.org/licenses/by/4.0/).

Abstract: The objective of this study is to increase the knowledge regarding school principals' work situations by examining the associations between various factors and the school principals' assessments of their ability or wish to work until 65 years of age or longer. The 1356 participating school principals in this study were aged between 50 and 64 years of age. Individual and work factors were evaluated in relation to two dichotomized outcomes: i.e., can work and want to work beyond 65 years of age, respectively. Generalized Estimating Equations (GEE) models were used to specify bivariate and multivariate cross-sectional logistic regression models that accounted for repeated measurements. The results showed that, both in 2018 and 2019, about 83% of the school principals stated that they could work and about 50% stated that they wanted to work until 65 years of age and beyond. School principals' exhaustion symptoms and experiences of an excessive burden were statistically significantly associated with whether they both could not and did not want to work beyond 65 years of age. Additionally, the school principals' experiences of support from the executive management in the performance of their managerial duties was of primary importance for whether the school principals wanted to work until 65 years of age and beyond. To conclude, it is important that school principals receive sufficient support from the management to cope with their often very stressful leadership tasks so that they have the opportunity to be able and willing to continue working their entire working life. The study strengthens the robustness of the theoretical SwAge model regarding the investigated factors related to determinant factors for a sustainable working life and as a basis for developing practical tools for increased employability for people of older ages.

Keywords: principals; organisation; mental; psychosocial; burnout; work environment; health; work ability; work engagement; swage-model; older workers; senior employees

1. Introduction

The increasing number of older citizens in society is widely seen as one of the most significant threats to global wealth, due to the tensions that impact the welfare systems through potentially profound economic consequences and social effects [1]. In 2080, it is estimated that for every person of working age (20–64 years), there will be 0.6 people who are 65 years of age or older in the countries that are part of the Organisation for Economic Cooperation and Development (OECD) [1]. This means that every pensioner (if the retirement is set to age 65 years of age) will need to be supported by fewer than two people active in the labour force. This can be compared, for example, with the fact that in the Swedish pension system in 1950, six people in the labour force supported every pensioner [1]. In order to achieve sufficient financial sustainability and to maintain pension systems, many countries are postponing the retirement age in order to make a larger amount of people work for an extended working life and thus contribute to the national economy. Accordingly, there are both societal and organisational interests in increasing the knowledge concerning people's beliefs and assessments regarding whether they can extend their working life, as well as if they want to extend their working life. Presumably, this knowledge will facilitate the possibilities of taking appropriate organisational measures that will increase the possibility of an extended working life [2–7].

In Sweden, school principals have a key role in society with responsibilities entailing, for example, the implementation of governmental directives and the responsibility for teachers' and pupils' local work environments as well as educational development (i.e., the responsibility for production, operation and organisation) [8,9]. However, and even if research on principals' work environments is limited, recent Swedish research has shown that role conflicts, resource deficits and harboring co-workers' frustrations are demands that many principals frequently face in their managerial position [10]. According to the Teaching and Learning International survey from 2018, principals in Sweden are particularly stressed by excessive administrative tasks, understaffing and working with students with special needs [11]. It has been estimated that approximately 25% of the principals in Sweden are at risk of developing poor mental health if their situation becomes long-lasting [12]. In addition, principal turnover is considered a problem in Sweden—it has been estimated that approximately one in four principals switched schools in the semesters 2011/12, 2012/13 and 2014/15 [13]. Indeed, a high turnover rate may disrupt school development, affect student learning and require the school to recruit new people to fill vacant leadership positions. Nevertheless, compared to many other countries, the cause for principal turnover is less studied in a Swedish context, and turnover rates may differ between age groups, school level and type of municipality (e.g., urban or rural) [14]. Like turnover, retirement also risks disrupting school development, creating a need to fill vacant leadership positions and impacting student learning and the working conditions of staff at the school. However, to date, no study seems to have examined the factors and circumstances associated with principals' withdrawal from their working life—in other words, their retirement.

In the case of high withdrawal from workplaces, measures need to be taken. It is therefore important to detect problems in the work situation and identify what needs to be improved to support healthy and sustainable employability. The SwAge model is a theoretical model that acknowledges areas of employability and states nine impact and determinant areas connected to sustainable healthy working life and whether individuals can and want to work or not [2–7]. Those nine determinant areas are sorted into four spheres based on research on individuals' consideration of leaving the workplace or being able to stay:

➢ The health effects of the work environment, which include the following areas of determination:
   (1) Self-rated health, diagnoses and diverse physical and mental health functionalities in work, in relation to
   (2) Physical work environment and work accidents;
   (3) Mental work environment with risk of stress and fatigue syndrome, threats of violence; and
   (4) Working hours, work pace and recuperation during and between work shifts.

Working life affects biological aging, and adequate health is a prerequisite for employability and to be included in working life [2–7].

➢ Financial incentives for organisations and workplace finances determine which equipment and techniques can be used to facilitate a more sustainable work environment, thus increasing long-term employability and the staffing ratio, as well as sick leave, unemployment and early retirement, not least in bad times.

(5) The effects of personal financial situations on issues regarding individuals' needs and willingness to work due to the possibility of working in relation to the individual employees' health situation, skills, etcetera, affecting their employability [2–7].

➢ Relationships and participation concern whether the individual receives sufficient social support from the environment when needed or is included or excluded in the group due to attitudes in the social context. The sphere includes the following areas of determination:

(6) The effects of the personal social environment, with a family, friends and leisure context; and

(7) The social work environment with leadership, discrimination and the significance of the employment relationship context for individuals' work.

The relationships and social supports relate to the individuals' social age and affect the individuals' opportunities and willingness to work [2–7].

➢ Execution of tasks and activities at work can be a source of motivation, stimulation and joy, but it can also be a source of boredom, dissatisfaction and stagnation. Employability also concerns the employees' ability to meet the requirements in terms of knowledge and skills to execute the activities and tasks and depends also on instrumental support [2–7]. The sphere includes the following areas of determination:

(8) Motivation, appreciation, satisfaction and stimulation in the execution of work tasks; and

(9) Knowledge, competence and the importance of competence development for the individual's work.

The SwAge model is based on and was developed through the grounded theory method and is based on quantitative and qualitative empirical studies, register data and literature reviews regarding factors of employability and the importance of a healthy and sustainable working life for all ages. The SwAge model also addresses areas of importance for both being able and wanting to work and choosing to leave or stay at a workplace. In addition, the SwAge model also describes how aging relates to various factors in the work environment and work situation. For this reason, the SwAge model is used as a reference framework in the discussion of the analysis results in this study.

Aim

The objective of this study was to increase the knowledge regarding school principals' work situations by examining the associations between various individual factors and factors in the work situation and the school principals' assessment of their ability or wish to work until 65 years of age or longer. Specifically, we asked the following research questions:

- To what extent do Swedish school principals report that they can and want to work beyond 65 years of age?
- How strongly are indicators for (a) exhaustion symptoms; (b) mental resources, work engagement and work ability as well as (c) supportive and demanding managerial circumstances related to principals' statements of whether they (a) can and (b) want to work until 65 years of age or beyond.

Presumably, this knowledge could inform various stakeholders (e.g., supervisors and politicians) and help to tailor initiatives that allow principals to extend their working life in a gainful way and thus prolong their possibilities of contributing to society.

2. Materials and Methods

2.1. Study Design

The present explorative longitudinal study entailed two assessments one year apart: in the autumn of 2018 and in the autumn of 2019. The data were collected through a web survey. The participants were recruited from a list of e-mail addresses including participants from the compulsory principal education and training programs during the period of 2008–2017, funded and arranged by the Swedish National Agency for Education. The e-mail list had a nationwide reach and entailed 9900 e-mail addresses. Of the 9900 invited, 4640 potential respondents either accepted (n = 2 633) or declined (n = 2007) to participate. In the end, 2317 respondents completed the entire questionnaire of the first survey in 2018 (i.e., a 50% response rate among those who actively responded yes or no to participation). One year after the first survey, in the autumn of 2019, all except one retiree were once again invited to participate in the second part of the study. Of the 2316 re-invited individuals, 202 could not be reached through their e-mail address anymore (i.e., terminated employment, etc.), 42 refrained from participation, and 544 did not respond to the second survey (66% response rate among those who participated in 2018). In addition, 468 principals participated in 2019, but not in 2018. In total, 1992 principals participated in 2019, and 2781 principals participated in either 2018, 2019 or both. For the analyses carried out in the present paper, only participants aged 50 to 64 years of age at the time of the questionnaire (2018 or 2019) were selected, ending up in a final study sample consisting of 1356 principals (1102 women, 250 men and 4 participants who did not disclose their gender). In this sample, 342 persons participated only in 2018, 307 persons participated only in 2019 and 707 persons participated in both surveys.

2.2. Outcome Measures

The outcome measures constituted two single-item measures that have been used in previous studies investigating factors associated to retirement, public health and a sustainable working life until an older age [15–21]. The first item read "My experience is that I CAN work in my profession until age … ". The second item read "I WANT to withdraw from my professional work when I am … years of age". Both items were responded to using an eight-step categorical scale indicating the expected age for one's own retirement in years: 55–60, 61–62, 63–64, 65, 66–67, 68–69, 70–72 and 73 years or older. The response options were dichotomized at 65 years of age (i.e., working until <65 versus ≥65 years of age). The reason for this is because 65 years is the most common retirement age in Sweden, as in many other countries [1], and to withdraw from working life before this age is perceived as an early retirement age.

2.3. Stress and Exhaustion Symptoms

The Lund University Checklist for Incipient Exhaustion (LUCIE) was used to measure early manifestations of stress and exhaustion [22,23]. The 28 items of the checklist cover 6 dimensions: sleep and recovery (3 items), separation between work and leisure time (4 items), sense of community and support in the workplace (2 items), managing work duties and personal capabilities (5 items), personal life and leisure time activities (3 items) and health complaints (11 items) [22,23]. The items are responded to on a four-point scale: 1 = not at all, 2= somewhat, 3 = quite a bit, and 4 = very much. The scoring builds two separate but supplementary scales: the Stress Warning Scale (SWS) and the Exhaustion Warning Scale (EWS). Specifically, SWS is sensitive to milder signs of incipient exhaustion, whereas the Exhaustion Warning Scale (EWS) reflects more severe signs of exhaustion. The SWS and EWS are in practice combined into a four-step ranking of incremental stress symptomatology, with the highest level possibly being indicative of ED: Step 1—GG (SWS green zone and EWS green zone), Step 2—YG (SWS yellow zone and EWS green zone), Step 3—RG (SWS red zone and EWS green zone), and Step 4—RR (SWS red zone and EWS red zone). Thus, increasing scores reflect a larger amount of stress symptoms. In the present study, low levels of indications and warnings of demanding stress and exhaustion were used as a reference (Step 1) versus moderate to high (Steps 2–4) indications and warnings of demanding stress and exhaustion symptoms.

Additionally, the Karolinska Exhaustion Disorder Scale (KEDS) was used to assess exhaustion symptoms [24]. KEDS comprises nine items regarding ability to concentrate, memory, physical stamina, mental stamina, recovery, sleep, hypersensitivity to sensory impressions, experience of demands and irritation and anger (24). Each item is responded to on a seven-point scale (0–6). Short descriptive verbal phrases serve as anchors for the scale steps 0, 2, 4 and 6, but not for 1, 3 and 5. Higher scores reflect a more severe exhaustion symptomatology. In the present study, the mean KEDS sum score (range 0 to 54) was used as an outcome. A score ≥ 19 indicates possible exhaustion disorder [24].

2.4. Personal Mental Resources

Mental resources were assessed with three items from the Work Ability Index (WAI) [25,26]. The three items were WAI 7a. Have not been able to enjoy daily activities lately; WAI 7b. Have not felt alert and spirited lately; WAI 7c. Have not felt hopeful for the future lately. The items were responded to on a five-point scale: 1 = often, 2 = fairly often, 3 = sometimes, 4 = seldom, 5 = never. For the purposes of analysis, each item was dichotomized into 0 = sometimes, seldom and never and 1 = often and fairly often and used individually in the statistical analyses.

2.5. Work Ability

Items from the Work Ability Index (WAI) [25] were used to measure the school principals' perceptions of their work ability. The used items were as follows: WAI 1a was used to measure the optimistic assessment of the current work ability in comparison to the lifetime best work ability and was responded to with an 11-step Likert type scale with verbal anchors at the endpoints (0 = completely unable to work and 10 = work ability at its best). In addition, WAI 2a was used to measure poor work ability in comparison with the physical needs in the work environment, and WAI 2b was used to measure poor work ability in comparison to the mental needs in the work environment. Both WAI2 items were responded to on a five point scale: 1 = very good, 2 = rather good, 3 = moderate, 4 = rather poor, 5 = very poor. For the purposes of analysis, each item was dichotomized into 0 = moderate, rather poor, very poor and 1 = rather good and very good and used individually in the statistical analyses. Finally, WAI 6 was used to measure whether health is too poor to cope with the current profession in two years from now, based on present health status, and was responded to with a three-step scale: 1 = yes, relatively certain, 2 = not certain and 3 = no, it is unlikely. For the purposes of analysis, the was dichotomized into 0 = yes, relatively certain and 1 = not certain and no it is unlikely.

2.6. Work Engagement

The Utrecht Work Engagement Scale comprises nine items (UWES-9) [26]. UWES-9 entail three aspects of engagement: vigor (experience of good energy and enthusiasm for the work), dedication (experience of happiness and inspiration for the work) and absorption (experience of flow in work and pride of work performance). Each aspect encompass three items and responses are made on a seven-point scale (0–6): 0 = never, 1 = almost never, a few times a year or less, 2 = rarely, once a month or less, 3 = sometimes, a few times a month, 4 = often, once a week, 5 = very often, a few times a week and 6 = always, every day. Following the manual, results are reported as the mean value of each aspect. Higher scores indicate increasingly frequent experiences of work engagement.

2.7. Demanding and Supportive Managerial Circumstances

A brief version of the Gothenburg Manager Stress Inventory (GMSI) [27] was used to assess demanding and supportive managerial circumstances. The brief version includes 32 items. Demanding managerial circumstances encompass 22 items covering eight organisational areas: resource deficits, organisational control deficits, role conflicts, role demands, group dynamics, buffer function, co-workers and container function. The items were responded to using a five-point scale: 1 = never, almost never, 2 = rarely, 3 = sometimes, 4 = often, 5 = always, almost always. Supportive managerial circumstances encompass 10 items and cover four organisational areas as well as one area concerning personal life: supportive management, co-operation with co-workers, supportive leader colleagues, supportive organisational structures and supportive personal life. The items were responded to on a five-point scale indicating the participant's level of agreement: 1 = applies very poorly, 2 = applies poorly, 3 = applies to some extent, 4 = applies well and 5 = applies very well. For both demanding and supportive factors, the mean score was used as an indicator. A higher mean score indicates experiencing demands more frequently or perceiving less support.

2.8. Statistical Analysis

To investigate the association between the items, Generalized Estimating Equations (GEE) models were used to specify a repeated measures model with two different dichotomous outcome variables (binary logistic regression) and multiple independent factors. GEE:s were chosen because parameter estimates are, under mild regularity conditions, consistent even when the covariance structure is mis-specified, which make them attractive to use in the present setting. The first dichotomous outcome comprised the item that assessed whether the school principals stated they were able to work until 65 years of age or not. The second dichotomous outcome comprised the item that assessed whether the school principals reported they wanted to work until 65 years of age or beyond or not.

Data from the initial 2018 survey were combined with data from the second survey in 2019, considering dependent observations since many study subjects had participated in both surveys. Data are presented as odds ratios (ORs) with their 95% confidence intervals (CIs), meaning that p-values < 0.05 were considered as statistically significant. Univariate analysis was estimated for all analyses to investigate the association between the independent and the dependent variables. There was an interest in analysing possible demanding and supporting managerial circumstances regarding whether principals' assessed that they can or want to work until 65 years of age and beyond. To cater to this, multivariate analyses were performed to investigate which items were mostly statistically significantly associated to whether the school principals stated they could or wanted to work in an extended working life. Additionally, the analyses were stratified by sex. First, the univariate analyses were executed, and independent factors with p-values < 0.1 in the main analyses (men and women) were selected for a multivariate analysis in the GMSI analysis [28] and entered at the same time. All statistical analyses were performed using SPSS version 25.0 software.

3. Results

3.1. Occurrence of Statements concerning the Ability and Wish to Work beyond 65 Years of Age

A larger proportion of school principals stated they could work until 65 years of age or beyond when compared with those who stated that they wanted to work until 65 years of age or beyond (Table 1). There were no major differences between the years 2018 and 2019.

Table 1. School principals' statements regarding whether they "Can work" or "Want to work" until 65 years of age and beyond in 2018 and in 2019. (no = can/want only to work until 55 to 64 years of age; yes = I can/want to work 65 years or beyond).

	School Principals' Statements			
	Can Work until 65 Years or beyond		Want to Work until 65 Years or beyond	
	No	Yes	No	Yes
2018	16.8%	83.2%	49.5%	50.5%
2019	17.3%	82.7%	48.8%	51.2%

The next step of the analysis was to investigate factors associated with why school principals assessed that they were able to and wanted to work until 65 years of age and beyond.

3.2. Associations between Principals' Assessments regarding Whether They Believe They Would Not Be Able to or Would Not Want to Work until 65 Years of Age or beyond, and Their Experience of Mental Health and Exhaustion Symptoms

The findings showed a statistically significant association between school principals' elevated risk of exhaustion disorder and whether they stated that they were not able to and did not want to keep working beyond 65 years of age (Table 2). Furthermore, there was a statistically significant association between whether the principals reported that they were able to and wanted to work until 65 years of age and beyond and whether their health was too poor to cope with their current profession, as well as whether they experienced a lack of work ability. When separate analyses were carried out among men and women, the variables regarding indications and warnings of demanding stress and exhaustion proved to be statistically significant and negatively associated with whether female principals were able to work for an extended working life (i.e., exhaustion symptoms, not having been able to enjoy daily activities lately, not having felt alert and spirited lately, not having felt hopeful for the future lately, perceiving poor work ability in comparison to the physical and mental needs in the work environment). However, for male principals, the only statistically significant association was with the variable "poor work ability in comparison to the needs in the work environment". However, except for men regarding the variable "poor work ability in comparison to the physical needs in the work environment", both sexes showed statistically significant associations with all the variables that indicated demanding stress and exhaustion symptoms and whether they did not want to work until 65 years of age.

Table 2. Univariate estimates from multiple binary logistic regression with repeated measurements on school principals' assessment of whether they "cannot work" or "do not want to work" until 65 years of age and beyond in association with the school principals' experience of health problems in their situation for the total study population and stratified by sex. The results are presented as odds ratios (OR) with accompanying 95% confidence intervals (CI) and *p*-values.

Outcome Variables Independent Variables	Group	Cannot Work until 65 Years of Age or beyond			Do Not Want to Work until 65 Years of Age or beyond		
		OR	95% CI	*p*-Value	OR	95% CI	*p*-Value
Indications and warnings of demanding stress and exhaustion symptoms (LUCIE)	Total	1.99	1.53–2.59	<0.0001	1.68	1.36–2.07	<0.0001
	Women	1.99	1.50–2.62	<0.0001	1.62	1.28–2.05	<0.0001
	Men	1.88	0.85–4.16	0.12	1.81	1.24–2.65	0.002
Exhaustion disorder indications (KEDS)	Total	1.92	1.51–2.45	<0.0001	1.57	1.29–1.91	<0.0001
	Women	1.88	1.45–2.43	<0.0001	1.47	1.18–1.83	0.0007
	Men	2.02	0.97–4.20	0.06	1.96	1.34–2.86	0.0005
My health is too poor to cope with the current profession, based on my current health status (WAI_6)	Total	6.01	3.70–9.76	<0.0001	2.80	1.72–4.56	<0.0001
	Women	7.66	4.44–13.20	<0.0001	2.79	1.59–4.88	0.0003
	Men	2.20	0.66–7.47	0.20	2.93	1.10–7.79	0.03
Have not been able to enjoy daily activities lately (WAI_7a)	Total	1.96	1.25–3.07	0.003	1.47	1.24–0.45	0.08
	Women	2.03	1.25–3.28	0.004	1.47	0.90–2.38	0.12
	Men	1.68	0.46–6.13	0.44	1.58	0.67–3.73	0.29
Have not felt alert and spirited lately (WAI_7b)	Total	2.75	1.97–3.84	<0.0001	2.13	1.59–2.85	<0.0001
	Women	2.80	1.94–4.02	<0.0001	1.93	1.40–2.65	<0.0001
	Men	2.72	1.13–6.51	0.03	3.55	1.75–7.22	0.0005
Have not felt hopeful for the future lately (WAI_7c)	Total	2.36	1.61–3.47	<0.0001	1.50	1.08–2.08	0.01
	Women	2.38	1.58–3.60	<0.0001	1.31	0.91–1.88	0.15
	Men	2.58	1.01–6.59	0.05	2.93	1.41–6.10	0.004

Table 2. Cont.

Outcome Variables Independent Variables	Group	Cannot Work until 65 Years of Age or beyond			Do Not Want to Work until 65 Years of Age or beyond		
		OR	95% CI	p-Value	OR	95% CI	p-Value
Poor work ability in comparison to the physical needs in the work environment (WAI_2a)	Total	4.21	2.03–8.74	0.0001	2.60	1.27–5.13	0.01
	Women	4.13	1.90–8.97	0.0003	2.60	0.76–0.87	0.02
	Men	4.37	0.41–37.76	0.23	2.36	0.37–14.90	0.36
Poor work ability in comparison to the mental needs in the work environment (WAI_2b)	Total	3.46	2.38–5.04	<0.0001	2.01	1.46–2.79	<0.0001
	Women	3.36	2.22–5.10	<0.0001	1.97	1.36–2.86	0.0003
	Men	4.35	1.86–10.15	0.0007	2.21	1.18–4.12	0.01

3.3. Associations between School Principals' Assessment regarding Whether They Cannot or Do Not Want to Work until 65 Years of Age or beyond and Their Mental Resources, Work Engagement and Work Ability

The logistic regression results regarding whether school principals experience a good energy and enthusiasm for work, their experience of happiness and inspiration in work and their experience of flow in work and pride of their work performance showed a statistically significant association with whether school principals could and wanted to work until 65 years of age or beyond for both men and women (Table 3). Stratification by sex concerning the same question proved statistically significant associations for almost all variables. However, an optimistic assessment of the current work ability in comparison to the lifetime best work ability was statistically significant only for whether female school principals experienced that they could work for an extended working life.

Table 3. Univariate estimates from multiple binary logistic regression with repeated measurements on school principals' assessment of whether they "cannot work" or "do not want to work" until 65 years of age and beyond in association with the school principals' experience of enthusiasm (continuous variables), for the total study population and stratified by sex. The results are presented as odds ratios (OsR) per one unit increase in the independent variables with accompanying 95% confidence intervals (CsI) and p-values.

Outcome Variables Independent Variables	Group	Cannot Work until 65 Years of Age or beyond			Do Not Want to Work until 65 Years of Age or beyond		
		OR	95% CI	p-Value	OR	95% CI	p-Value
Optimistic assessment of the current work ability in comparison to the lifetime best work ability (WAI_1)	Total	0.80	0.75–0.85	<0.0001	0.82	0.78–0.87	<0.0001
	Women	0.77	0.72–0.83	<0.0001	0.81	0.76–0.87	<0.0001
	Men	0.91	0.78–1.06	0.21	0.86	0.78–0.95	0.003
Experience of good energy and enthusiasm for work (UWES_Vigor)	Total	0.61	0.54–0.69	<0.0001	0.69	0.62–0.76	<0.0001
	Women	0.59	0.52–0.68	<0.0001	0.68	0.61–0.77	<0.0001
	Men	0.65	0.46–0.93	<0.0001	0.70	0.57–0.86	0.0006
Experience of happiness and inspiration in work (UWES_Dedication)	Total	0.61	0.52–0.72	<0.0001	0.64	0.56–0.70	<0.0001
	Women	0.59	0.50–0.71	<0.0001	0.63	0.54–0.74	<0.0001
	Men	0.67	0.43–1.03	0.07	0.62	0.47–0.84	0.0016
Experience of flow in work and pride of work performance (UWES_Absorbtion)	Total	0.72	0.63–0.84	<0.0001	0.71	0.62–0.80	<0.0001
	Women	0.59	0.58–0.81	<0.0001	0.71	0.62–0.83	<0.0001
	Men	0.73	0.53–1.00	0.05	0.61	0.63–0.78	0.0001

3.4. Associations between School Principals' Assessments regarding Whether They Believe They Could Not or Did Not Want to Work until 65 Years of Age or beyond and Their Experience of Demanding and Supporting Managerial Circumstances

In order to measure demands and support in working life and the association with whether the school principals thought that they were able to or wanted to remain working for an extended working life until or beyond 65 years of age, we used the GMSI questionnaire. The univariate estimates in the binary logistic regression analyses with repeated measurements showed statistically significant associations between whether the school principals in the total group stated that they were able to work until 65 years of age or beyond and the following areas of analysis: demanding role requirements, container function, supportive management, supportive organisational resources, buffer issues, resource imbalance, organisational deficiencies, logic conflicts, supportive colleagues and a supportive personal life (Table 4).

However, the multivariate modelling only proved a statistically significant association ($p < 0.05$) for 1 of 13 variables. In particular, role demands—that is, burdensome role requirements (i.e., the experience of the burden in terms of the responsibility to be a manager)—proved statistically significant and associated (OR 1.43) with whether the school principals experienced that they could work for an extended working lif, and was more likely for female school principals (OR 1.44). However, this relationship proved not to be statistically significant for male school principals when stratified for sex. Furthermore, the multivariate model proved that supportive colleagues—i.e., support from managers' colleagues in performing the managerial duties (OR 1.04)—was found to be nearly statistically significantly ($p < 0.06$) associated with whether school principals were able to work for an extended working life.

In the analysis of whether various areas in the school principals' work situations were associated with wanting to work for an extended working life, the univariate estimates of the areas of demanding role requirements, group dynamic issues, container function, supportive management, supportive colleagues, supportive organisational resources, buffer issues, resource imbalance, organisational deficiencies and logic conflicts all showed statistically significant associations (Table 4). The multivariate modelling finally stated that 2 of 13 investigated variables were found to be statistically significant and associated with whether the school principals wanted to work for an extended working life. In particular, role demands—that is, burdensome role requirements—proved to be statistically significant and associated with whether the school principal wanted to work until 65 years of age or beyond (in the total group: OR 1.44; women: OR 1.35, men: OR 1.52).

Table 4. Univariate and multivariate estimates from multiple binary logistic regression with repeated measurements on school principals' assessments of whether they "cannot work" or "do not want to work" until 65 years of age and beyond in association with demanding and supporting managerial circumstances (GMSI variables), for the total study population and stratified by sex. The results are presented as odds ratios (ORs) with accompanying 95% confidence intervals (CIs) and p-values.

Scale Name	Explanation	Group	Cannot Work until 65 Years of Age or beyond						Do Not Want to Work until 65 Years of Age and beyond					
			Univariate Estimates			Multivariate Model			Univariate Estimates			Multivariate Model		
			OR	95% CI	p-Value	OR	95% CI	p-Value	OR	95% CI	p-Value	OR	95% CI	p-Value
Demanding circumstances														
Resource deficits	Resource imbalance, i.e., financial imbalance	Total	1.18	1.06–1.32	0.004	1.03	0.91–1.18	0.6292	1.11	1.02–1.21	0.018	1.03	0.90–1.18	0.6495
		Women	1.19	1.05–1.34	0.0077				1.07	0.97–1.17	0.1936			
		Men	1.15	0.89–1.48	0.2765				1.31	1.08–1.59	0.0052			
Organisational control	Organisational deficiencies, i.e., lack of transparency and communication from management	Total	1.21	1.07–1.37	0.0027	1.02	0.86–1.20	0.9916	1.13	1.03–1.25	0.0145	1.02	0.86–1.20	0.8597
		Women	1.21	1.06–1.39	0.0044				1.11	1.00–1.24	0.0605			
		Men	1.18	0.86–1.62	0.2967				1.20	0.94–1.52	0.1407			
Role conflicts	Logic conflicts, i.e., imbalance between administration and practical management work	Total	1.32	1.15–1.52	<0.0001	1.00	0.83–1.21	0.9916	1.22	1.11–1.36	0.0001	1.01	0.84–1.22	0.9055
		Women	1.30	1.11–1.52	0.0010				1.22	1.09–1.37	0.0007			
		Men	1.37	1.00–1.86	0.0473				1.18	0.95–1.45	0.1292			
Role demands	Burdensome role requirements, i.e., the experience of the burden in terms of the responsibility to be the manager	Total	1.63	1.40–1.89	<0.0001	1.43	1.17–1.75	0.0005	1.48	1.31–1.67	<0.0001	1.44	1.18–1.77	0.0004
		Women	1.60	1.36–1.89	<0.0001	1.44	1.16–1.79	0.0009	1.45	1.26–1.66	<0.0001	1.35	1.13–1.62	0.0008
		Men	1.76	1.17–2.58	0.0064	1.44	0.76–2.75	0.2667	1.57	1.24–2.01	0.0002	1.52	1.09–2.14	0.0146
Group dynamics	Group dynamic issues, i.e., employees' acceptance of the principal as manager	Total	1.10	0.94–1.28	0.2196				1.08	0.96–1.22	0.2199			
		Women	1.08	0.92–1.27	0.3645				1.06	0.93–1.21	0.4046			
		Men	1.30	0.88–1.91	0.7908				1.14	0.87–1.49	0.3513			
Buffer function	Buffer issues, i.e., being caught between management and employees	Total	1.21	1.06–1.37	0.0039	0.96	0.80–1.14	0.6106	1.18	1.08–1.29	0.0004	0.96	0.80–1.14	0.6432
		Women	1.16	1.01–1.32	0.0302				1.16	1.05–1.28	0.0048			
		Men	1.67	1.11–2.50	0.0136				1.27	1.03–1.56	0.0256			
Co-workers	Employee issues, i.e., supporting employees in their work tasks	Total	1.10	0.94–1.29	0.2464				1.16	1.04–1.30	0.0095	0.89	0.74–1.08	0.2315
		Women	1.01	0.85–1.20	0.9240				1.15	1.01–1.30	0.0339			
		Men	1.65	1.02–2.65	0.0369				1.11	0.89–1.40	0.3604			

Table 4. Cont.

Scale Name	Explanation	Group	Cannot Work until 65 Years of Age or beyond						Do Not Want to Work until 65 Years of Age and beyond					
			Univariate Estimates			Multivariate Model			Univariate Estimates			Multivariate Model		
			OR	95% CI	p-Value	OR	95% CI	p-Value	OR	95% CI	p-Value	OR	95% CI	p-Value
Container function	Container function i.e., partly therapeutic role in employees' (work) stress	Total	1.38	1.18–1.60	<0.0001	1.16	0.96–1.39	0.1272	1.28	1.15–1.43	<0.0001	1.20	0.99–1.47	0.0680
		Women	1.32	1.12–1.56	0.0009				1.28	1.13–1.45	<0.0001			
		Men	1.62	1.09–2.42	0.0180				1.19	0.96–1.48	0.1122			
Supportive circumstances														
Supportive management	Lack of supportive management, i.e., support from executive management to perform the managerial duties	Total	1.16	0.95–1.30	0.0052	1.04	0.91–1.19	0.5485	1.20	1.12–1.32	<0.0001	1.04	0.91–1.19	0.5636
		Women	1.16	1.04–1.32	0.0090				1.19	1.30–1.87	<0.0001			
		Men	1.20	0.89–1.61	0.2639				1.32	1.10–1.56	0.0029			
Cooperating co-workers	Lack of collaboration with co-workers, i.e., support from the employees to perform managerial duties	Total	1.09	0.92–1.30	0.3308				1.02	0.89–1.15	0.8034			
		Women	1.05	0.88–1.27	0.5661				1.00	0.87–1.15	0.9923			
		Men	1.35	0.80–2.27	0.2609				1.02	0.78–1.34	0.8977			
Supportive (manager) colleagues	Lack of supportive colleagues, i.e., support from managers' colleague to perform managerial duties	Total	1.16	1.04–1.30	0.0067	1.09	0.96–1.23	0.1824	1.11	1.02–1.21	0.0130	1.09	0.96–1.24	0.102
		Women	1.16	1.04–1.32	0.0089				1.08	0.99–1.18	0.0994			
		Men	1.20	0.84–1.72	0.3123				1.27	1.05–1.54	0.0136			
Supportive personal life	Lack of supportive personal life, i.e., support from family and personal network to perform managerial duties	Total	1.14	0.56–0.94	0.0437	1.02	0.90–1.16	0.7599	1.09	0.99–1.19	0.0960	1.02	0.89–1.16	0.7819
		Women	1.10	0.96–1.25	0.1741				1.06	0.99–1.18	0.0994			
		Men	1.41	0.97–2.04	0.0717				1.14	0.91–1.43	0.2542			
Supportive organisational structures	Lack of supportive organisational resources, i.e., support and legacy in the organisation to perform managerial duties	Total	1.22	1.09–1.37	0.0007	1.06	0.93–1.22	0.3547	1.11	1.00–1.22	0.0560	1.08	0.93–1.23	0.3006
		Women	1.19	1.05–1.35	0.0048				1.06	0.95–1.19	0.2860			
		Men	1.47	1.01–2.08	0.0423				1.22	0.95–1.56	0.1184			

4. Discussion

Due to the demographic challenge, a larger number of people need to extend their working life [1]. Furthermore, it takes time to build leadership experiences, and there are too few individuals with the competence of being a school principal in society; therefore, we need to retain competence and experience within organisations [8,9]. However, there is a difference between being able to execute work tasks and wanting to do so— i.e., whether individuals can and/or want to work for an extended working life—as shown by earlier research and stated in the theoretical SwAge model regarding a sustainable working life for all ages [2–7,14–18,29]. In this study, the results showed that 83.5% of the school principals stated that they were able to work until 65 years of age and beyond, though only 51.0% wanted to keep working until 65 years of age and beyond. This could be compared to another study, conducted in 2018, which stated that 72.6% of Swedish teachers (n = 682) thought they were able to work until 65 years of age and beyond, though only 43.0% of the participants wanted to keep working until 65 years of age and beyond [19]. Additionally, according to another study with Swedish managers in different sectors (except school principals), 86.3% of the included managers (n = 153) stated that they were able to work until 65 years of age and beyond, though only 39.9% of the participants wanted to keep working until 65 years of age and beyond [18]. Despite the difference between whether the school principals stated that they were able to and whether they wanted to work in an extended working life, their willingness to remain working proved to be higher than other professions in the same occupational area [18].

4.1. School Principals' Risk of Exhaustion Disorders and Poor Health That Affect Their Possibility of Being Able to and Wanting to Work for an Extended Working Life

The results of this study suggest that school principals with signs of stress and exhaustion and risk of developing mental health problems related to their work situation showed an increased risk of assessing that they were not able to or wanted to keep working for an extended working life, especially for female school principals. In previous research, the school principal profession has been described as a risk group regarding the stated connections between work environment and stress-related mental disorders; e.g., depression, anxiety and fatigue [10,11]. Today, the school principal profession is female-dominated, with about 70% female school principals in Sweden. The school principal is controlled and based on political decisions, although the work is executed closest to the citizen, and the role is often caught between these two aspects in their duties [30,31]. Additionally, many school principals in Sweden have reached a mature age, and many will withdraw from working life for retirement within some years [32]. It is apparent that many school principals today, in their roles as leaders, must deal with the consequences of several school reforms that have resulted in major changes in the governance of schools. Moreover, school principals often work based on very varied conditions in terms of organisational and operational responsibilities [9,33]. Work tasks require school principals to manage structural problems (e.g., insufficient resources and organisational governance deficiencies), value conflicts (e.g., different values and norm systems that may collide) and staff problems (e.g., sick leave and staffing) [34]. The work situation of school principals also risks having secondary effects on others, such as impacts on the employees' work environment and on students' work environment as well as educational results [35]. Therefore, it is important to make the school principals' work situation more sustainable through health-promoting organisational strategies and policies, due to the influence and possible effects on many other aspects and people in society. For example, previous research and the SwAge model state that health, personal financial situation and social environments have a profound impact on the individuals' attitudes towards their ability and willingness to participate in an extended working life or not [2–7]. Additionally, the individual's physical work environment, mental work environment, work schedule, work pace and possibility of recuperation, as well as knowledge, skills and competence development in relation to work demands might be key determinants for whether an individual decides that they can remain working for an extended working life or not. Furthermore, the workplace social environment and the experience of motivation, stimulation and meaningfulness in the work tasks seem to be major determinant areas that affect an individual's willingness to keep working in an extended working life or not [2–7].

4.2. The School Principals' Strategies to Cope with Their Work Situation in Association with Whether They Can and Want to Work for an Extended Working Life

Most of the principals participating in this study reported a fair work engagement and work ability, which proved to be statistically significant and associated with whether they assessed that they were able to and wanted to work for an extended working life. However, in an earlier study based on the current dataset, which also entailed principals below 50 years of age, we observed that approximately 25% of the participating principals seemed to be in a state of mental distress according to their ratings in two inventories that are used in clinical practice: LUCIE and KEDS. [12]. If measures are not taken to counteract further declines in health, this could risk decreasing their capacity to work, their employability and ability to function as school principals, consequently forcing them into early retirement. In previous studies, work ability has been suggested to be a good predictor for future absence due to sickness and early retirement [36,37]. An optimistic assessment of the current work ability in comparison to the lifetime best work ability proved a statistically significant association with wanting to work in an extended working life in this study. However, that association only proved to be statistically significant for women and not for men. The possibility to remain employable and work is a complex issue. The theoretical SwAge model (sustainable working life for all ages) states that employability and whether people can and want to work depend on four spheres: A. the health impacts of the work environment, including the determinant areas of (1) self-rated health, diagnoses and functional diversity; (2) physical work environment and prevention of injuries; (3) mental work environment, stress, effort/reward balance, violence and threats and (4) working hours, work pace and time for recuperation; B. financial incentives, including the determinant area of (5) personal finance; C. social support and participation, including the determinant areas of (6) personal social environment and (7) social work environment; D. self-fulfilment through work tasks, including the determinant areas of (8) motivation, stimulation and self-crediting tasks, the core of work and work satisfaction and (9) competence, skills, knowledge and opportunities for development [2–7,29,38,39]. Regardless of profession, all nine determinant areas based on the theories in the SwAge model are important to examine in order to promote an individual's assessments of whether they can and want to keep working in an extended working life. Additionally, management tools and measurement activities may be needed to increase the school principals' abilities and wishes to extend their working life.

4.3. The School Principals' Vulnerability in Their Tasks and Roles as Principals in Association with Whether They Can and Want to Work for an Extended Working Life

The multivariate modelling in this study regarding whether school principals' experiences that they could work for an extended working life proved statistically significant associations with their experience of burdens in terms of the responsibilities in the role of a manager, as well as the support from the managers' colleagues in their performance of their managerial duties. The role of a school principal includes the need for skills, knowledge and competence development to cope with and execute the work tasks as a manager and in the role of a leader. Otherwise, if school principals do not have adequate or full knowledge of how to cope with their role as a manager, the role of a school principal, with a great deal of responsibility, will be mentally demanding and may make the school principals' personal stress harder to cope with and control. Furthermore, previous research into other professions and the SwAge model state that both adequate knowledge to manage work tasks and the mental work environment, with a balance of demand and control, are important for individuals' assessments of whether they can work for an extended working life or not [2–7,29,38].

The other multivariate modelling in this study—whether school principals wanted to work until 65 years of age or beyond—also proved a statistically significant association with their experience of burdens in terms of the responsibilities of the role of being a manager but was also related to the support from executive management in performing their managerial duties. These results are in accordance with previous studies on other professions, which state the need for support and confirmation from their managers and from the management in order to see their own work effort as an important part and their own role as a part of the organisation's purpose; otherwise, the work can be perceived as meaningless [2–7,29,38]. Social and instrumental support, coherence and inclusion in a group are important determinant factors that affect whether individuals want to stay in the workplace and keep working until an older age, as shown in the SwAge model [2–7,14–18,29,38].

4.4. Limitations

A limitation of this study was that the survey mostly focused on the mental and organisational issues of school principals' work situations and did not investigate all nine determinant areas for a sustainable working life stated in the SwAge model [2–7,14–18,29,38]. However, the difficulties and complexities in the school principals' work situations are probably, to a large extent, contingent on mental and organisational workloads and to a lesser extent on the physical workload. Another limitation could be that the study used questions from previous studies and did not investigate the school principals' retirement considerations in depth. However, the questions used in the survey were validated and reliability controlled in previous studies, providing robustness to the present study. Additionally, the opportunities of this dataset, being based on a follow-up study and using the same participating respondents in two consecutive years, increase the robustness of the results. This investigation included Swedish school principals throughout the country, from north to south, including principals working at schools in small villages and large cities and school principals from pre-school to high school and adult school. Although framed in a Swedish context, we presume that school principals in other countries and cultures might share similar challenges in their work situations and perceived health due to the occupational similarity of schools; however, the organisations of school systems could be quite different.

5. Conclusions

The results show that circa 17% of Swedish school principals do not perceive that they can work until 65 years of age or beyond, and circa 49% do not want to work until 65 years or beyond. In addition, most indicators that covered exhaustion symptoms, poor health, poor mental resources and low work ability in relation to the physical and mental demands of work were positively associated with reports of not being able to work or not wanting to work until 65 years of age or beyond. In contrast, reporting a high workability in relation to respondents' lifetime best performance and expressing a higher work engagement decreased the probability of reporting being unable or not wanting to work until or beyond 65 years of age. Furthermore, among the organisational variables assessing demanding and supportive circumstances, the multivariate analysis showed that role demands seem to be the best indicator for reporting not being able to work as well as not wanting to work until 65 years of age or beyond. Collectively, the present results seem to suggest that interventions that aim to improve school principals' individual health and well-being and strive to reduce their role demands are likely to be beneficial for the principals and thus for the school organisation they manage. However, the results also suggest that it might be worthwhile in future research to address the question of school principals' withdrawal from the labour market from a more comprehensive theoretical framework such as the SwAge model; i.e., that employability and whether people can and want to work depend on four spheres: the health impacts of the work environment, financial resources, social support and experiences of social participation and self-fulfilment through work tasks. In order to increase the likelihood and capacity to function as a school principal, a work environment with a positive impact on health— that is, with a sense of community in the organisation, trust and social support, acceptance from the employees' executive management and a generally manageable stress exposure—appears to be an important determinant. This could probably reduce the risk of developing health problems. Furthermore, such interventions may likely increase school principals' willingness and ability to work for an extended working life. A work situation experienced as healthy, supportive and trustful, as well as stimulating and meaningful for individuals' professional roles and duties, is likely a good way to inspire school principals to keep working for an extended working life.

Author Contributions: Conceptualisation, K.N., A.O., I.A., C.H., K.Ö., U.L. and R.P.; methodology, K.N., and A.O.; formal analysis, A.O. and K.N., original draft preparation, K.N.; writing, review and editing, K.N., A.O., I.A., C.H., K.Ö., U.L. and R.P.; funding acquisition, R.P. All authors have read and agreed to the published version of the manuscript.

Funding: This research was funded by AFA Insurances Sweden, grant number 170094.

Institutional Review Board Statement: The study was conducted according to the guidelines of the Declaration of Helsinki and approved by The Regional Ethical Review Board in Lund, Sweden (reg. no. 2018/247). Written informed consent statements were obtained from all subjects involved in the study.

Informed Consent Statement: Informed consent was obtained from all subjects involved in the study.

Data Availability Statement: In accordance with the ethical approval by the Regional Ethical Review Board, crude data are not to be published on the internet. Consistent with the study protocol, anonymised data are stored locally at the Division of Occupational and Environmental Medicine, Lund University, Lund, Sweden. Access to data will be granted to eligible researchers wanting to audit our research. Requests should be directed to the corresponding author.

Acknowledgments: The authors wish to thank all participants who responded.

Conflicts of Interest: The authors declare no conflict of interests. The funders had no role in the design of the study; in the collection, analyses, or interpretation of data; in the writing of the manuscript, or in the decision to publish the results.

References

1. OECD. *Pensions at a Glance 2019: OECD and G20 Indicators*; OECD Publishing: Paris, France, 2019. [CrossRef]
2. Nilsson, K. A sustainable working life for all ages–The SwAge-model. *Appl. Ergon.* **2020**, *86*, 103082. [CrossRef] [PubMed]
3. Nilsson, K. Conceptualization of ageing in relation to factors of importance for extending working life—A review. *Scand. J. Public Health* **2016**, *44*, 490–505. [CrossRef] [PubMed]
4. Nilsson, K.; Rignell-Hydbom, A.; Rylander, L. Factors influencing the decision to extend working life or to retire. *Scand. J. Work Environ. Health* **2011**, *37*, 473–480. [CrossRef] [PubMed]
5. Nilsson, K. When is work a cause of early retirement and are there any effective organisational measures to combat this? A population-based study of perceived work environment and work-related disorders among employees in Sweden. *BMC Public Health* **2020**, *20*, 716. [CrossRef] [PubMed]
6. Nilsson, K. The Influence of Work Environmental and Motivation Factors on Seniors' Attitudes to an Extended Working Life or to Retire. A Cross Sectional Study with Employees 55–74 Years of Age. *Open J. Soc. Sci.* **2017**, *5*, 30–41. Available online: http://file.scirp.org/pdf/JSS_2017071013594273.pdf. (accessed on 11 July 2017). [CrossRef]
7. Nilsson, K.; Nilsson, E. Organisational Measures and Strategies for a Healthy and Sustainable Extended Working Life and Employability—A Deductive Content Analysis with Data Including Employees, First Line Managers, Trade Union Representatives and HR-Practitioners. *Int. J. Environ. Res. Public Health* **2021**, *18*, 5626. [CrossRef] [PubMed]
8. Hoppey, D.; McLeskey, J. A case study of principal leadership in an effective inclusive school. *J. Spec. Educ.* **2013**, *46*, 245–256. [CrossRef]
9. The Swedish Schools Inspectorate. *Rektors Ledarskap Med Ansvar För Den Pedagogiska Verksamheten. [School Principal's Leadership with Responsibility for The Educational Activities]*; The Swedish Schools Inspectorate: Stockholm, Sweden, 2012.
10. Persson, R.; Leo, U.; Arvidsson, I.; Håkansson, C.; Nilsson, K.; Österberg, K. Prevalence of exhaustion symptoms and associations with school level, length of work experience and gender: A nationwide cross-sectional study of Swedish principals. *BMC Public Health* **2021**, *21*, 331. [CrossRef] [PubMed]

11. Skolverket [Swedish National Agency for Education]. En studie om lärares och rektorers arbete i grund- och gymnasieskolan. Delrapport 2. [A study on the work of teachers and school leaders in compulsory and upper secondary school. Part 2]. In OECD. *Organisation for Economic Co-Operation and Development (OECD) and International Association for the Evaluation of Educational Achievement (IEA) Teaching and Learning International Survey (TALIS Part 2) Principal Questionnaire 2018*; Skolverket [Swedish National Agency for Education]: Stockholm, Sweden, 2020.
12. Skolverket [Swedish National Agency for Education]. *Beskrivande Data 2015. Förskola, Skola Och Vuxenutbildning. [Descriptive Data 2015. Preschool, School and Adult Education.]*; Skolverket [Swedish National Agency for Education]: Stockholm, Sweden, 2016.
13. Thelin, K. Principal turnover: When is it a problem and for whom? Mapping out variations within the swedish case. *Res. Educ. Adm. Leadsh.* **2020**, *5*, 417–452. [CrossRef]
14. Nilsson, K. Pension Eller Arbetsliv? [Pension or Working Life?]. Ph.D. Thesis, National Institute in Working Life, Malmö, Sweden, 2005; pp. 1–280.
15. Nilsson, K. Vem kan och vill arbeta till 65 år eller längre? En studie av anställda inom hälso- och sjukvården. [Who can and want to work until 65 years or beyond? A study with employed in health and medical care]. In *Arbete Och Hälsa*; Arbetslivsinstitutet: Stockholm, Sweden, 2005; Volume 14, pp. 1–35. Available online: https://gupea.ub.gu.se/bitstream/2077/4345/1/ah2005_14.pdf. (accessed on 28 April 2021).
16. Nilsson, K. *Hållbart Arbetsliv Inom Hälso- Och Sjukvården–Studie Om Hur 11 902 Medarbetare Upplever Sin Arbetssituation [Sustainable Working Life in Health Care–Survey on How 11 902 Employees Experience Their Work Situation]*; Arbets- och miljömedicin & Lunds universitet: Lund, Sweden, 2017; Volume 17, pp. 1–83.
17. Löfqvist, L.; Nilsson, K. *Medarbetare Inom Hållbart Arbetsliv För Alla Åldrar I Helsingborgs Stad: Rapport nr 12/2019*; Arbets- och miljömedicin Syd & Lund University: Lund, Sweden, 2019; Volume 12, pp. 1–102.
18. Löfqvist, L.; Nilsson, K. *Chefer–Hållbart Arbetsliv I Helsingborgs Stad: Rapport nr 17/2019*; Arbets- och Miljömedicin Syd & Lund University: Lund, Sweden, 2019; Volume 17, pp. 1–72.
19. Nilsson, K. *Situationen Under COVID-19 Pandemin För 7 781 Hälso- Och Sjukvårdsanställda: Enkätsvar Vid Uppföljningsstudien: Hållbart Arbetsliv Inom Hälso- Och Sjukvården 2020. [The Situation During The COVID-19 Pandemic for 7781 Health and Medical Care Employees: Questionnaire Responses to The Follow-Up Study: Sustainable Working Life in Health and Medical Care 2020.]*; Arbets- och miljömedicin Syd: Lund, Sweden, 2020; Volume 14, pp. 1–45.
20. Scania Public Health Cohort. Available online: https://www.lupop.lu.se/scania-public-health-cohort (accessed on 28 April 2021).
21. Persson, R.; Österberg, K.; Viborg, N.; Jonsson, P.; Tenenbaum, A. The Lund University Checklist for Incipient Exhaustion-a cross-sectional comparison of a new instrument with similar contemporary tools. *BMC Public Health* **2016**, *16*, 350. [CrossRef] [PubMed]
22. Persson, R. Österberg, K. Viborg, N. Jonsson, P. Tenenbaum, A. Two Swedish screening instruments for exhaustion disorder: Cross-sectional associations with burnout, work stress, private life stress, and personality traits. *Scand. J. Public Health* **2017**, *45*, 381–388. [CrossRef] [PubMed]
23. Beser, A.; Sorjonen, K.; Wahlberg, K.; Peterson, U.; Nygren, A.; Asberg, M. Construction and evaluation of a self-rating scale for stress-induced exhaustion disorder, the Karolinska Exhaustion Disorder Scale. *Scand. J. Psychol.* **2014**, *55*, 72–82. [CrossRef] [PubMed]
24. Ilmarinen, J.; Tuomi, K.; Klockars, M. Changes in the work ability of active employees over an 11-year period. *Scand. J. Work Environ. Health* **1997**, *23*, 49–57. [PubMed]
25. Tuomi, K.; Jarvinen, E.; Eskelinen, L.; Ilmarinen, J.; Klockars, M. Effect of Retirement on Health and Work Ability among Municipal Employees. *Scand. J. Work Environ. Health* **1991**, *17*, 75–81. [PubMed]
26. Schaufeli, W.B.; Bakker, A.B. *UWES-Utrecht Work Engagement Scale*; Preliminary Manual Version 1.1.; Occupational Health Psychology Unit Utrecht University: Utrecht, The Netherlands, 2004; Volume 26. [CrossRef]
27. Eklöf, M.; Pousette, A.; Dellve, L.; Skagert, K.; Ahlborg, G., Jr. *Utveckling Av Ett Variations- Och Förändringskänsligt Frågeinstrument För Mätning Av Stressorexponering, Coping Beteende Och Coping Resurser Bland 1:A Och 2:A Linjens Chefer Inom Offentlig Vård Och Omsorg. [The Development of A Variation- and Change Sensitive Question Instrument for Measuring Stressor Exposure, Coping Behavior and Coping Resources Among 1st and 2nd Line Managers in Public Health Care]*; ISM-Rapport 7; Institutet för Stressmedicin: Göteborg, Sweden, 2010.
28. Bursac, Z.; Gauss, C.H.; Williams, D.K.; Hosmer, D.W. Purposeful selection of variables in logistic regression. *Sour. Code Biol. Med.* **2008**, *3*, 17. [CrossRef] [PubMed]
29. Nilsson, K. *Attraktivt Och Hållbart Arbetsliv På Människors Villkor-Arbete, Hälsa Och Ledarskap Med SwAge-Modellen I Teori Och Praktik. [Attractive and Sustainable Working Life on Human Terms-Work, Health and Leadership with The SwAge Model in Theory and Practice]*; Studentlitteratur: Lund, Sweden, 2021; pp. 1–420.
30. Johansson, R. Vid Byråkratins ränser: Om Handlingsfrihetens Organisatoriska Begränsningar I Klientrelaterat Arbete. [At The Limits of Bureaucracy: The Freedom Om Actions' Organizational Constraints in Client-Related Work]. Ph.D. Thesis, Studentlitteratur, Lund, Sweden, 1992. (In Swedish).
31. Lipsky, M. *Street Level Bureaucracy–Dilemmas of The Individual in Public Services*; Russell Sage Foundation: New York, NY, USA, 1980; Volume 10. [CrossRef]

32. Sveriges Kommuner och Regioner. Möt Välfärdens Kompetensutmaning–Rekryteringsrapport 2020. [Meet the Welfare States Skills Challenges-Recruitment Report 2020]. Available online: https://rapporter.skr.se/mot-valfardens-kompetensutmaning.html (accessed on 1 February 2021).
33. Pollitt, C.; Bouckaert, G. *Public Management Reform: A Comparative Analysis-New Public Management, Governance, and the Neo-Weberian State*, 3rd ed.; Oxford University Press: Oxford, UK, 2011. [CrossRef]
34. Leo, U. Ledning av iinre organisation för lärande–att synliggöra professionella normer. In *Skolledare I Mötet Mellan Nationella Mål Och Lokal Policy. [School Leaders in The Meeting Between National Goals and Local Policy]*; Nihlfors, E., Johansson, O., Eds.; Gleerups: Malmö, Sweden, 2014; pp. 141–159. (In Swedish)
35. Swedish Work Environment Authority. *Rektorers Arbetsmiljö. Tillsynsinsats Genomförd Av Arbetsmiljöverket Göteborgsdistrikt 2009–2010. [Principals' Work Environment. Supervisory Effort Carried Out by The Swedish Work Environment Authority Gothenburg District 2009–2010]*; Arbetsmiljöverket: Gothenburg, Sweden, 2011.
36. Tuomi, K.; Hauuntanen, P.; Nykyri, E.; Ilmarinen, J. Promotion of work ability, the quality of work and retirement. *Occup. Med.* **2001**, *51*, 318–324. [CrossRef] [PubMed]
37. Lundin, A.; Leijon, O.; Vaez, M.; Hallgren, M.; Torgen, M. Predictive validity of the Work Ability Index and its individual items in the general population. *Scand. J. Public Health* **2017**, *45*, 350–356. [CrossRef] [PubMed]
38. Nilsson, K. Why work beyond 65? Discourse on the decision to continue working or retire early. *Nordic J. Work. Life Stud.* **2012**, *2*, 7–28. Available online: http://www.nordicwl.com/nilsson-2012-why-work-beyond-65-discourse-on-the-decision-to-continue-working-or-retire-early/ (accessed on 28 April 2021). [CrossRef]
39. Homepage for the Theoretical SwAge-Model. Available online: https://swage.org/en.html (accessed on 28 April 2021).

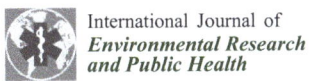

International Journal of
Environmental Research and Public Health

Article

Should I Stay or Should I Go? Associations between Occupational Factors, Signs of Exhaustion, and the Intention to Change Workplace among Swedish Principals

Inger Arvidsson [1,*], Ulf Leo [2], Anna Oudin [1,3], Kerstin Nilsson [1,4], Carita Håkansson [1], Kai Österberg [5] and Roger Persson [1,5]

1 Division of Occupational and Environmental Medicine, Lund University, SE-223 81 Lund, Sweden; anna.oudin@med.lu.se (A.O.); kerstin.nilsson@med.lu.se (K.N.); carita.hakansson@med.lu.se (C.H.); roger.persson@psy.lu.se (R.P.)
2 Centre for Principal Development, Umeå University, SE-901 87 Umeå, Sweden; ulf.leo@umu.se
3 Department of Public Health and Clinical Medicine, Umeå University, SE-901 87 Umeå, Sweden
4 Department of Public Health, Kristianstad University, SE-291 88 Kristianstad, Sweden
5 Department of Psychology, Lund University, SE-221 00 Lund, Sweden; kai.osterberg@psy.lu.se
* Correspondence: Inger.Arvidsson@med.lu.se; Tel.: +46-46-173175

Citation: Arvidsson, I.; Leo, U.; Oudin, A.; Nilsson, K.; Håkansson, C.; Österberg, K.; Persson, R. Should I Stay or Should I Go? Associations between Occupational Factors, Signs of Exhaustion, and the Intention to Change Workplace among Swedish Principals. *IJERPH* **2021**, *18*, 5376. https://doi.org/10.3390/ijerph18105376

Academic Editor: Paul B. Tchounwou

Received: 13 April 2021
Accepted: 11 May 2021
Published: 18 May 2021

Publisher's Note: MDPI stays neutral with regard to jurisdictional claims in published maps and institutional affiliations.

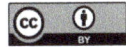

Copyright: © 2021 by the authors. Licensee MDPI, Basel, Switzerland. This article is an open access article distributed under the terms and conditions of the Creative Commons Attribution (CC BY) license (https://creativecommons.org/licenses/by/4.0/).

Abstract: A high turnover among principals may disrupt the continuity of leadership and negatively affect teachers and, by extension, the students. The aim was to investigate to what extent various work environment factors and signs of exhaustion were associated with reported intentions to change workplace among principals working in compulsory schools. A web-based questionnaire was administered twice, in 2018 and in 2019. Part I of the study involved cross-sectional analyses of the associations 2018 (n = 984) and 2019 (n = 884) between occupational factors, signs of exhaustion, and the intention to change workplace, using Generalized Estimating Equations models. Part II involved 631 principals who participated in both surveys. The patterns of intended and actual changes of workplace across two years were described, together with associated changes of occupational factors and signs of exhaustion. Supportive management was associated with an intention to stay, while demanding role conflicts and the feeling of being squeezed between management and co-workers (buffer-function) were associated with the intention to change workplace. The principals who intended to change their workplace reported more signs of exhaustion. To increase retention among principals, systematic efforts are probably needed at the national, municipal, and local level, in order to improve their working conditions.

Keywords: psychosocial working conditions; mental health; school leader

1. Introduction

The leadership of principals is of great importance for the school. The reports of a high turnover among principals are worrying [1–4], since it may disrupt the continuity of the leadership and negatively impact the school climate [5]. Long-term relationships are required to build mutual trust within the organization [6,7], which forms the basis for being able to offer support and adequate development opportunities for teachers [8]. It has been observed that frequent changes of principals results in lower teacher retention, which is particularly harmful for low-achieving schools with many inexperienced teachers [1]. Moreover, associations between principal turnover and student performance have been observed [1–3]. In a Swedish context, the National Agency for Education [9] and the Swedish schools-inspectorate [10] have expressed concerns that a high principal turnover may impair opportunities for students to achieve their goals. According to The Teaching and Learning International Survey (TALIS) [11], the median number of years working at their current school was three years for Swedish principals. Corresponding values in the Nordic countries ranged between four and six years, and the median value was five years across all 48 countries participating in TALIS 2018. It thus seems as if a problematic principal turnover occurs to a large extent in Sweden and it is therefore important to improve the understanding of its underlying factors.

There may be a variety of reasons why principals decide to change workplaces. One reason may be that the change represents a natural career move, for example, from being an assistant principal to principal. Other reasons may have more practical and private origins. Anyhow, complex and demanding working conditions among principals have been reported [12–15], which may be of importance for the principals' inclination to stay or change workplaces. In a review of principal-turnover research [2], it was pointed out that inadequate preparation and professional development, poor working conditions, and a lack of decision-making authority were some of the reasons why principals leave their jobs. In addition, in Sweden, large variations in principal turnover have been observed between schools and municipalities [3], as well as between different school forms [10]. These indicate variable conditions depending on both external factors (e.g., socioeconomic factors) and the working conditions within the organizations.

While work environment factors and stress-related health among teachers have gained a large interest among researchers [16–20], less scientific studies have focused on the work environment and health among principals [13,21,22]. Anyhow, evidence has been provided of an association between principals' satisfaction with their work characteristics and their mental health status [12]. Furthermore, several sources of occupational stress have been identified, for example work overload, handling relationships with staff, teacher climate, lack of resources and personal characteristics [13,23,24]. As a leader of the school, the principals' work is associated with a wide range of responsibilities and roles comprising pedagogical development, staffing, finances, premises, and work environment issues, to name a few. Furthermore, the principal may experience numerous expectations from the school owner, superintendents, the schools-inspectorate, co-workers, parents, and students [14]. Whether these demanding organizational and social work environment factors are balanced by supportive management, supportive manager colleagues, or organizational structures, is most likely of great importance for their well-being and intention to stay in the organization [25]. A previous literature review of studies in different occupational groups has shown that risk factors such as high demands, low job control, and a high workload, increased the risk for exhaustion and poor mental health [26]. The association between burnout and high job demands and low job control also applied to Swedish teachers [19,20]. In a previous study of the present study population [22], 29% of the principals and assistant principals in compulsory school met the exhaustion criteria according to Karolinska Exhaustion Disorder Scale (KEDS) [27]. This prevalence rate is almost twice as large as the prevalence rate observed in a highly educated but occupationally diverse study sample [28]. Since a clear association has been found between a high level of stress and the intention to change jobs among teachers [29], it is of interest to find out whether this is true also among principals. Furthermore, to gain knowledge for preventive actions, there is a need to identify which specific occupational factors are of importance for the principals' intention to stay at, or leave, their current workplace.

Aims

The aims of the present study were twofold. The first aim (Part I) was to identify which occupational factors (organizational structures and work environmental factors) were associated with the intention to stay or the intention to change workplace, among principals and assistant principals in Swedish compulsory schools. The second aim (Part II) was to describe the patterns of intended and actual change of workplace across two years (2018 and 2019), and the associations with occupational factors and signs of exhaustion.

2. Materials and Methods

2.1. Study Design

The present study was a part of a longitudinal study of working conditions and health among principals in 277 municipalities in Sweden that included two web-based questionnaires using the software Textalk Textalk (Mölndal/Gothenburg, Sweden; www.textalk.com/products/websurvey/ accessed on 11 November 2019). The questionnaires were administered with a one-year interval in September/October 2018 and in September/October 2019.

In the present study, both cross-sectional and longitudinal analyses were performed, and the study comprised two parts. Part I involved cross-sectional analyses of the associations of year 2018 (n = 984) and year 2019 (n = 884) between occupational factors, signs of exhaustion, and the intention to change workplace, among principals and assistant principals working in compulsory schools. The cross-sectional analyses accounted for the fact that some participants had responded to the survey on both occasions and thus had repeated measurements (see statistical analyses).

Part II was a longitudinal analysis comprising 631 principals and assistant principals who participated in both surveys and who worked in compulsory schools in 2018. The patterns of intended and actual changes of workplace across two years (2018 and 2019) were described. Analyses were performed of associations between changes of the intention to stay, or leave the current workplace between 2018 and 2019, and changes of occupational factors and signs of exhaustion during the same period (with all actual workplace changes taken into account).

2.2. Participants

The participants in the longitudinal study were recruited via e-mail address by principals who had participated in training programs for principals funded and arranged by the Swedish National Agency for Education, during the period 2008–2017. In 2018, 9900 principals potentially working in pre-schools, compulsory schools, upper secondary schools, or adult education were invited to participate in the study. Of these, 4640 individuals either accepted (n = 2633) or declined (n = 2007) participation. Eventually, 2317 completed the entire questionnaire in 2018. The response rate was 50%, based on the principals that responded yes and also completed the survey, versus no-responders and those that did not complete the survey. In 2019, the second questionnaire was directed to the 2316 presumed still occupationally active responders in the first survey, of which 1528 responded. Furthermore, the participants who did not answer in the first assessment round (in 2018) were re-invited to the second round. Out of the 5149 previously silent individuals, 3350 were seemingly reached without technical problems (i.e., bouncing e-mail), of which 464 decided to complete the second questionnaire. Thus, the second survey comprised a total of 1992 principals. The study was approved by the Regional Ethical Review Board in Lund, Sweden, Dnr 2018/247.

Part I included principals and assistant principals working in compulsory schools, which comprised 1000 out of the 2316 respondents in 2018, and 901 out of the 1992 respondents in 2019. Participants who stated "other title" were omitted from the study (n = 15 in both years 2018 and 2019). Due to internal missing values, another three individuals (one in 2018 and two in 2019) were omitted. Thus, the present study sample comprised 984 principals (720 women and 264 men; mean age 49; range 30–67 years old) who responded to the first questionnaire and 884 principals (649 women and 235 men) who responded to the second one. Among these, 633 responded to both questionnaires. In total, 1235 principals had completed at least one of the questionnaires.

Part II involved the principals and assistant principals who participated in both surveys and worked in compulsory schools in 2018, irrespective of any change to another school-level in 2019 (n = 651). Twenty participants who stated that they would retire in 2018 or 2019 were excluded from the study, resulting in a study sample of 631 individuals.

2.3. Outcome Measure

In Part I, the outcome of the study was based on the question "Do you intend to change workplace within the coming two years?" with the response alternative 1: Yes definitely; 2: Yes, probably; 3: No; and 4: I will retire. The dichotomous outcome consisted of 1: No (i.e., intention to stay) vs. 2: yes, probably/yes, definitely (i.e., intention to leave). Participants who responded that they would retire were omitted.

2.4. Independent Factors

The data collection, for both Part I and Part II, comprised questions on gender, age, and occupational factors, i.e., job title (principal/assistant principal), school owner (municipality/other organization), seniority as principal, the number of co-workers and the number of students the principal was responsible for. Furthermore, information was collected on the staff availability (1: Full staff or more than full staff; 2: somewhat or very understaffed), overtime work (1: Once a week or less often, 2: a few times a week or every day; 3: No agreed working hours), and perceived physical working environment (1: Adequate, good or very good; 2: poor or very poor).

Demanding and Supportive organizational and social work environment factors were measured with Gothenburg Manager Stress Inventory (GMSI). GMSI-mini is a brief version of GMSI [30], which has been has been shortened by one of the authors (KÖ), in consultation with the developers Mats Eklöf and Anders Pousette. The selected items showed the highest correlation with the corresponding subscale in the original GMSI, which have been analyzed in two different samples. Demanding work environment factors were assessed in relation to the preceding six months, by 22 items distributed along eight dimensions, i.e., Resource deficits, Organizational control, Role conflicts, Role demands, Group dynamics, Buffer-function, Co-workers, and Container-function (i.e., dealing with co-workers' problems and frustrations). In each dimension, all questions were answered along a five-point scale with the options 1: "never/almost never"; 2: "Rarely"; 3: "Sometimes"; 4: "Often" and 5: "Always/almost always". The supportive organizational and social work environment factors were assessed with 10 items distributed along five dimensions, i.e., Supportive management, Cooperating co-workers, Supportive manager colleagues, Supportive private life, and Supportive organizational structures. The responses to each item were given along a five-point scale, indicating the level of agreement with various statements about supportive factors; 1: "Applies very poorly", 2: "Applies poorly", 3: "Applies to some extent", 4: "Applies well", and 5: "Applies very well". For both demanding and supportive factors, the mean score in each dimension was calculated for each individual. A higher mean score indicated more frequent experience with actual demands, and the perception of better support. In Supplementary Table S1, the number of items and a description of the included questions are given for each GMSI-dimension (this information has previously been presented in [15]).

In study specific questions, the participants were asked about "To what extent do you perceive stressful external expectations" from the following eight actors: the Swedish schools-inspectorate, the National Agency for Education, the school owner, Superintendent, immediate manager, co-workers, parents, and students. Each of the eight questions was answered along a seven-point scale ranging from 0 (verbalized as "not stressful at all") to 6 (very stressful). Thereafter, in Part I of the study, the scales were dichotomized into low (<4 points) and high (≥4 points) stressful external expectations. In Part II, the mean value on each scale was calculated for comparisons within and between specific groups of principals (see further description below).

Signs of exhaustion were measured with The Karolinska Exhaustion Disorder Scale (KEDS) [27], which includes 9 items that refer to the last 2 weeks, comprising the following domains: (1) ability to concentrate, (2) memory, (3) physical resistance, (4) mental resistance, (5) recovery, (6) sleep, (7) hypersensitivity to sensory impressions, (8) experience with demands, and (9) irritation and anger. Each item was answered on a 7-point scale (0–6). The sum score was calculated for each individual (0–54 possible) and higher values reflected more severe symptoms. The mean value, as well as the prevalence of a score ≥ 19 points, which indicated signs of exhaustion/possible exhaustion disorder [25], was calculated for specific groups of principals.

The participants were also asked, "How many times have you changed workplace during the past five years?" (2018) and "How many times have you changed workplace during the past 12 months" (2019), with the response alternatives "none", "once", "twice", or "three times or more". The latter question was used in Part II of the study where "None" indicated no change of workplace (=No), and once or more indicated that the principal had changed workplace (=Yes).

In Table 1, descriptive estimates for the occupational factors, signs of exhaustion, and intended and actual changes of workplace are presented for 2018 and 2019, for the participants included in Part I of the study.

Table 1. Characteristics among participants included in Part I of the study, regarding reported conditions at work in the years 2018 (N = 984) and 2019 (N = 884). The number of participants who responded to both questionnaires was 633.

	Categories/Scale	2018 N = 984	2019 N = 884
School owner; N (%)	Municipality	853 (87)	762 (86)
	Other organization	131 (13)	122 (14)
Job title; N (%)	Principal	717 (73)	665 (75)
	Assistant principal	267 (27)	219 (25)
Seniority as principal; N (%)	<3 years	202 (21)	177 (20)
	3–10 years	554 (56)	676 (76)
	>10 years	228 (23)	31 (4)
Number of co-workers; N (%)	0–20	180 (18)	146 (17)
	21–30	273 (28)	259 (29)
	31–40	294 (30)	260 (29)
	41–130	235 (24)	219 (25)
Staff access/availability; N (%)	Full staff	571 (58)	578 (65)
	Very or somewhat understaffed	413 (42)	306 (35)
Number of students; N (%)	0–200	343 (35)	283 (32)
	201–400	466 (47)	446 (50)
	401–600	139 (14)	115 (13)
	601–1377	35 (4)	40 (5)
Overtime work; N (%)	Once a week or less often	164 (17)	177 (20)
	Every day or a few days/week	779 (79)	676/(76)
	No agreed working hours	41 (4)	31 (4)
Perceived physical working environment; N (%)	Adequate, good or very good	762 (77)	700 (79)
	Poor or very poor	222 (23)	184 (21)
Demanding organizational and social work environment; mean (SD)			
Resource deficits	Scale 1–5	3.5 (0.9)	3.5 (1.0)
Organizational Control	Scale 1–5	2.6 (0.9)	2.6 (0.9)
Role conflicts	Scale 1–5	3.8 (0.8)	3.7 (0.8)
Role demands	Scale 1–5	3.1 (0.8)	3.1 (0.8)
Group dynamics	Scale 1–5	2.3 (0.7)	2.3 (0.7)
Buffer-function	Scale 1–5	2.9 (0.9)	2.9 (0.9)
Co-workers	Scale 1–5	2.9 (0.7)	2.8 (0.7)
Container- function	Scale 1–5	3.4 (0.8)	3.3 (0.8)
Supportive organizational and social work environment; mean (SD)			
Supportive management	Scale 1–5	3.1 (1.1)	3.1 (1.1)
Cooperating with co-workers	Scale 1–5	4.3 (0.6)	4.3 (0.6)
Supportive manager colleagues	Scale 1–5	3.9 (1.0)	3.8 (1.0)
Supportive private life	Scale 1–5	3.8 (1.0)	3.9 (1.0)
Supportive organizational structures	Scale 1–5	3.6 (0.9)	3.6 (0.9)

Table 1. Cont.

	Categories/Scale	2018 N = 984	2019 N = 884
Stressful external expectations; N (%) [a]			
The National Agency of Education	Score ≥ 4	322 (33)	250 (28)
The Swedish schools-inspectorate	Score ≥ 4	599 (61)	519 (59)
School owner	Score ≥ 4	440 (45)	385 (44)
Super intendent	Score ≥ 4	312 (32)	260 (29)
Immediate supervisor	Score ≥ 4	288 (29)	257 (29)
Co-workers	Score ≥ 4	484 (49)	374 (42)
Parents	Score ≥ 4	544 (55)	505 (57)
Students	Score ≥ 4	181 (18)	166 (19)
Karolinska Exhaustion disorders scale (KEDS)			
Mean score (SD)	Score 0–54	14 (8)	14 (9)
Possible exhaustion disorder; N (%)	Score ≥ 19 points	290 (29)	232 (26)
Change of workplace in the past five years; N (%)	None	385 (39)	n.a.
	Once	393 (40)	
	Twice	121 (12)	
	Three times or more	85 (9)	
Change of workplace in the past twelve months; N (%)	None	n.a.	797 (90)
	Once		82 (9)
	Twice		4 (0.5)
	Three times or more		1 (0.1)
Intention to change workplace within two years; N (%)	Yes, definitely	98 (10)	96 (11)
	Yes, probably	304 (31)	271 (31)
	No	559 (57)	495 (56)
	I will retire	23 (2)	22 (2)

[a] The seven-point scales (0–6) were dichotomized into low (<4 points) and high (≥4 points). Bold faces may help the reader to identify the different categories of dimensions.

2.5. Part II: Longitudinal Patterns of Intended and Actual Change of Workplace

The patterns of intention to change workplace in the year 2018 and year 2019 (no vs. yes, probably/yes, definitely), together with the actual change of workplace reported in 2019, are described in Figure 1.

A large proportion of the principals remained at their workplace and had no intention of changing workplace, neither in 2018 nor in 2019. However, some principals had changed their mind concerning the intention of changing, or staying at the present workplace between 2018 and 2019. This may of course be due to the fact that they had actually changed workplace during the year, and of natural reasons had other working conditions. However, the reason for them to change their mind may also be due to changes of their working conditions and/or stress-related health at the present workplace, which is of interest to study.

To distinguish the groups, the participants were first divided into two groups based on the reports in 2018: those who intended to stay and those who intended to change workplace within the next two years. In the next step, the two groups were divided into four, based on the question in the survey in 2019 "Have you changed workplace during the past twelve months?" (No vs. Yes). In the third step, these four groups were divided into 8 groups, based on their intention to stay or leave their current workplace in 2019. This revealed eight different paths:

1. Intention to stay 2018—No change of workplace—Intention to stay 2019 (Stay/No change/Stay)
2. Intention to stay 2018—No change of workplace—Intention to leave 2019 (Stay/No change/Leave)
3. Intention to stay 2018—Change of workplace—Intention to stay 2019 (Stay/Change/Stay)

4. Intention to stay 2018—Change of workplace—Intention to leave 2019 Stay/Change/Leave)
5. Intention to leave 2018—No change of workplace—Intention to stay 2019 (Leave/No change/Stay)
6. Intention to leave 2018—No change of workplace—Intention to leave 2019 (Leave/No change/Leave)
7. Intention to leave 2018—Change of workplace—Intention to stay 2019 (Leave/Change/Stay)
8. Intention to leave 2018—Change of workplace—Intention to leave 2019 (Leave/Change/Leave)

As an indicator of stress-related health in each of the groups, the prevalence of a sum score $\geq$ 19 points (signs of exhaustion; KEDS [24]) is shown in Figure 1.

For in-depth analyses of factors that may be of importance for the intention to change workplace, we chose to perform pairwise comparisons of occupational factors and signs of exhaustion in years 2019 and 2018, within and between Group 1 (Stay/No change/Stay) and Group 2 (Stay/No change/Leave), within and between Group 5 (Leave/No change/Stay) and Group 6 (Leave/No change/Leave), and within and between Group 7 (Leave/Change/Stay) and Group 8 (Leave/Change/Leave) (Supplementary Table S2). The Groups 3 (Stay/Change/Stay) and 4 (Stay/Change/Leave) were not involved in these in-depth analyses, because they comprised a limited number of participants (N = 16 and N = 4, respectively). Longitudinal patterns of intended and actual change of workplace are shown in Figure 1, which is placed further ahead in the results (Section 3.2).

2.6. Statistical Analyses

All statistical analyses were performed with IBM SPSS software, version 24 (IBM Corp.). p-values $\leq$ 0.05 (two-tailed) were considered statistically significant.

To estimate the associations between gender, age, occupational factors, and signs of exhaustion, and the intention to change workplace (No vs. yes, probably/yes, definitely) Generalised Estimating Equation (GEE) models were used to specify a repeated measure model with a dichotomous outcome (binary logistic regression). Thus, survey data from 2018 were combined with survey data from 2019, taking into account that 633 out of 1235 study subjects had participated in both surveys (dependent observations). The intention to change workplace was first estimated in bivariate GEE models for all variables (gender, age, occupational factors, and signs of exhaustion) by Odds ratios (ORs) and their 95% confidence intervals (CIs). In the next step, ORs for intention to change workplace were estimated using multivariate GEE, for all variables with bivariate p-values < 0.1. In the multivariate GEE model, five variables concerning stressful external expectations were omitted from the analyses (i.e., expectations from the Swedish schools-inspectorate, National Agency of Education, school owner, superintendent, and immediate supervisor), due to a conceptual overlap with the variables in GMSI regarding demanding organizational and social work environment factors.

In Part II of the study, analysis within the groups (2019 vs. 2018) were done using the Wilcoxon Signed Rank Test for continuous variables and McNemar's test for dichotomous variables. Comparisons between the groups were performed using the nonparametric Mann–Whitney U-test for continuous variables and Fisher's exact test for dichotomous variables.

3. Results

3.1. Part I

In 2018, 98 principals out of 984 (10%) reported that they definitely intended to change workplace within the coming two years, and 304 (31%) that they probably would do so (Table 1). Corresponding values for the 884 participants in 2019 were 96 (11%) and 271 (31%), respectively.

3.1.1. Bivariate Analyses of Associations between Occupational Factors, Gender, Age, and Signs of Exhaustion, and the Intention to Change Workplace

Younger age, assistant principal, understaffing, and a perceived poor physical working environment were all associated with an intention to change workplace (Table 2). In addition, for all of the demanding organizational and social work environment factors in GMSI, high scores were statistically significantly associated with the intention to change workplace. The same was true for stressful external expectations from the school owner, superintendent, immediate manager, co-workers, and parents. Furthermore, a high sum-score on the exhaustion scale (KEDS) was associated with the intention to change workplace.

For all of the supportive organizational and social work environment factors, except for a Supportive private life, high scores were significantly associated with the intention to stay at the current workplace (Table 2). There were no statistically significant associations between the intention to change workplace, and gender, school owner, seniority, number of students and co-workers, and overtime work.

Table 2. Cross-sectional bivariate and multivariate binary logistic regression analysis between occupational factors, gender age, and signs of exhaustion and the dichotomous outcome of intention to change workplace (no vs. yes, probably/yes, definitely) in the total study sample, taking repeated assessments in the years 2018 (N = 984) and 2019 (N = 884) into account. Odds ratio (OR) and 95% confidence intervals (CI) are presented, which in continuous variables (GMSI and KEDS) are associated with a one-unit increase/decrease in mean score on the scale. Results in bold face are statistically significant.

Independent Factors	Categories/Scale	Bivariate OR (CI 95%)	Multivariate [a] OR (CI 95%)
Gender	Female	1	-
	Male	1.15 (0.91–1.46)	
Age	years	**0.97 (0.96–0.99)**	**0.97 (0.96–0.99)**
School owner	Municipality	1	-
	Other organization	0.93 (0.67–1.28)	
Job title	Principal	1	1
	Assistant principal	**1.39 (1.09–1.76)**	**1.43 (1.10–1.84)**
Seniority as principal	<3 years	1	-
	3–10 years	1.19 (0.89–1.59)	
	>10 years	1.18 (0.84–1.66)	
Number of co-workers	0–20	1	-
	21–30	1.25 (0.92–1.71)	
	31–40	1.15 (0.84–1.57)	
	41–130	1.22 (0.88–1.68)	
Staff access/availability	Full staff	1	1
	Very or somewhat understaffed	**1.31 (1.07–1.60)**	0.94 (0.76–1.16)
Number of students	0–200	1	-
	201–400	1.09 (0.87–1.37)	
	401–600	1.08 (0.78–1.49)	
	601–1377	1.31 (0.73–2.33)	
Overtime	Once a week or less often	1	-
	Every day or a few days/week	0.98 (0.75–1.27)	
	No agreed working hours	0.88 (0.49–1.58)	
Physical working environment	Adequate, good or very good	1	1
	Poor or very poor	**1.54 (1.22–1.95)**	1.10 (0.85–1.42)
Demanding organizational and social work environment			
Resource deficits	Score 1–5	**1.21 (1.09–1.34)**	0.93 (0.82–1.07)
Organizational Control	Score 1–5	**1.48 (1.31–1.67)**	1.00 (0.85–1.18)
Role conflicts	Score 1–5	**1.57 (1.37–1.80)**	**1.22 (1.03–1.46)**
Role demands	Score 1–5	**1.41 (1.23–1.61)**	0.85 (0.70–1.03)
Group dynamics	Score 1–5	**1.54 (1.34–1.78)**	1.13 (0.93–1.36)
Buffer-function	Score 1–5	**1.61 (1.43–1.81)**	**1.27 (1.08–1.50)**
Co-workers	Score 1–5	**1.45 (1.26–1.68)**	1.14 (0.95–1.37)
Container-function	Score 1–5	**1.35 (1.19–1.54)**	0.86 (0.72–1.02)

Table 2. Cont.

Independent Factors	Categories/Scale	Bivariate OR (CI 95%)	Multivariate [a] OR (CI 95%)
Supportive organizational and social work environment			
Supportive management	Score 1–5	**0.67 (0.61–0.74)**	**0.79 (0.71–0.89)**
Cooperating with co-workers	Score 1–5	**0.69 (0.59–0.81)**	0.96 (0.79–1.17)
Supportive manager colleagues	Score 1–5	**0.70 (0.63–0.77)**	**0.83 (0.74–0.94)**
Supportive private life	Score 1–5	0.92 (0.83–1.01)	**1.17 (1.04–1.31)**
Supportive organizational structures	Score 1–5	**0.71 (0.63–0.79)**	0.95 (0.83–1.09)
Stressful external expectations			
The National Agency of Education	Score < 4	1	
	≥4	0.90 (0.73–1.12)	
The Swedish schools-inspectorate	Score < 4	1	
	≥4	0.98 (0.80–1.19)	
School owner	Score < 4	1	-
	≥4	**1.40 (1.15–1.70)**	
Super Intendent	Score < 4	1	-
	≥4	**1.32 (1.07–1.63)**	
Immediate supervisor	Score < 4	1	-
	≥4	**1.73 (1.39–2.14)**	
Co-workers	Score < 4	1	-
	≥4	**1.64 (1.35–2.00)**	
Parents	Score < 4	1	1
	≥4	**1.57 (1.28–1.91)**	**1.32 (1.05–1.65)**
Students	Score < 4	1	1
	≥4	1.24 (0.97–1.59)	1.02 (0.77–1.34)
Karolinska Exhaustion disorder scale (KEDS)	Score 0–54	**1.05 (1.04–1.06)**	**1.03 (1.02–1.05)**

[a] The variables stressful external expectations from school owner, super intendent, immediate supervisor, and co-workers were omitted from the multivariate analyses due to a conceptual overlap with the demanding and supporting dimensions in GMSI. Bold faces are remained to indicate which factors that are statistically significant (as stated in the Table text).

3.1.2. Multivariate Analyses of Associations between Occupational Factors, Age, and Signs of Exhaustion, and the Intention to Change Workplace

In the multivariate analyses, younger age and assistant principal remained statistically significantly associated with the intention to change workplace (Table 2). The same was true for high scores of stressful external expectations from parents. Among the demanding organizational and social work environment factors (GMSI), Role conflicts, (OR 1.22 (CI 1.03–1.46), associated with a one unit increase in mean score, on the scale 1–5) and Buffer-function, OR 1.27 (CI 1.08–1.50) remained statistically significant, while Resource deficits, Organizational Control, Role demands, Group dynamics, Co-workers and Container-function did not. Furthermore, a high score of a Supportive private life was associated with the intention to change workplace. The strongest association with an intention to change workplace was found for a high sum-score on the exhaustion scale (KEDS) (OR 1.03 (CI 1.02–1.05), associated with a one unit increase in mean score, on the scale 0–54].

High scores of Supportive management (OR 0.79 (CI 0.71–0.89), associated with a one unit decrease in mean score, on the scale 1–5) and Supportive manager colleagues remained statistically significantly associated with the intention to stay at the current workplace, while Cooperating with co-workers and Supportive organizational structures did not (Table 2).

3.2. Part II: Longitudinal Patterns of Intended and Actual Change of Workplace

As described in the methods section, and illustrated in Figure 1, the longitudinal analysis revealed eight different paths of intended and/or actual changes of workplace during 2018 and 2019.

3.2.1. Group 1 (Stay/No Change/Stay) and Group 2 (Stay/No Change/Leave)

The principals in Group 1 (N = 274) had no intention to change workplace neither in 2018 nor in 2019, and reported no change of workplace in the survey in 2019 (Figure 1).

The longitudinal results within the group showed generally better working conditions in 2019 compared to 2018 (Table 3).

The principals in Group 2 (N = 99) had no intention to change workplace in 2018. In 2019, no actual change of workplace was reported, but they now reported that they had the intention to change workplace within the next two years (Figure 1). The longitudinal results within Group 2 showed statistically significantly impaired scores in 2019 compared to 2018, in terms of Resource deficits, Buffer-functions, and Supportive management (Table 3).

Differences between Group 1 and Group 2: Already in 2018, the principals in Group 1 reported generally better working conditions than the principals in Group 2 (Table 3). In 2019, most of the differences were accentuated. Group 2 reported statistically significantly higher scores in external expectations from school owners, immediate supervisors and co-workers, and in all of the demanding organizational dimensions. Group 2 also reported less Supportive Management and less Supportive organizational resources than Group 1. A higher proportion of the principals in Group 1 were employed in an organization other than in the municipality and they were responsible for a higher number of students. Group 2 reported significantly higher scores on the exhaustion scale (KEDS) in 2018, and the difference between the groups was accentuated in 2019.

3.2.2. Group 5 (Leave/No Change/Stay) and Group 6 (Leave/No Change/Leave)

In 2018, the principals in Group 5 (N = 52) reported that they had the intention to change workplace within the next two years. In 2019, no actual change of workplace was reported, and they no longer had the intention to change workplace (Figure 1). In 2019, they reported generally better working conditions compared to 2018 (Table 4). The scores of stressful external expectations from the superintendent and the immediate supervisor declined, and the same was true for Role conflicts and Container functions. Group 5 also reported statistically significantly lower scores on the exhaustion scale (KEDS) in 2019 compared to 2018.

Table 3. Changes of reported exposures (2018 vs. 2019) within Group 1 (Stay/No change/Stay) and within Group 2 (Stay/No change/Leave) (Figure 1); and comparison of exposures between Group 1 and Group 2.

Independent Factors	Categories/Scale	Group 1 (Stay/No Change/Stay) N = 274		2018 vs. 2019; p-Value [B]	Group 2 (Stay/No Change/Leave) N = 99		2018 vs. 2019; p-Value [B]	Difference between Group 1 and Group 2 p-Value [A]	
		2018	2019		2018	2019		2018	2019
Gender (2018); N (%)	Female	207 (76)			68 (69)			0.19	
	Male	67 (24)			31 (31)				
Age (2018); mean (SD)	years	50 (7)			47 (7)			<0.001	
School owner; N (%)	Municipality	229 (84)	229 (84)	1.00	91 (92)	90 (91)	1.00	0.04	0.09
	Other organization	45 (16)	45 (16)		8 (8)	9 (9)			
Job title; N (%)	Principal	205 (76)	207 (76)	0.51	72 (73)	72 (73)	1.00	0.69	0.59
	Assistant principal	69 (25)	66 (24)		27 (27)	27 (27)			
	Other title [C]	-	1 (0.4)		-	0			
Number of co-workers; mean (SD)		34 (16)	34 (15)	0.77	34 (12)	33 (12)	0.56	0.98	0.93
Staff access/availability	Full staff	166 (61)	192 (70)	<0.01	56 (57)	64 (65)	0.22	0.55	0.32
	Very or somewhat understaffed	108 (39)	82 (30)		43 (43)	35 (35)			
Number of students; mean (SD)		277 (166)	286 (166)	<0.01	270 (136)	252 (136)	0.52	0.65	0.05
Overtime	Once a week or less often	44 (16)	60 (22)	<0.01	11 (11)	19 (19)	0.09	0.25	0.67
	Every day or a few days/week	215 (78)	206 (75)		85 (86)	76 (77)			
	No agreed working hours [D]	15 (5)	8 (3)		3 (3)	4 (4)			
Physical working environment; N (%)	Adequate, good or very good	229 (84)	222 (81)	0.39	72 (73)	73 (74)	1.00	0.03	0.15
	Poor or very poor	45 (16)	52 (19)		27 (27)	26 (26)			
Demanding organizational and social work environment; mean (SD)									
Resource deficits	Score 1-5	3.4 (0.9)	3.4 (1.0)	0.33	3.6 (0.9)	3.8 (0.9)	0.01	0.21	<0.001
Organizational Control	Score 1-5	2.5 (0.9)	2.4 (0.9)	0.66	2.6 (0.8)	2.7 (0.8)	0.23	0.15	0.02
Role conflicts	Score 1-5	3.6 (0.8)	3.5 (0.9)	<0.01	3.9 (0.8)	3.8 (0.8)	0.35	<0.01	<0.01
Role demands	Score 1-5	3.0 (0.8)	3.0 (0.8)	0.41	3.2 (0.8)	3.2 (0.8)	0.17	0.06	0.02
Group dynamics	Score 1-5	2.2 (0.7)	2.1 (0.7)	0.02	2.4 (0.7)	2.4 (0.7)	0.98	0.02	<0.001
Buffer-function	Score 1-5	2.7 (0.9)	2.7 (0.9)	0.87	2.9 (0.9)	3.2 (0.9)	0.001	0.05	<0.001
Co-workers	Score 1-5	2.8 (0.7)	2.7 (0.7)	0.19	2.9 (0.7)	2.9 (0.7)	0.80	0.05	0.03
Container-function	Score 1-5	3.3 (0.8)	3.2 (0.8)	0.02	3.5 (0.7)	3.4 (0.9)	0.12	0.04	0.04

Table 3. Cont.

Independent Factors	Categories/Scale	Group 1 (Stay/No Change/Stay) N = 274		2018 vs. 2019; p-Value [B]	Group 2 (Stay/No Change/Leave) N = 99		2018 vs. 2019; p-Value [B]	Difference between Group 1 and Group 2 p-Value [A]	
		2018	2019		2018	2019		2018	2019
Supportive organizational and social work environment; mean (SD)									
Supportive management	Score 1–5	3.4 (1.1)	3.4 (1.1)	0.44	3.1 (1.1)	2.9 (1.2)	0.01	**0.03**	**<0.001**
Cooperating with co-workers	Score 1–5	4.4 (0.6)	4.4 (0.6)	0.55	4.2 (0.7)	4.2 (0.7)	0.88	0.06	0.06
Supportive manager colleagues	Score 1–5	**4.0 (0.9)**	**3.9 (1.0)**	**0.05**	3.9 (1.0)	3.8 (0.9)	0.39	0.33	0.26
Supportive private life	Score 1–5	3.8 (1.0)	3.9 (1.0)	0.18	3.6 (1.1)	3.7 (1.0)	0.40	0.19	0.18
Supportive organizational structures	Score 1–5	**3.7 (0.9)**	**3.8 (0.9)**	**0.03**	3.6 (0.9)	3.5 (0.9)	0.52	0.24	**<0.01**
Stressful external expectations; mean (SD)									
The National Agency of Education	Score 1–7	3.5 (1.8)	3.3 (1.8)	0.27	3.5 (1.8)	3.3 (1.9)	0.40	0.81	0.90
The Swedish schools-inspectorate	Score 1–7	4.9 (1.8)	4.7 (1.9)	0.19	4.9 (1.8)	4.6 (2.0)	0.06	0.85	0.45
School owner	Score 1–7	4.0 (1.5)	3.9 (1.7)	0.32	4.2 (1.6)	4.3 (1.6)	0.48	0.18	**0.03**
Super Intendent	Score 1–7	3.4 (1.6)	3.3 (1.7)	0.17	3.8 (1.7)	3.6 (1.7)	0.49	0.11	0.11
Immediate supervisor	Score 1–7	3.2 (1.6)	3.1 (1.7)	0.19	3.4 (1.6)	3.7 (1.6)	0.26	0.23	**<0.01**
Co-workers	Score 1–7	4.1 (1.4)	3.8 (1.5)	<0.01	4.5 (1.6)	4.4 (1.6)	0.62	<0.01	**<0.001**
Parents	Score 1–7	4.4 (1.7)	4.4 (1.7)	0.90	4.8 (1.6)	4.7 (1.5)	0.49	0.05	0.16
Students	Score 1–7	2.9 (1.5)	2.9 (1.6)	0.89	3.0 (1.6)	3.1 (1.8)	0.26	0.53	0.42
Karolinska Exhaustion Disorder Scale									
Mean score (SD)	Score 0–54	13.1 (7.7)	12.7 (8.0)	0.08	15.0 (7.9)	15.9 (8.0)	0.18	**0.04**	**<0.001**
Possible exhaustion disorder; N (%)	Score ≥ 19 points	66 (24)	57 (21)	0.21	29 (29)	34 (34)	0.40	0.35	**<0.01**

[A]. The Mann–Whitney U-test was used for continuous variables, and Fisher's exact test was used for dichotomous variables. [B]. The Wilcoxon Signed Rank Test was used for continuous variables, and McNemar's test for dichotomous variables. [C]. One person with "other title" in 2019 was excluded from the statistical analysis. [D]. Participants with "No agreed working hours" were excluded from the statistical analysis.

Table 4. Change of reported exposures in the year 2018 vs. in the year 2019, within and between Group 5 (Leave/No change/Stay) and Group 6 (Leave/No change/Leave) (Figure 1).

Independent factors	Categories/Scale	Group 5 N = 52			Group 6 N = 146			Difference between Group 5 and Group 6 p-Value [A]	
		2018	2019	2018 vs. 2019; p-Value [B]	2018	2019	2018 vs. 2019; p-Value [B]	2018	2019
Gender (2018); N (%)	Female	42 (81)			113 (77)			0.70	
	Male	10 (19)			33 (23)				
Age (2018); mean (SD)	years	51 (6)			48 (7)			0.02	
School owner; N (%)	Municipality	45 (87)	45 (87)	1.00	123 (84)	123 (84)	1.00	0.82	0.82
	Other organisation	7 (13)	7 (13)		23 (16)	23 (16)			
Job title; N (%)	Principal	38 (73)	41 (79)	0.12	95 (65)	97 (66)	0.62	0.31	0.08
	Assistant principal	14 (27)	10 (19)		51 (35)	49 (34)			
	Other title [C]	-	1 (1.9)		-	0			
Number of co-workers; mean (SD)		33 (12)	34 (16)	0.95	35 (16)	34 (17)	0.60	0.62	0.92
Staff access/availability	Full staff	28 (54)	31 (60)	0.65	90 (62)	89 (61)	1.00	0.33	0.87
	Very or somewhat understaffed	24 (46)	21 (40)		56 (38)	57 (39)			
Number of students; mean (SD)		256 (136)	287 (184)	0.07	303 (197)	307 (202)	0.12	0.19	0.49
Overtime	Once a week or less often	7 (13)	12 (23)	0.06	29 (20)	32 (22)	0.72	0.40	1.00
	Every day or a few days/week	43 (83)	39 (75)		111 (76)	107 (73)			
	No agreed working hours [D]	2 (4)	1 (2)		6 (4)	7 (5)			
Physical working environment; N (%)	Adequate, good or very good	40 (77)	42 (81)	0.77	114 (78)	110 (75)	0.56	0.85	0.57
	Poor or very poor	12 (23)	10 (19)		32 (22)	36 (25)			
Demanding organisational and social work environment; mean (SD)									
Resource deficits	Score 1-5	3.6 (1.0)	3.6 (1.0)	0.62	3.5 (1.0)	3.6 (1.0)	0.35	0.33	0.64
Organisational Control	Score 1-5	2.8 (0.8)	2.8 (0.9)	0.83	2.7 (0.8)	2.7 (0.9)	0.59	0.28	0.52
Role conflicts	Score 1-5	4.0 (0.8)	3.6 (0.8)	0.001	3.9 (0.8)	3.9 (0.8)	0.79	0.72	0.02
Role demands	Score 1-5	3.2 (0.8)	3.0 (0.7)	0.07	3.2 (0.8)	3.2 (0.8)	0.39	0.76	0.11
Group dynamics	Score 1-5	2.3 (0.8)	2.3 (0.8)	0.95	2.4 (0.7)	2.4 (0.7)	0.42	0.52	0.92
Buffer-function	Score 1-5	3.1 (0.9)	3.1 (1.0)	0.52	3.1 (0.9)	3.1 (0.9)	0.48	0.96	0.40
Co-workers	Score 1-5	2.8 (0.8)	2.6 (0.8)	0.07	3.0 (0.7)	3.0 (0.7)	0.34	0.22	0.02
Container-function	Score 1-5	3.6 (0.8)	3.3 (0.9)	0.02	3.5 (0.8)	3.4 (0.8)	0.45	0.21	0.39

Table 4. Cont.

Independent factors	Categories/Scale	Group 5 N = 52			Group 6 N = 146			Difference between Group 5 and Group 6 p-Value [A]	
		2018	2019	2018 vs. 2019; p-Value [B]	2018	2019	2018 vs. 2019; p-Value [B]	2018	2019
Supportive organisational and social work environment; mean (SD)									
Supportive management	Score 1–5	3.0 (1.1)	3.0 (1.0)	0.69	2.9 (1.0)	2.9 (1.1)	0.81	0.74	0.56
Cooperating with co-workers	Score 1–5	4.2 (0.6)	4.2 (0.6)	0.94	4.2 (0.7)	4.2 (0.6)	0.45	0.63	0.65
Supportive manager colleagues	Score 1–5	3.8 (0.8)	3.9 (1.0)	0.87	3.6 (1.1)	3.6 (1.0)	0.67	0.35	0.20
Supportive private life	Score 1–5	3.8 (1.1)	3.9 (1.0)	0.16	3.8 (1.1)	3.9 (1.0)	0.74	0.88	0.84
Supportive organisational structures	Score 1–5	3.5 (0.9)	3.8 (0.9)	0.07	3.6 (1.0)	3.5 (1.0)	**0.03**	0.29	0.17
Stressful external expectations; mean (SD)									
The National Agency of Education	Score 1–7	3.7 (1.9)	3.3 (1.8)	0.16	3.4 (1.8)	3.5 (1.8)	0.41	0.40	0.44
The Swedish schools-inspectorate	Score 1–7	4.9 (2.0)	5.0 (1.8)	0.95	4.8 (1.8)	4.9 (1.8)	0.69	0.49	0.77
School owner	Score 1–7	4.3 (1.8)	4.1 (1.6)	0.47	4.4 (1.6)	4.4 (1.6)	0.81	0.80	0.35
Super intendent	Score 1–7	4.1 (1.6)	3.4 (1.7)	**0.007**	3.8 (1.6)	3.8 (1.7)	0.82	0.22	0.18
Immediate supervisor	Score 1–7	3.8 (1.8)	3.2 (1.7)	**0.02**	3.8 (1.8)	3.8 (1.8)	0.88	0.99	**0.04**
Co-workers	Score 1–7	4.2 (1.5)	3.8 (1.6)	0.13	4.7 (1.5)	4.4 (1.5)	**0.01**	0.06	**0.04**
Parents	Score 1–7	4.9 (1.5)	4.8 (1.7)	0.72	5.0 (1.6)	5.0 (1.6)	0.90	0.62	0.49
Students	Score 1–7	2.9 (1.5)	3.0 (1.8)	0.80	3.3 (1.6)	3.3 (1.7)	0.19	0.19	0.19
Karolinska Exhaustion Disorder Scale									
Mean score (SD)	Score 0–54	15 (7.2)	12 (7.6)	<**0.001**	16 (8.9)	16 (9.1)	0.51	0.49	**0.006**
Possible exhaustion disorder; N (%)	Score ≥ 19 points	15 (29)	10 (19)	0.18	55 (38)	50 (34)	0.44	0.31	0.05

[A] The Mann–Whitney U-test was used for continuous variables, and Fisher's exact test was used for dichotomous variables. [B] The Wilcoxon Signed Rank Test was used for continuous variables, and McNemar's test for dichotomous variables. [C] One person with "other title" in 2019 was excluded from the statistical analysis. [D] Participants with "No agreed working hours" were excluded from the statistical analysis.

The principals in Group 6 (N = 146) reported both in 2018 and in 2019 that they had the intention to change workplace within the next two years, but no actual change of workplace was reported in 2019 (Figure 1). Within the group, there were only minor changes of the reported working conditions and signs of exhaustion in 2019 compared to 2018 (Table 4).

Differences between Group 5 and Group 6: In the survey in 2018, there were no statistically significant differences between Group 5 and Group 6, neither in occupational factors nor in exhaustion (Table 4). In 2019, the principals in Group 5 reported better conditions with regards to stressful external expectations from the immediate supervisor and co-workers, and lower scores regarding Role conflicts and Co-workers' problems, compared to Group 6. Furthermore, in 2019, Group 5 reported significantly lower scores on the KEDS exhaustions scale, compared to Group 6.

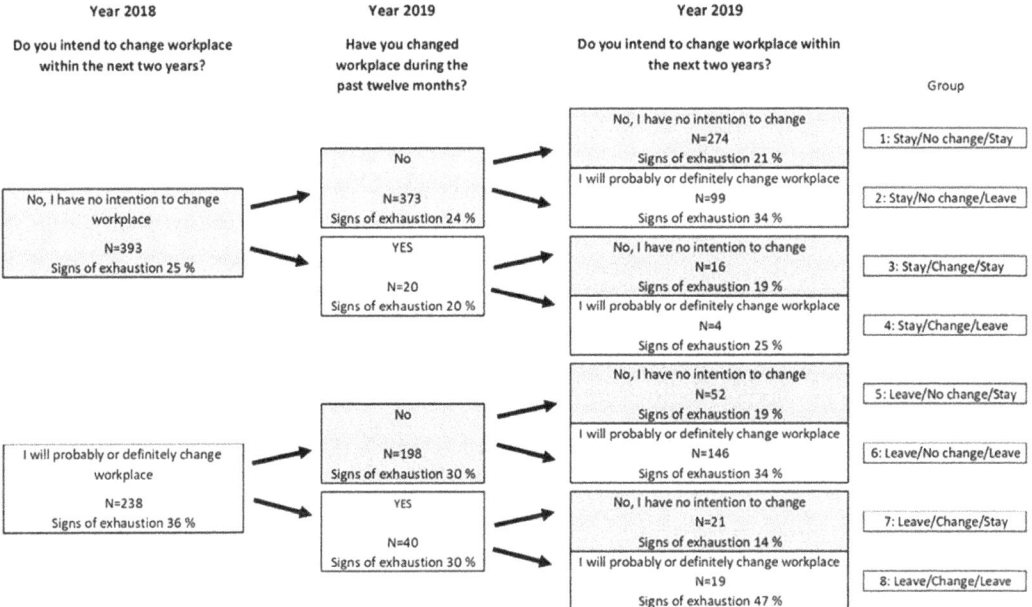

Figure 1. Longitudinal patterns of intended and actual change of workplace and its association with signs of exhaustion among 631 principals in compulsory schools.

3.2.3. Group 7 (Leave/Change/Stay) and Group 8 (Leave/Change/Leave)

The pairwise comparisons of occupational factors and signs of exhaustion in 2019 and 2018, within and between Group 7 (N = 21) and Group 8 (N = 19), are given in Supplementary Table S2.

4. Discussion

4.1. Principal Findings

A general finding based on both parts of the study is that most of the principals with the intention to stay at the present workplace reported better working conditions and a lower mean sum score on the exhaustion scale (i.e., KEDS), compared to those who had the intention to change workplace.

The multivariate analyses indicated that the occupational factors that were most strongly associated with the intention to change workplace, were a demanding buffer-function between management and co-workers, demanding role conflicts, and a perception of high external expectations from parents. Furthermore, an increased score on the KEDS exhaustion scale was associated with the intention to change workplace. An intention to stay at the current workplace was most strongly associated with Supportive management and Supportive manager colleagues.

In Part II of the study, the longitudinal analyses indicated that changes in the intention to stay at, or leave, the present workplace showed associations with changes in the working conditions and the level of exhaustion. For example, the principals in Group 2 (Stay/No change/Leave) had no intention to change workplace 2018, but they did have such an intention in 2019. At the same time, they reported an increased Buffer-function, increased Resource deficits, and less Supportive management, compared to 2018. The principals in Group 5 (Leave/No change/Stay) had the intention to change workplace in 2018, but did not report any actual change in 2019. In 2019, they no longer intended to change workplace and also reported reduced Role conflicts, reduced Container functions, less stressful external expectations from the superintendent and the immediate supervisor, and markedly improved scores on the exhaustion scale, compared to 2018. Thus, the present results point to the need for improved working conditions among principals, for their well-being and for a reduction in their turnover. The most important preventive measures seem to be improving managerial support, reducing the demanding Buffer-function between management and co-workers, and reducing Role conflicts.

4.2. Methodological Considerations

A strength of the study is that it involved principals from 277 out of 290 municipalities in Sweden, comprising principals in cities, villages, and schools of all sizes. In this respect, the present participants are likely to be fairly representative of the entire population of principals in Swedish compulsory schools. Whether the conditions reported can be extrapolated to the working conditions among principals in an international context is more uncertain, and probably mostly due to specific circumstances in various countries and cultural settings.

Another strength of the study is the use of multiple methods to address the research questions, i.e., cross-sectional analyses with repeated measurements, together with an analysis of the longitudinal patterns in subgroups of principals with varying intentions to stay, or leave, the workplace. The fact that similar results were found in both parts of the study strengthens its validity.

The present study included principals who participated in training programs for principals funded and arranged by the Swedish National Agency for Education, during the period 2008–2017. Thus, both principals who participated in the training programs before 2008 (most likely older than the average for the study sample), and those who still had not passed the training program (most likely younger than the average) were not included. However, since the study sample is representative of Swedish principals concerning age [31], this might be a minor problem. Another concern is that principals who are better prepared for the positions are supposed to be less stressed and stay longer at the workplace [2]. Thus, the present selection of only trained principals may have resulted in an underestimation of the signs of both exhaustion and the principal turnover.

In the original study sample of principals at all school-levels, 2317 out of the 9900 who were invited responded to the questionnaire, which generated a response rate of 23 percent. However, as the invitation list included principals who participated in the training program in 2008–2017, there may have been an unknown fraction of principals who had left the profession before the first survey in 2018, and thus did no longer belong to the target group. Among the 4640 principals who were successfully contacted, 50 percent responded to the questionnaire. Although similar low response rates are common in large-scale surveys [23,32], this is a limitation of the study. Another limitation is that all of the data were self-reported. Furthermore, although it is likely that adverse working conditions in many cases may have preceded the intention to change workplace, the limitations of the study design preclude a definite statement on causal relationships.

In Part II of the study, the described patterns of intended and actual changes of workplace resulted in eight different scenarios/groups. Because some of the scenarios were less common, some of the groups had a limited number of participants. This was the case in particular for Groups 3 and 4, and they were therefore omitted from further analyses. Additionally, the analyses within and between Groups 7 and 8 suffered from a low power, which limited the possibility to detect statistically significant differences, if any were present.

4.3. Signs of Exhaustion

Several previous studies have shown associations between work environment factors and burnout/signs of exhaustion (e.g., [26,33]), which most likely apply also to the principals in the present study. Thus, it is reasonable to assume that the associations between signs of exhaustion and the intention to change workplace, to a large extent, are mediated through demanding circumstances in the work environment.

4.4. Should I Stay at the Present Workplace . . . ?

A high score of Supportive management, i.e., that the principals trust that superiors, when needed, will help them solve problems and that they express a genuine interest for the principals' work and leadership, was strongly associated with the intention to stay at the present workplace. As a leader, the principal is the one that is supposed to give support to the staff [34], but the principal, in turn, needs support and guidance from the superintendent or the school owner [14]. Furthermore, a high score of Supportive manager colleagues was associated with the intention to stay. Thus, the present results confirm previous findings that support from colleagues and managers belongs to the factors that are decisive for the will to continue working in the workplace [25,35]. That supportive leadership is an important work environment issue is also confirmed by its protective effect against exhaustion and burnout [19,20,26]. Of course, due to the nature of the data, low scores in the demanding organizational and social work environment factors presented below also represent factors that were associated with the intention to stay.

4.5. . . . Or Should I Go?

Among the occupational factors, the strongest association with the intention to change workplace was found for a high score of Buffer-function, i.e., that the principals perceived themselves to be squeezed between co-workers and higher levels in the organization, and that superiors expect them to be understanding and committed to accepting decisions that were bad for them and the organization, and to advocate for such decisions towards their subordinates [30]. The challenge of acting as a buffer function may be related to other factors that were associated with the intention to change workplace, i.e., low managerial support and stressful external expectations from the superintendent and immediate manager. Insufficient managerial support is often reflected in a lack of trust between principals and the actors in the local governance chain [14]. The Buffer-function may also be related to a lack of decision-making authority, (i.e., deficient influence, control, or autonomy to shape decisions and solutions in the school) which has been emphasized to be one of the most important reasons for principal turnover in a US context [2]. Additionally, Resource deficits, reflected by lacking resources due to decisions by superiors, politicians, or governmental authorities, can be closely related to the Buffer-function.

Burdensome Role conflicts among principals may have to do with frictions between administrative work tasks, organizational development, being a pedagogical leader, and taking part in daily activities in interactions with co-workers. Overall, this may result in an excessive workload. Thus, besides a possible perceived sense of inadequacy among principals, the association between Role conflicts and intention to change workplace may be influenced by the complexity of the job and the amount of time needed to complete all necessary activities [2].

A perception of stressful external expectations from parents was associated with the intention to change workplace. According to Leo et al. [14], most parents are supportive. However, among complaints from parents that were reported to the Swedish schools-inspectorate, a majority concerned children and students who did not receive the support they needed, according to their parents. Responding to complaints was perceived as a stressful and time-consuming task for the principals [14]. The present finding of a high score of stressful external expectations from the Swedish schools-inspectorate can most likely be, and largely is, related to their handling of complaints from parents [14].

The intention to change workplace was more frequent among younger principals than among older ones, and more frequent among assistant principals than in principals. This may partly be explained by young assistant principals accepting an interim and challenging period of hard work as a stepping-stone in order to display merit for a future position as full principal.

Moreover, the dimension Supportive private life comprised questions on the opportunities to rest and to relax from work during leisure time. No statistically significant association was found in the bivariate analysis, but in the multivariate analyses, a high score turned out to be associated with the intention to change workplace. A possible explanation is that a supportive private life might give a principal the inner strength to decide to leave a workplace associated with difficult working conditions and declining well-being and health.

4.6. Possible Implications

Due to the fact that an unstable management function is associated with a high teacher turnover [1], which in turn may lead to poor results for the students, the situation for principals poses an important societal issue. In order to increase retention among principals, systematic efforts to establish improved working conditions for principals seem to be sorely needed. It is likely that a joint effort along the entire governance chain, i.e., at the national, municipal, and local level, intending to improve working conditions for principals, would be a fruitful endeavor.

5. Conclusions

A general finding was the clear association between the principals' working conditions and their intention to stay at or leave their current workplace. Poor working conditions in terms of, primarily, a lack of support from management, the feeling of being squeezed between management and co-workers (Buffer-function), and demanding Role conflicts were associated with a consideration to change workplace. At the same time, principals who intended to change workplace reported more signs of exhaustion.

Supplementary Materials: The following are available online at https://www.mdpi.com/article/10.3390/ijerph18105376/s1, Supplementary Table S1: Description of the scales in the 32-item Gothenburg Manager Stress Inventory (GMSI)-Mini, Supplementary Table S2: Comparisons of occupational factors and signs of exhaustion in 2019 and 2018, within and between Group 7 and Group 8.

Author Contributions: Conceptualization, I.A., U.L., A.O., K.N., C.H., K.Ö. and R.P.; methodology, I.A. and A.O.; software, R.P., K.Ö. and I.A.; validation, I.A., U.L., A.O., K.N., C.H., K.Ö. and R.P.; formal analysis, A.O. and I.A.; investigation, I.A., K.Ö. and R.P.; resources, R.P.; data curation, I.A., R.P. and K.Ö.; writing—original draft preparation, I.A.; writing—review and editing, I.A., U.L., A.O., K.N., C.H., K.Ö. and R.P.; visualization, I.A.; supervision, R.P.; project administration, R.P. and I.A.; funding acquisition, R.P. All authors have read and agreed to the published version of the manuscript.

Funding: This research was funded by AFA Insurances, grant number 170094.

Institutional Review Board Statement: The study was conducted according to the guidelines of the Declaration of Helsinki, and approved by The Regional Ethical Review Board in Lund, Sweden (reg. no. 2018/247).

Informed Consent Statement: Written informed consent was obtained from all subjects involved in the study.

Data Availability Statement: Consistent with the study protocol approved by the Regional Ethical Review Board, anonymized data are stored locally at the Division of Occupational and Environmental Medicine, Lund University, Lund, Sweden. In accordance with the ethical approval, crude data are not to be published on the internet. Access to data will be granted to eligible researchers wanting to audit our research. Requests should be directed to the corresponding author.

Acknowledgments: The authors wish to thank all participants who responded to the questionnaire.

Conflicts of Interest: The authors declare no conflict of interests. The funders had no role in the design of the study; in the collection, analyses, or interpretation of data; in the writing of the manuscript, or in the decision to publish the results.

References

1. Béteille, T.; Kalogrides, D.; Loeb, S. Stepping stones: Principal career paths and school outcomes. *Soc. Sci. Res.* **2012**, *41*, 904–919. [CrossRef] [PubMed]
2. Levin, S.; Bradley, K. Understanding and Addressing Principal Turnover. A Review of the Research. National Association of Secondary School Principals (NASSP). 2019. Available online: https://learningpolicyinstitute.org/sites/default/files/product-files/NASSP_LPI_Principal_Turnover_Research_Review_REPORT.pdf (accessed on 1 April 2021).
3. Thelin, K. Principal Turnover: When is it a problem and for whom? Mapping out Variations within the Swedish case. *Res. Educ. Adm. Leadersh.* **2020**, *5*, 417–452.
4. Boyce, J.; Bowers, A.J. Principal turnover: Are there different types of principals who move from or leave their schools? A latent class analysis of the 2007–2008 Schools and Staffing Survey and the 2008–2009 Principal Follow-Up Survey. *Leadersh. Policy Sch.* **2016**, *15*, 237–272. [CrossRef]
5. Meyer, M.J.; Macmillan, R.B.; Northfield, S. Principal succession and its impact on teacher morale. *Int. J. Leadersh. Educ.* **2009**, *2*, 171–185. [CrossRef]
6. Erdogan, B.; Bauer, T.N. Leader-member exchange (LMX) theory: The relational approach to leadership. In *Oxford Library of Psychology. The Oxford Handbook of Leadership and Organizations*; Day, D.V., Ed.; Oxford University Press: Oxford, UK, 2014; pp. 407–433.
7. Tschannen-Moran, M.; Gareis, C.R. Faculty trust in the principal: An essential ingredient in high-performing schools. *J. Educ. Adm.* **2015**, *53*, 66–92. [CrossRef]
8. Fullan, M. *Leading in a Culture of Change*; Jossey-Bass: San Francisco, CA, USA, 2001.
9. Skolverket [The National Agency for Education]. *TALIS 2018. En Studie om Lärares och Rektorers Arbete i Grund-och Gymnasieskolan. Delrapport 1. [A Study on Teachers and Principals Work in Compulsory and High Schools. Interim Report 1]*; Skolverket: Stockholm, Sweden, 2020.
10. Skolinspektionen [The Swedish Schools Inspectorate]. *Huvudmannens Arbete för Kontinuitet på Skolor Med Många Rektorsbyten. Tematisk Kvalitetsgranskning. [The School Owners Work for Continuity in Schools with Frequent Changes of Principals. Thematic Quality Review]*; Skolinspektionen: Stockholm, Sweden, 2019.
11. OECD: Organisation for Economic Co-operation and Development (OECD). Teaching and Learning International Survey (TALIS) 2018. Principal questionnaire. In *Organisation for Economic Co-operation and Development (OECD)—International Consortium, International Association for the Evaluation of Educational Achievement (IEA), The Netherlands and Germany; Australian Council for Educational Research (ACER), Australia*; Statistics Canada: Ottawa, ON, Canada, 2018.
12. Dewa, C.S.; Dermer, S.W.; Chau, N.; Lowrey, S.; Mawson, S.; Bell, J. Examination of factors associated with the mental health status of principals. *Work* **2009**, *33*, 439–448. [CrossRef]
13. Darmody, M.; Smyth, E. Primary school principals' job satisfaction and occupational stress. *Int. J. Educ. Manag.* **2016**, *30*, 115–128. [CrossRef]
14. Leo, U.; Persson, R.; Arvidsson, I.; Håkansson, C. External expectations and well-being, fundamental and forgotten perspectives in school leadership: A study on new leadership roles, trust and accountability. In *Re-Centering the Critical Potential of Nordic School Leadership Research*; Moos, L., Nihlfors, E., Merok Paulsen, J., Eds.; Springer Educational Governance Research: Berlin/Heidelberg, Germany, 2020; Volume 14, pp. 209–228.
15. Persson, R.; Leo, U.; Arvidsson, I.; Nilsson, K.; Österberg, K.; Håkansson, C. Supporting and demanding managerial circumstances and associations with excellent workability: A cross-sectional survey of Swedish principals. submitted.
16. Travers, C.J.; Cooper, C.L. Teachers under pressure. In *Stress in the Teaching Profession*; Routledge: London, UK, 1996.
17. Scott, C.; Stone, B.; Dinham, S. "I love teaching but . . . ": International patterns of teacher discontent. *Educ. Policy Anal. Arch.* **2001**, *9*, 1–7.
18. Dicke, T.; Stebner, F.; Linninger, C.; Kunter, M.; Leutner, D. A longitudinal study of teachers' occupational well-being: Applying the job demands-resources model. *J. Occup. Health Psychol.* **2018**, *23*, 262–277. [CrossRef] [PubMed]
19. Arvidsson, I.; Håkansson, C.; Karlson, B.; Björk, J.; Persson, R. Burnout among Swedish school teachers—A cross-sectional analysis. *BMC Public Health* **2016**, *6*, 823. [CrossRef] [PubMed]
20. Arvidsson, I.; Leo, U.; Larsson, A.; Håkansson, C.; Persson, R.; Björk, J. Burnout among school teachers: Quantitative and qualitative results from a follow-up study in southern Sweden. *BMC Public Health* **2019**, *19*, 55. [CrossRef]

21. Dicke, T.; Marsh, H.W.; Riley, P.; Parker, P.D.; Guo, J.S.; Horwood, M. Validating the Copenhagen psychosocial questionnaire (COPSOQ-II) using set-ESEM: Identifying psychosocial risk factors in a sample of school principals. *Front. Psychol.* **2018**, *9*, 584. [CrossRef] [PubMed]
22. Persson, R.; Leo, U.; Arvidsson, I.; Håkansson, C.; Nilsson, K.; Österberg, K. Prevalence of exhaustion symptoms and associations with school level, length of work experience and gender: A nationwide cross-sectional study of Swedish principals. *BMC Public Health* **2021**, *21*, 331. [CrossRef]
23. Cooper, C.L.; Kelly, M. Occupational stress in head teachers—A national Uk study. *Brit. J. Educ. Psychol.* **1993**, *63*, 130–143. [CrossRef] [PubMed]
24. Bedi, I.K.; Kukemelk, H. School principals and job stress: The silent dismissal agent and forgotten pill in the United Nations sustainable development goal 4*. *US-China Educ. Rev. B* **2018**, *8*, 357–364.
25. Nilsson, K. A sustainable working life for all ages—The swAge-model. *Appl. Ergon.* **2020**, *86*. [CrossRef]
26. Aronsson, G.; Theorell, T.; Grape, T.; Hammarström, A.; Hogstedt, C.; Marteinsdottir, I.; Skoog, I.; Träskman-Bendz, L.; Hall, C. A systematic review including meta-analysis of work environment and burnout symptoms. *BMC Public Health* **2017**, *17*, 1–13. [CrossRef] [PubMed]
27. Beser, A.; Sorjonen, K.; Wahlberg, K.; Peterson, U.; Nygren, A.; Åsberg, M. Construction and evaluation of a self rating scale for stress-induced exhaustion disorder, the Karolinska Exhaustion Disorder Scale. *Scand. J. Psychol.* **2014**, *55*, 72–82. [CrossRef]
28. Persson, R.; Österberg, K.; Viborg, N.; Jonsson, P.; Tenenbaum, A. The Lund University checklist for incipient exhaustion—A cross-sectional comparison of a new instrument with similar contemporary tools. *BMC Public Health* **2016**, *16*, 350. [CrossRef] [PubMed]
29. Skolverket [The National Agency for Education]. *TALIS 2018. En Studie om Lärares och Rektorers Arbete i Grund och. Gymnasieskolan. Delrapport 2, TALIS 2018. [A Study on Teachers and Principals Work in Compulsory and High Schools. Interim Report 2]*; Skolverket: Stockholm, Sweden, 2020.
30. Eklöf, M.; Pousette, A.; Dellve, L.; Skagert, K.; Ahlborg, G. *Gothenburg Manager Stress Inventory (GMSI). Utveckling av ett Variations- och Förändringskänsligt Frågeinstrument för Mätning av Stressor-Exponering, Copingbeteende och Copingresurser Bland 1:a och 2:a Linjens Chefer Inom Offentlig Vård och Omsorg [Development of a Variation- and Change-Sensitive Instrument for Measuring Stress Exposure, Coping Behaviour and Coping Resources among 1st and 2nd Line Managers in Public Health and Care]. ISM-Rappport 7*; Institutet för stressmedicin: Göteborg, Sweden, 2010.
31. SCB. *Yrkesregistret med Yrkesstatistik 2018. Yrkesstrukturen i Sverige. [The Swedish Occupational Register with Occupational Statistics 2018]*; SCB: Stockholm, Sweden, 2020.
32. Persson, R.; Cleal, B.; Jakobsen, M.O.; Viladsen, E.; Andersen, L.L. Reasons for using workplace wellness services: Cross-sectional study among 6000 employees. *Scand. J. Public Health* **2018**, *46*, 347–357. [CrossRef]
33. Theorell, T.; Hammarström, A.; Aronsson, G.; Träskman Bendz, L.; Grape, T.; Hogstedt, C.; Marteinsdottir, I.; Skoog, I.; Hall, C. A systematic review including meta-analysis of work environment and depressive symptoms. *BMC Public Health* **2015**, *15*, 738. [CrossRef]
34. Littrell, P.C.; Billingsley, B.S.; Cross, L.H. The Effects of Principal Support on Special and General Educators' Stress, Job Satisfaction, School Commitment, Health, and Intent to Stay in Teaching. *Remedial Spec. Educ.* **1994**, *15*, 297–310. [CrossRef]
35. Nilsson, K.; Rignell-Hydbom, A.; Rylander, L. Factors influencing the decision to extend working life or to retire. *Scand. J. Work Environ. Health* **2011**, *37*, 473–480. [CrossRef]

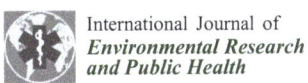

Article

Meetings are an Important Prerequisite for Flourishing Workplace Relationships

Sophie Schön Persson, Kerstin Blomqvist and Petra Nilsson Lindström *

Faculty of Health Sciences, Kristianstad University, 291 88 Kristianstad, Sweden; Sophie.schon@hkr.se (S.S.P.); Kerstin.blomqvist@hkr.se (K.B.)
* Correspondence: petra.nilsson@hkr.se; Tel.: +46-44-250-39-61

Abstract: Relationships among colleagues, managers, and care recipients are mutually important, and need to be highlighted in workplace health promotion. The aim was to explore prerequisites for flourishing workplace relationships in a municipal healthcare setting for old people. As part of this process, we explored the staff's suggestions on how work relationships could be improved. The study had a salutogenic and participatory approach, examining staff perceptions of what was required for flourishing relationships to be created, and their suggestions for the relationships to be more promotive. Four multi-stage focus groups, which met three times each, were conducted with staff (n = 26) in old age healthcare settings. A deductive analysis was performed, based on components of the flourishing concept: challenge, connectivity, autonomy, and competence. Informal and formal meetings at work were shown to build positively perceived relationships. The study describes meetings and relationships connected to the four components of flourishing. Suggestions for improving work relationships are also presented. This study contributes to workplace health promotion, and has a salutogenic and participatory focus on how to explore workplace relationships as a resource. The flourishing concept shows how workplace relationships can be explored as prerequisites for workplace health promotion.

Keywords: workplace relationships; flourishing; multi-stage focus groups; old age healthcare; participatory approach; workplace health promotion

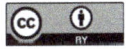

1. Introduction

In recent years, there has been an increase, albeit slow, in work-related studies adopting a salutogenic approach [1–5], i.e., focusing on maintaining and/or increasing health-promoting resources [6,7]. The opposite is to focus on risks of illness, which is a pathogenic approach, and studies that examine risk factors and why people feel bad through, e.g., their work. A significant factor in occupational health is relationships, and research focusing on negative work-related relationships that contribute to ill health is common [8–10]. Therefore, there is value in conducting studies with a salutogenic approach, that in different ways and from different theories examine the workplace as a health-promoting arena to understand which factors and processes can increase sustainable work-related relationships and employees' health [11–13].

Workplace health promotion focuses on factors and processes (resources) as prerequisites for doing well and feeling good at work [12]. One resource is relationships, and these could be among colleagues, managers, and, in a healthcare context, also the care recipients [3,4,14–17]. Studies about relationships at work from aspects of teamwork and communication, also in relation to a higher quality of care [18,19], are more common. However, the various interaction patterns that underlie the effects of relationships on individual health and well-being, the processes through which these effects occur [20,21], and which specific aspects of positive workplace relationships contribute to health appear to be less explored [2,15,22].

Therefore, the specific aspects of relationships at work need to be further explored. A salutogenic concept that could be used to understand which aspects contribute, in a deeper sense, to positive relationships at work, is flourishing. Flourishing, as a concept, has theoretically been described by several authors in recent years. At first, it was more individually focused and used in terms of the state a person achieves when attaining the highest levels of functioning in life and perceiving psychosocial health [23]. Seligman (2012) likewise focused on the individual's well-being as a key to flourishing, but also identified relationships as one of the key elements. He highlighted five key elements of well-being that people need in life to be able to flourish: positive emotions, engagement, relationships, meaning in life, and accomplishment (PERMA) [24]. McCormack and Titchen (2014) confirmed that relationships are an assisting and important factor for flourishing. They argued that it is the interconnections between a person's health experience (physical, psychical, social, spiritual), creativity, and purposeful interactions with others, that create flourishing [25].

Later, Gaffney (2015) described from a practical point of view how flourishing could be identified and developed, and presented four important components of flourishing. The first of these is challenge. A challenge can come from oneself or from another person; it may be positive or negative; and people have different approaches for meeting and managing a challenge depending on different factors in their lives. The second component is connectivity, which is about feeling connection to oneself, to one's surroundings, and/or with other people. The third component is autonomy, which is about feeling sufficient control and having a choice about things that matter to oneself. The last component is about using one's own competencies such as intelligence, strengths, and experiences gained from challenges. Flourishing has its foundation in the circumstances and situations that enable persons to meet challenges in life and that enable them to flourish by viewing upcoming situations with optimism [26].

A situation that many individuals find themselves in on a daily basis is the work situation. When Colbert et al. (2016) applied flourishing to a work situation, they saw that workplace relationships played a key role in promoting employee flourishing. Work relationships promoted personal growth through friendship, and the opportunity to give to and help others in a work situation. Positively experienced workplace relationships also increased job satisfaction and feelings of meaningfulness at work, supported overall life satisfaction, and had benefits for both individuals and organizations by creating flourishing [27]. However, the need to further investigate the flourishing components for employees in a workplace context has been highlighted [27,28].

From previous theoretical descriptions of the associations between flourishing and relationships [23–25], together with Gaffney's (2015) practical description [26], there is both a theoretical and a practical benefit to further investigating the specific aspects of positive work relationships with flourishing as a salutogenic concept.

In summary, the introduction has highlighted that there are limited health promotion studies with a salutogenic approach concerning (a) what is required for positive workplace relationships to develop, (b) how positive workplace relationships can be enhanced, and (c) what aspects of positive relationships are already provided in work. Thus, there is a gap to fill to extend the knowledge of how workplace relationships can improve employee health and thereby also the care of care recipients.

The aim of this study was to explore prerequisites for flourishing workplace relationships in a municipal old age healthcare setting. As part of this process, we also explored the staff's suggestions on how work relationships could be improved in their work situation.

2. Materials and Methods

2.1. Context and Participants

As the number of elderly people is increasing [29,30], it is important to be able to provide elderly care with competent staff in the future. Therefore, the current study was conducted in an elderly care context. In Swedish municipal old age care settings, nurse assistants work either on a day shift or night shift, and provide regular as well as palliative care. The managers, registered nurses (RNs), occupational therapists and physiotherapists at the residential care units usually work during the daytime on weekdays [29,30].

This study is the final part of a participatory action research (PAR) project, and was conducted in two similar general residential care units in the south of Sweden during the period 2015–2016. The selection of units for participation was made in consultation between researchers and managers. The two chosen residential care units together had about 39 residents. Altogether, four working groups, one day shift team and one night shift team from each unit, were asked to participate. The care units employed only assistant nurses, and it was those who worked in the units who were included in the study. Nurses and other care professions were employed in another department and were therefore not part of this study. All 31 assistant nurses in the four working groups were invited to participate in the study, and 26 took part. In the Results section and thereafter, we refer to the participants as "caring staff".

2.2. Procedure

With our salutogenic approach, we wanted the study to be participatory and emancipatory, to give advantage to the participants in their work situation by their participation. Therefore, the study was based on methodology for PAR. A participatory approach has the intention to enable participants to extend their understanding of issues and to empower them to use their new knowledge [31]. Previous studies in this research project also investigated workplace relationships using a salutogenic approach [3,14,15]. In these studies, the meaning and significance of workplace relationships were investigated in relation to staff, managers, and care recipients. The findings showed key aspects of relationships in the workplace, see Table 1.

Table 1. Examples of statements made in multi-stage focus group discussions about workplace relationships with care recipients, colleagues, and managers.

Positively Experienced Relationships with Care Recipients
There is a value in sharing one's own everyday events with the care recipients.
A deeper relationship allows for more trusting conversations and is important for understanding each other's situation better.
With a deeper relationship it is easier to meet and see the care recipient's needs.
Being appreciated by the care recipient makes me feel needed and makes my work feel meaningful.
Positively Experienced Relationships with Colleagues
I feel good about having an opportunity to air my views and feelings about matters concerning the work with my colleagues.
I get a lot out of being able to feel community (trust, pride, harmony) with my colleagues.
It is important that the work flows well, and that we have good cooperation and good understanding for each other.
It is important that I feel respected by my colleagues.
Positively Experienced Relationships with Managers
I appreciate it when the manager feels like "one of the group".
It is important to me that the manager is open (e.g., dares to ask for help; is open to new suggestions and questions).
It is important that the manager delegates or leaves new tasks to me, because then I develop.
It is important that the manager listens to me and sees my work, because then I feel security/trust.
It is important that the manager gives me encouragement and motivates me, because then I become engaged.
It is important that I can see that my work is a part of a greater whole (in the organization).

In the current study, we wanted to further explore how these findings could be used for a health-promoting purpose in practice. To put previous results to practical use for the participants themselves, multi-stage focus groups were formed [32]. The multi-stage focus group method is characterized by the same group exploring a question or phenomenon in depth over the course of several meetings. Letting the same group meet multiple times allows participants to get to know each other in a deeper sense. A sense of shared history develops, which distinguishes the multi-stage focus group from a normal focus group that usually meets only once. Through multiple meetings the discussions in the group can further expand and different problems can be addressed to achieve a higher level of abstraction. Multi-stage focus groups were chosen because the method itself can contribute to emancipation within the working group through ongoing discussions. Multi-stage focus groups can also be a way to create sustainable change in the workplace, as the method recognises the local context and uses the participants' experiences. Therefore, the method was considered suitable for PAR.

During information meetings in the spring of 2015, one of the researchers (S.S.P.) verbally invited potential participants to participate, informing them about the study and handing out written information. The intention of the information meetings was to increase interest in and motivation for participating in the multi-stage focus groups. The multi-stage focus groups were conducted from September 2015 to January 2016. Each group consisted of assistant nurses from the same working groups, as the intention was to enable dialogues in which the participants would describe experiences, share thoughts, and create suggestions for how to achieve improvements. Each group met three times and between two and nine persons attended each meeting. The focus groups lasted 70–120 min and were held in meeting rooms at the participants' workplaces. One problem with multi-stage focus groups is that it cannot be expected that all participants can attend all meetings [32]. To keep everyone updated on the process, each meeting began with a brief recap of what had been discussed last time. Those who had not attended the previous meeting were given a report of what had been discussed. However, all participants in this study attended at least two of the three meetings.

As a starting point, statements about positively experienced relationships with care recipients, colleagues, and managers were used (see Table 1). Our intention with this was to let the participants choose the subjects that were most important for them to discuss in relation to workplace relationships, rather than selecting subjects that we researchers found the most interesting. The statements were based on previous studies of positively experienced workplace relationships [3,14,15].

One researcher acted as a moderator and the other researcher (either P.N.L. or K.B.) acted as an observer. The moderator (S.S.P.) steered all the multi-stage focus group discussions by asking questions about experiences of what is required for workplace relationships to flourish, and by urging the participants to make suggestions for how to improve the workplace relationships. The observer made a written summary of the content and interaction in the group, asked for clarifications, and urged reflections in the group. Both researchers did their utmost to allow all participants to speak freely but still to guide the actual content of the discussion. At the end of each focus group, the researchers made a summary of the suggestions for improvements that had emerged, and this summary was followed by a discussion within the group about how the staff could proceed to realise their suggestions in their unit.

2.3. Analysis

Initially, all the researchers read the interviews several times and discussed them together. The interview material was thereafter read with a view to identifying different kinds of relationships: relationships between caring staff colleagues within the team; relationships between the day and night shift care workers; relationships between caring staff colleagues and other occupational groups such as RNs, occupational therapists, and physiotherapists; and relationships between caring staff colleagues and the manager. Upon further examination, we saw a pattern emerge, in that the specific relationships were connected to two types of meetings: informal and formal meetings. Therefore, the material was sorted into the two content areas: Informal meetings and Formal meetings.

After reading and discussing the material further, a deductive content analysis [33] was carried out, using a modified version of Gaffney's (2015) description of the four flourishing components [26]. We related the components of Gaffney to a work situation and workplace relationship processes as follows: (1) challenges, which refers to challenging situations in everyday work that have to be faced and managed to enhance relationships;

(2) connectivity, meaning concrete actions or suggestions needed for the work relationship to be mutual; (3) autonomy, which refers to the employee's self-determination and freedom to act in work situations; and (4) competence, which relates to an expression of feeling needed and able to use personal as well as professional skills at work.

Finally, within each kind of relationship, the four key components of the concept of flourishing were applied. To identify challenges, connectivity, autonomy and competence in each relationship, the following questions were asked when examining the material: Challenges: Which relational challenges are expressed? Connectivity: Which concrete actions or suggestions are expressed, and how are the mutual relationships described? Autonomy: How is the employees' job autonomy described? Competence: Which competence is described, and how can it be used?

2.4. Ethical Considerations

The written information given to the participants covered the aim of the study, the focus for the discussions in the multi-stage focus groups, and included an assurance that participation was voluntary and that data would be handled confidentially. The researchers emphasized the importance of the discussion within the focus groups remaining confidential. This information was given again at the start of each focus group.

The participants were given the opportunity to participate by their managers, but they also had the opportunity to decline without the manager knowing about it. The study was conducted in agreement with the Swedish Ethical Review Act, SFS 2003:460, and was approved by the Ethical Review Board of Lund, Sweden (dnr: 2015/565).

3. Results

In this section, the various workplace relationships at meetings are described and how they relate to the four components of Gaffney's (2015) concept of flourishing [26]. Two main categories emerged in the analysis: Informal meetings as a prerequisite for flourishing and Formal meetings as a prerequisite for flourishing. The staff described their experiences of what was required for positive workplace relationships to occur, and also made suggestions for how to improve workplace relationships. These suggestions are presented at the end of each workplace relationship.

3.1. Informal Meetings as a Prerequisite for Flourishing

Based on the participants' descriptions, informal meetings in daily work consisted of small talk and non-work-related conversation going on all the time between people. Informal meetings took place during work but also during breaks. Our results show that most informal meetings took place (1) between caring staff colleagues; (2) between the caring staff and the RNs; and (3) between the caring staff and the manager.

3.1.1. Informal Meetings between Caring Staff Colleagues

Informal meetings between caring staff colleagues mainly occurred during breaks but sometimes also during work. Regarding the relationship between caring staff colleagues, the participants described how the challenge was to maintain good interactions with and trust between each other. Connectivity was achieved when the caring staff felt they could be open with each other and that they were able to both give and take criticism. When there was good interaction between staff, the work had more flow. Everyone took more responsibility and became more self-motivated, which contributed to increased autonomy. When the colleagues in the group knew each other, they felt more confident in work situations, as everyone's competence was better used at work. The participants described good interaction between colleagues as a resource for high quality of care, allowing everyone to use their particular competence well.

Suggestions for quality improvement were to make time for joint breaks. The participants expressed how they longed for breaks with their colleagues as this was a time to air their views and feelings, talk about difficult work situations, and have a nice time and also talk about private matters.

3.1.2. Informal Meetings between Caring Staff and Registered Nurses

Informal meetings between the caring staff and RNs occurred mainly when the RN showed up at the ward. In the relationship between caring staff and the RN, the challenge was to organize informal meetings between the two. The caring staff often perceived the RN as absent from the daily work, so that informal meetings and conversation were hard to achieve. An example of a relationship as a resource was when the RN showed up at the ward just to ask if the caring staff had any questions or support needs. Another example was when the RN was available on the phone and the caring staff felt safe to call and ask about things. Such relationships between the RN and the caring staff were considered to contribute to connectivity. With stable connectivity in the relationship, the caring staff's autonomy was considered to increase; for instance, the caring staff would feel confident about making decisions on their own if required. When the RN involved the caring staff in decisions about care recipients, they felt that their competence in the organization was not only being used but also increased. By taking advantage of the staff's joint knowledge about the care recipients, the RN made the caring staff feel needed.

A suggestion from the caring staff was to introduce a notebook at the ward as an easy way to note and collect questions or information to the RN without having to leave the ward to ask the RN for advice in every single case.

3.1.3. Informal Meetings between Caring Staff and the Manager

Informal meetings between caring staff and the manager occurred mainly during breaks. Challenges in the relationship between the caring staff and the manager were to create mutual respect between the two, to make the manager understand the importance of being fair, and for the manager to treat everyone equally and to express their expectations clearly. The participants said that when the manager dared to be a manager with clear directives, and when expectations were clearly stated, this created connectivity between the caring staff and the manager. When the caring staff felt respected and taken seriously, and when the manager showed respect for the caring staff's thoughts by listening and being part of the work group, autonomy was strengthened. When the manager asked the caring staff for their opinions, the participants felt that their competence was put to use in the organization and that their knowledge was considered important.

A suggestion from the caring staff was that the manager should have more open discussions with the caring staff, for instance, about planning and routines for temporary staff.

3.2. Formal Meetings as a Prerequisite for Flourishing

According to the participants, formal meetings had a defined time and agenda. Formal meetings were staff meetings, care planning meetings. and daily report meetings. Formal meetings were held: (1) between the caring staff colleagues; (2) between day and night shift workers; (3) between the caring staff and other occupational groups; and (4) between the caring staff and the manager.

3.2.1. Formal Meetings between Caring Staff Colleagues

Formal meetings between caring staff colleagues were mainly staff meetings. One challenge was to plan formal meetings with time to talk about issues in the caring staff group's daily work and routines. In other words, the caring staff needed their own time to talk about matters that were important to them without the manager present. To have the opportunity to discuss freely was described to contribute to connectivity. By discussing work routines and their caring activities, the participants felt that they grew as professionals together. They also said that discussions between colleagues contributed to autonomy. It was described that the "any other matters" item on the agenda at staff meetings provided an opportunity to speak as a group, which increased the caring staff's ability to use their competence at work in a better way.

A suggestion from the participants was that they should have their own time at staff meetings, without the manager present, to be able to address issues that only concerned the caring staff.

3.2.2. Formal Meetings between Day and Night Shift Caring Staff

Formal meetings between day and night shift staff were mainly care planning meetings. However, they were difficult to arrange because of different working hours and therefore were rarely scheduled. A challenge between night and day staff was to be open to each other's different work situations. Many routines hindered an understanding of each other's different work circumstances, but also led to an unawareness of each other's work. Another challenge was to create a sense of belonging between the night and day shifters. Even if they were working in the same place and with the same care recipients, the participants did not really feel that they were a united team. When the overlap between night and day shift worked well and the groups sat down together to review what had happened during their shift, feelings of connectivity between the night and day staff arose. Autonomy was increased when the meeting between night and day staff provided an opportunity to talk about something that had happened and to explain, or get an understanding of, why a task (e.g., cleaning) had not been performed.

A suggestion was to arrange discussions between day and night staff to adopt common goals and missions and make everyone aware of the importance of a common approach, not only for their own wellbeing but also for the benefit of the care recipients. By discussing these issues, everyone's competence could be strengthened. A further suggestion from the participants, regarding how the relationship could be strengthened and used as a resource, was that working hours between shifts should overlap a bit more to give a better opportunity to meet and talk to each other, now this time was experienced as too short.

3.2.3. Formal Meetings between Caring Staff and Other Occupational Groups

Formal meetings between caring staff and other occupational groups largely consisted of care planning meetings. In the relationship between the caring staff group and other occupational groups such as RNs, coordinators, physiotherapists, occupational therapists, and staff at the hospital, the challenge was to create respectful verbal and also written communication. Cooperation and discussions with professionals from other occupational groups at formal meetings were found to contribute to connectivity.

Suggestions for how to improve connectivity were to have structured follow-ups and dialogues about the caring work together with other occupational groups. When these dialogues worked well, the feeling of participation and autonomy increased. The participants suggested, in addition, regular common discussions about how staff should act in difficult work situations, and clearly stated routines and values when the caring staff had to make their own decisions in challenging work situations. The participants expressed a desire to use their caring competence by cooperating with other occupational groups and believed this would be a way to improve the quality of care.

Other suggestions from the caring staff were to preserve and develop the meetings with the RN on a weekly basis, focusing on individual care recipients, and that the RN should be present in the mornings at the overlap meetings between night and day shifters.

3.2.4. Formal Meetings between Caring Staff and the Manager

Formal meetings between the caring staff and the manager mainly took place at staff meetings. The challenge in formal meetings with the manager was to save meeting time during staff meetings to talk about important matters, mainly relating to how to improve the care of the care recipients. However, the participants said that much time during these meetings was spent on financial and information issues, which was not always perceived as the most important by the caring staff. Another challenge was to get the manager to stick to decisions and provide the same information to all the working groups, as they did not have staff meetings together. A manager who took the experience of the staff into consideration during discussions was regarded as contributing to connectivity between them. When they felt listened to, the participants experienced that their autonomy was strengthened. If the manager discussed their work and work situation with them, their skills could be better used in their work and they thereby felt that their competence was used.

A suggestion from the caring staff was that the manager could provide more written information instead of oral information during staff meetings. This would make more time available for important discussions between the manager and the caring staff about the care recipients and the daily caring work and aspects of the work situation.

In summary, a methodological result of the study process with multi-stage focus group meetings is that this method had an emancipatory effect, as all participating groups decided to proceed with their own suggestions and tried to put them into action at their wards. In order to give an overview on concrete examples of improvements, we condensed all the staff's suggestions and related them to the various relationships, and informal or formal meeting type (see Table 2).

Table 2. The two categories of meetings that lead to flourishing of different work relationships, and participants' (condensed) suggestions for improvement work.

Categories	Improvement Suggestions
Informal meetings:	
Between caring staff colleagues	There should be time for joint breaks, as these allowed time for the staff to air their views and feelings about what needed to be talked about.
Between caring staff and RNs	An information notebook should be introduced at the ward as an easy way for staff to access information.
Between caring staff and the manager	The manager should coordinate with the caring staff, for instance, about planning and routines for temporary staff.
Formal meetings:	
Between caring staff colleagues	The caring staff should have their own time at staff meetings, without the manager present.
Between day and night shift caring staff	Working hours should overlap more, to give the opportunity for dialogue.
Between caring staff and other occupational groups	Meetings about the caring work should be held on a weekly basis with focus on individual care recipients, with structured follow-ups.
Between caring staff and the manager	The manager should provide more written information to give time for discussions about the care recipients and the daily work.

Note: Registered nurses (RNs).

4. Discussion

Positive relationships characterized by challenge, connectivity, autonomy, and competence could have an enhancing effect on employees' health and could be useful as a starting point in workplace health promotion to develop a flourishing workplace for care professionals. To achieve this, conditions need to be created for both informal and formal meetings based on the staff's experience.

Informal and formal meetings with colleagues, other occupational groups and the manager are important for enhancing employee health. While the informal meetings in this study group were important for the ability to exchange information and make everyday decisions, the formal meetings had a predetermined agenda and gave an opportunity to discuss issues relating to the care recipients. A common factor in informal and formal meetings was the experience of support and belonging, and being able to exchange thoughts and share feelings in the different meetings. This was important, not only for job performance, but also for well-being at work. This supports previous research suggesting that a workplace atmosphere that allows open-mindedness and a positive social climate is a resource for making work comprehensive, manageable, and meaningful [2]. Furthermore, in order to create sustainable workplaces and an organization with flourishing individuals, it is important to build a work structure based on positive relationships [13,27,34,35]. To achieve this, well-thought-out strategies for informal and formal meetings in the workplace are required.

Strong relationships with colleagues and managers and positive relationships with care recipients are closely linked. Our results showed that positive informal and formal meetings seemed to have a dual purpose. They made the staff themselves flourish at their workplace, but they were also a prerequisite for providing good care and having positive relationships with care recipients, which was also central to their own well-being. In the focus groups, the caring staff rarely talked about relationships with care recipients. Instead, they spoke about relationships with colleagues, professionals from other occupations, and managers. The caring staff chose to talk about their workplace relationships, not primarily to improve their own well-being but to achieve improved relationships with care recipients as a way of providing better care, which ultimately improved their own well-being. In human care professions, when employees are faced with high emotional demands [34], awareness of types of work relationships and why they function as a resource and as a prerequisite for flourishing is valuable.

A salutogenic approach to workplace health needs to emphasise positive relationships based on respect, security, and reciprocity. One interpretation of our study results is that there existed more of a "we-feeling" between caring colleagues working the same shift and more of an "us-and them feeling" between people from different shifts and representing different care professions. The we-feeling contributed to togetherness among the caring staff and created flow and confidence at informal meetings. This "we-feeling" of togetherness also contributed to good formal meetings because of respect, security, and strong reciprocity. Such a sense of belonging and security has also been shown in previous research [3] to contribute to well-being as well as recognition of self-worth. On the other hand, the results in this study also showed more of an "us-and-them feeling" in the relationships with caring staff from other shifts, the manager, and other occupational care groups. Hence, a major part of the challenge of turning the relationships with the manager and other occupational care groups into a resource seemed to lie with the organizational structure, as physical meetings in daily situations were sometimes considered inadequate. If an organization relies on interactions between people, relationships should be emphasized as more important to the organization than, for instance, organizational principles and structures [36]. By using the relationships as a tool for the development of the organization and by having a less hierarchical structure—a structure that is based on a democratic mindset between different professions—everyone's competence can be anchored in the overall organization and everyone can work towards the same goal [35]. This salutogenic approach may in turn benefit the flourishing of the individuals, and the organization [27,28].

4.1. Practical and Theoretical Implications

In this study with a salutogenic and a participatory design, practical and theoretical implications where deeply intertwined. A theoretical implication is that the concept of flourishing, and its four specific components, can be used in practice to identify, interpret, and explain positive relationships, and situations and elements of a workplace that affect employee health. The components of flourishing have links to the three components of motivational needs in Ryan and Deci's Self-Determination Theory (2000): autonomy, competence, and belongingness [37]. These three components create inner motivation for the individual to act in situations or in relationships that are important for health experience and well-being. There is also a connection between the concept flourishing and the model of person-centredness [28]. Person-centredness is usually discussed in relation to care, but an organization can also work in a person-centred manner with its employees and in the organization of work. Different dimensions of relationships at work become important to understand and improve, as relationships are vital for flourishing. Healthful relationships among employees may thereby also contribute to a person-centredness culture.

A practical implication is to use meetings, both formal and informal, as a means to enhance relationships in everyday practice. Conditions for meetings provide the opportunity for people to share experiences and get to know each other in the work group, which in itself contributes to a health-promoting workplace [14,15,38]. Using the concept of flourishing both in the planning of work tasks and in issues concerning the psychosocial work environment, could contribute to a flourishing and sustainable workplace. Using the four components in formal meetings enables the creation of a clear model to show what challenges and suggestions have emerged, and thus makes it possible to develop connectivity, autonomy, and use of competence in an optimal way. The identified challenges and suggestions for improvements can, for instance, undergo process evaluation at the staff meetings, in order to make the relationships a resource for the flourishing of individuals and the organization alike. It is advantageous to base dialogues on the four flourishing components to highlight both the salutogenic aspects and the challenges to creating a sustainable workplace that causes the individual workers to flourish. Previous research about using dialogue as a tool has shown that a structured dialogue model makes it easier to notice what is happening in daily work relations and provides the possibility to work in a promoting way [38].

Furthermore, a practical implication of informal meetings is to create conditions for things such as joint breaks. Conditions for informal meetings contribute to the opportunity for the staff to share their thoughts and feelings about different work situations. This promotes social relationships and the opportunity to give each other more support in everyday practice. Relationships can function as a job resource that helps employees to manage strain and job demands [39]. Especially in human-related work, such as healthcare, work tasks are often challenging and energy-draining, on the one hand, and energy-giving through daily human meetings, on the other [34].

Regardless of the subject, dialogue is essential in research with a salutogenic and participatory approach. In this study the dialogues in the multi-stage focus groups developed during the study process and had the effect that all groups decided to proceed with the suggestions and try to put them into action. Our interpretation is that the groups themselves, based on the participatory approach, were an enhancing action for the workplace relationships among the healthcare staff. This further justifies dialogue as useful in improvement work to achieve a health-promoting workplace. This should be taken into account in public health and workplace health promotion, considering society's rationalisation efforts, according to which, meetings should be minimized and must be effective and production-oriented.

4.2. Limitations and Trustworthiness

The methodological aspects of credibility, dependability, and transferability need to be considered for a study to be seen as trustworthy [40]. From a credibility perspective, multi-stage focus groups were considered appropriate for this study, as it was hoped they would create a reflective environment for the participants, be emancipatory, and yield detailed data. Although a situation where the participants know each other very well can lead to a lack of discussion, a sense of security within the group facilitates a trustful discussion where participants feel free to share their feelings, thoughts, and perceptions [41]. If the study is to be repeated in the future, the focus group method may need to be modified according to any current pandemic restrictions, for example, by offering digital participation or smaller group sizes. Results obtained using a deductive analysis approach can be questioned from a credibility point of view [40], as the deductive analysis brings a risk that unexpected results may be neglected. However, the participants' reflections and suggestions were often unexpected. Among the unexpected results was the large gap in the relationship between night and day staff. We were also surprised that the relationship with care recipients was hardly discussed. At the meetings, the participants instead focused on the relationship with their colleagues since a good relationship with their colleagues and the manager was a prerequisite for good care and a positive relationship with their care recipients. Being a study with a participatory approach, the weakest part is perhaps the lack of follow-up of whether the participants' suggestions for changes were introduced and how they turned out. This weakness was due to limited time for the project.

The researchers have nursing and public health backgrounds, which strengthens the credibility as it enhanced the possibility to see things from different perspectives. The fact that all researchers participated in the analysis and that there was high agreement between them also strengthens the study's credibility. Similar issues were discussed in the four focus groups, which demonstrates dependability. The transferability of the results is enhanced by descriptions of the study context, the participants, and the procedure and analysis process [40].

5. Conclusions

In view of the increased rationalization in society, in which meetings are minimized and are required to be strictly effective and production-oriented, our results regarding the importance of informal and formal meetings and work relationships need to be taken into account if we aim to create sustainable health-promoting workplaces. This study contributes to workplace health promotion research with its salutogenic and participatory approach and represents a new opportunity to explore and understand workplace relationships as a resource by strengthening, or maintaining, positive activities and processes. It is therefore vital to develop dialogues about relationship processes, and raise awareness of the importance of different relationships for improving the work situation and healthcare. The study also shows that the components of flourishing could be used to create a model for such dialogues. Taking the employees' own experiences into account in group dialogues seems to improve employee engagement and could be a fruitful way to conduct workplace health promotion interventions. However, further studies are required to explore the utility of our results in intervention studies, in various workplace settings, between night and day shifts, and among different occupational groups.

Author Contributions: Conceptualization, S.S.P., K.B. and P.N.L.; methodology, S.S.P., K.B. and P.N.L.; formal analysis, S.S.P., K.B. and P.N.L.; writing—original draft preparation, S.S.P.; writing—review and editing, K.B. and P.N.L.; supervision, K.B. and P.N.L. All authors have read and agreed to the published version of the manuscript.

Funding: This research received no external funding.

Institutional Review Board Statement: The study was conducted according to the guidelines of the Declaration of Helsinki, and approved by the Ethical Review Board of Lund, Sweden (dnr: 2015/565).

Informed Consent Statement: Informed consent was obtained from all subjects involved in the study.

Data Availability Statement: Not applicable.

Acknowledgments: We would like to thank all the healthcare staff who participated in this study. We would also like to thank the research platform Collaboration for Health at Kristianstad University, Kristianstad, Sweden, for financial support.

Conflicts of Interest: The authors declare no conflict of interest.

References

1. Lindmark, U.; Wagman, P.; Wåhlin, C.; Rolander, B. Workplace health in dental care—A salutogenic approach. *Int. J. Dent. Hyg.* **2016**, *16*, 103–113. [CrossRef]
2. Nilsson, P.; Andersson, I.; Ejlertsson, G.; Troein, M. Workplace health resources based on sense of coherence theory. *Int. J. Work. Health Manag.* **2012**, *5*, 156–167. [CrossRef]
3. Persson, S.S.; Lindström, P.N.; Pettersson, P.; Andersson, I. Workplace relationships impact self-rated health: A survey among Swedish municipal healthcare employees. *WORK J.Prev. Assess. Rehabil.* **2017**, *60*, 85–94. [CrossRef]
4. Bringsén, Å.; Andersson, I.; Ejlertsson, G.; Troein, M. Exploring workplace related health resources from a salutogenic perspective. *WORK J.Prev. Assess. Rehabil.* **2012**, *42*, 403–414.
5. Häusser, J.A.; Mojzisch, A.; Niesel, M. Ten years on: A review of recent research on the Job Demand-Control (-Support) model and psychological well-being. *Work Stress* **2010**, *24*, 1–35. [CrossRef]

6. Antonovsky, A. The salutogenic model as a theory to guide health promotion. *Health Promot. Int.* **1996**, *11*, 11–18. [CrossRef]
7. Bauer, G.; Davies, J.K.; Pelikan, J. The EUHPID Health development model for the classification of public health indicators. *Health Promot. Int.* **2006**, *21*, 153–159. [CrossRef] [PubMed]
8. Clausen, T.; Tufte, P.; Borg, V. Why are they leaving? Causes of actual turnover in the Danish eldercare services. *J. Nurs. Manag.* **2014**, *22*, 583–592. [CrossRef] [PubMed]
9. Heinen, M.M.; van Achterberg, T.; Schwendimann, R.; Zander, B.; Matthews, A.; Kózka, M.; Ensio, A.; Sjetne, I.S.; Casbas, T.M.; Ball, J.; et al. Nurses' intention to leave their profession: A cross sectional observational study in 10 European countries. *Int. J. Nurs. Stud.* **2013**, *50*, 174–184. [CrossRef]
10. Kouvonen, A.; Oksanen, T.; Vahtera, J.; Stafford, M.; Wilkinson, R.; Schneider, J.; Väänänen, A.; Virtanen, M.; Cox, S.J.; Pentti, J.; et al. Low workplace social capital as a predictor of depression: The Finnish public sector study. *Am. J. Epidemiol.* **2008**, *167*, 1143–1151. [CrossRef]
11. Schaufeli, W.B.; Bakker, A.B.; Salanova, M. The measurement of work engagement with a short questionnaire. A cross-national study. *Educ. Psychol. Meas.* **2006**, *66*, 701–716. [CrossRef]
12. Jenny, G.J.; Bauer, G.F.; Vinje, H.F.; Vogt, K.; Torp, S. The Application of Salutogenesis to Work. In *The Handbook of Salutogenesis*; Mittelmark, M.B., Sagy, S., Eriksson, M., Bauer, G.F., Pelikan, J.M., Lindström, B., Espnes, G.A., Eds.; Springer: Cham, Switzerland, 2017; pp. 197–210.
13. Nilsson, K. A sustainable working life for all ages—The swAge-model. *Appl. Ergon.* **2020**, *86*, 103082. [CrossRef] [PubMed]
14. Persson, S.S.; Nilsson Lindström, P.; Pettersson, P.; Andersson, I.; Blomqvist, K. Relationships between healthcare employees and managers as a resource for well-being at work. *Soc. Health Vulnerability* **2018**, *9*, 1547035. [CrossRef]
15. Persson, S.S.; Nilsson Lindström, P.; Pettersson, P.; Nilsson, M.; Blomqvist, K. Resources for work-related well-being: A qualitative study about healthcare employees' experiences of relationships at work. *J. Clin. Nurs.* **2018**, *27*, 4302–4310. [CrossRef]
16. Dutton, J.E.; Ragins, B.R. *Exploring Positive Relationships at Work: Building a Theoretical and Research Foundation*; Psychology Press: Hove, UK, 2007.
17. Rousseau, D.M.; Ling, K. Commentary: Following the resources in positive organizational relationships. In *Exploring Positive Relationships at Work: Building a Theoretical and Research Foundation*; Dutton, J.E., Ragins, B.R., Eds.; Lawrence Erlbaum and Associates: Mahwah, NJ, USA, 2007; pp. 373–384.
18. Gharaveis, A.; Hamilton, D.K.; Pati, D. The impact of environmental design on teamwork and communication in healthcare facilities: A systematic literature review. *HERD* **2018**, *11*, 119–137. [CrossRef] [PubMed]
19. Orrung-Wallin, A.; Jakobsson, U.; Edberg, A.-K. Job satisfaction and associated variables among nurse assistants working in residential care. *Int. Psychogeriatr.* **2012**, *24*, 1904–1918. [CrossRef]
20. Feeney, B.C.; Collins, N.L. A new look at social support: A theoretical perspective on thriving through relationships. *Personal. Soc. Psychol. Rev.* **2014**, *19*, 113–147. [CrossRef]
21. Nappo, N. Job stress and interpersonal relationships cross country evidence from the EU15. A correlation analysis. *BMC Public Health* **2020**, *20*. [CrossRef] [PubMed]
22. Tourangeau, A.; Cranley, L.; Laschinger, H.K.S.; Pachis, J. Relationships among leadership practices, work environments, staff communication and outcomes in long-term care. *J. Nurs. Manag.* **2010**, *18*, 1060–1072. [CrossRef]
23. Keyes, C.L.M. Promoting and protecting mental health as flourishing. *Am. Psychol.* **2007**, *62*, 95–108. [CrossRef]
24. Seligman, M.E. *Flourish: A Visionary New Understanding of Happiness and Well-Being*; Free Press: New York, NY, USA, 2012.
25. McCormack, B.; Titchen, A. No beginning, no end: An ecology of human flourishing. *Int. Pract. Dev. J.* **2014**, *4*, 2. [CrossRef]
26. Gaffney, M. *Flourishing: How to Achieve a Deeper Sense of Well-Being, Meaning and Purpose—Even When Facing Adversity*; Penguin: London, UK, 2015.
27. Colbert, A.E.; Bono, J.E.; Purvanova, R.K. Flourishing via workplace relationships: Moving beyond instrumental support. *Acad. Manag. J.* **2016**, *59*, 1199–1223. [CrossRef]
28. Dewing, J.; McCormack, B. Creating flourishing workplaces. In *Person-Centred Practice in Nursing and Health Care: Theory and Practice*, 2nd ed.; McCormack, B., McCance, T., Eds.; John Wiley & Sons, Ltd.: Hoboken, NJ, USA, 2017; pp. 150–161.
29. Swedish Association of Local Authorities and Regions. *Öppna Jämförelser 2020. Vård Och Omsorg Om Äldre*; Socialstyrelsen: Stockholm, Sweden, 2021. (In Swedish)
30. Socialstyrelsen. *Tillståndet Och Utvecklingen Inom Hälso- Och Sjukvård Och Socialtjänst: Lägesrapport 2015*; Socialstyrelsen: Stockholm, Sweden, 2015. (In Swedish)
31. Stringer, E.; Genat, W. *Action Research in Health*; Merrill Prentice Hall: Hoboken, NJ, USA, 2004.
32. Hummelvoll, J.K. The multistage focus group interview: A relevant and fruitful method in action research based on a co-operative inquiry perspective. *Nor. Tidsskr. Sykepl.* **2008**, *10*, 3–14.
33. Elo, S.; Kyngäs, H. The qualitative content analysis process. *J. Adv. Nurs.* **2008**, *62*, 107–115. [CrossRef] [PubMed]
34. Sias, P.M. *Organizing Relationships: Traditional and Emerging Perspectives on Workplace Relationships*; Sage Publications Inc.: Thousand Oaks, CA, USA, 2009.
35. Cohen, S.; Gottlieb, B.; Underwood, L. Social relationships and health. In *Measuring and Intervening in Social Support*; Cohen, S., Underwood, L., Gottlieb, B., Eds.; Oxford University Press: Oxford, UK, 2000; pp. 3–25.
36. Hobfoll, S.E. Social and psychological resources and adaptation. *Rev. Gen. Psychol.* **2002**, *6*, 307–324. [CrossRef]

37. Ryan, R.M.; Deci, E.L. Self-determination theory and the facilitation of intrinsic motivation, social development, and well-being. *Am. Psychol.* **2000**, *55*, 68–78. [CrossRef]
38. Nilsson, P.; Andersson, H.I.; Ejlertsson, G.; Blomqvist, K. How to make a workplace health promotion questionnaire process applicable, meaningful, and sustainable. *J. Nurs. Manag.* **2011**, *19*, 906–914. [CrossRef]
39. Bakker, A.B.; Demerouti, E. The Job Demands-Resources model: State of the art. *J. Manag. Psychol.* **2007**, *22*, 309–328. [CrossRef]
40. Graneheim, U.H.; Lundman, B. Qualitative content analysis in nursing research: Concepts, procedures and measures to achieve trustworthiness. *Nurse Educ. Today* **2004**, *24*, 105–112. [CrossRef]
41. Krueger, R.; Casey, M. *Focus Groups A Practical Guide for Applied Research*; Sage Publications: Thousand Oaks, CA, USA, 2009.

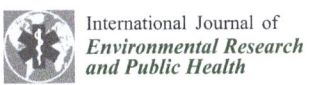

International Journal of
Environmental Research and Public Health

Article

Nurses' Work-Related Mental Health in 2017 and 2020—A Comparative Follow-Up Study before and during the COVID-19 Pandemic

Cicilia Nagel [1,2,*] and Kerstin Nilsson [1,2]

1. Division of Occupational and Environmental Medicine, Department of Laboratory Medicine, Lund University, 22184 Lund, Sweden
2. Division of Public Health, Kristianstad University, 29128 Kristianstad, Sweden
* Correspondence: cicilia.nagel@hkr.se; Tel.: +46-402-503-623

Abstract: The COVID-19 pandemic put a lot of strain on healthcare organizations. Nurses account for over 50% of healthcare staff, and how nurses perform in their work is influenced by a number of human and work environmental factors. However, to our knowledge, there has not been a previous study with the intention to look at all areas that affect a sustainable working life and how these impact nurses' mental well-being. The aim of this study is to investigate the association between, and the effect of, different factors in nurses' work situations associated with nurses' work-related mental-health diagnoses, before and during the COVID-19 pandemic. A questionnaire was sent out to all 9219 nurses in the Swedish county of Skane in the spring of 2017 and during wave two of the COVID-19 pandemic in the fall of 2020. The data were analyzed through logistic regression analysis. The results showed that lack of joy in the daily work, an increased workload and lack of support from co-workers had an increased association with work-related mental-health diagnoses. Future research regarding the long-term impact of COVID-19 on all areas of nurses' professional and personal lives is needed.

Keywords: work-related; mental-health diagnoses; work situation; work environment; nurses

1. Introduction

Healthcare workers around the world, primarily the nurses, were on the frontline of the Coronavirus pandemic that started in 2019 [1]. The second wave of the pandemic in Sweden occurred during the fall/winter 2020, the most serious wave of the pandemic regarding the burden on the healthcare sector. The pandemic has been described as a gigantic strain experiment on healthcare organizations, especially on healthcare staff due to exposure to hazards, such as psychological distress, fatigue, and trauma [1–5]. Healthcare workers had to perform their duties and face higher risks to their own health, such as the risk of infection [1]. Many nurses were afraid to become ill and die of COVID-19, which was incredibly stressful [6].

Nurses comprise half of the global health workforce [7,8]; however, for much of the general public, it is not fully understood what nurses do. Being a nurse includes promoting health, preventing illness as well as caring for people who are ill, disabled and dying. Advocating patients' rights, promoting a safe environment, conducting and/or taking part in research and education are also key nursing roles [9]. Nurses are often the first healthcare staff that the patient encounters. Their roles may vary depending on workplace, but often include triage, early recognition of life-threatening conditions, administration of medications, performance of life-saving procedures and initiation of early referral [7]. Despite nurses being a common profession in healthcare, there is an increasing demand for nurses worldwide [8]. According to the World Health Organization (WHO) [7], one out of six of the world's nurses are expected to retire in the next 10 years. Several countries experienced

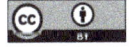

a lack of healthcare workers prior to the pandemic and many nurses are considering leaving the profession [10]. There is a serious nursing shortage in most European countries, which is insufficient to meet current healthcare demands [11,12]. Due to an ageing population, healthcare demands are predicted to increase, resulting in an estimated worldwide shortage of almost 6 million nurses by 2035 [7]. The ageing segment of the population is rapidly expanding and, thus, consuming more health services. Unfortunately, fewer new nurses are entering the work force; therefore, providing a healthy work environment to retain nurses in their workplace is essential for sustaining the profession [13].

Being able to work has a significant positive impact on people's health, and healthy workplaces are beneficial not only for employees but also for organizations and for society [14]. Decent work is one of the UN Global Goals for sustainable society development [15]. A sustainable work situation for employees is significant for a healthy organization that attracts people to work as well as promoting better health for employees, thus, also giving a better possibility for employability to an increased age [16–19]. Working in a hospital can be complicated due to the interaction between patients, nurses and the organization. This can, under normal circumstances, cause problematic work situations, but during the pandemic this was likely even more of a factor. It is, therefore, important to detect problems and shortcomings in the work situation in order to improve and support healthy and sustainable employability and understand what measures need to be taken. Areas of employability, and whether individuals can and want to work or not, has been stated as nine impact and determinant areas connected to sustainable healthy working life in the SwAge-model [6,16–19], i.e., (1) the employees self-rated health and diagnoses; (2) factors in the physical work environment; (3) factors in the mental work environment; (4) having time for recuperation within the employees' working hours, breaks and work pace; (5) the personal financial situation; (6) the employees' personal social environment outside of work; (7) the work social environment at the workplace, with leadership, colleagues, etcetera; (8) factors related to whether the employee experiences stimulation and motivation within work tasks and appreciation from the organization/work place regarding their performed tasks; (9) if the employees' have the right competence, skills and possibility for knowledge development in work.

As earlier mentioned, nurses play a key role in delivering care to patients [11]. How the nurses perform in their work environment is influenced by a number of human and environmental factors, including the type of information available, work experience, ambiguity, unpredictability, conflicting goals and time pressure [20]. Nurses face a higher risk of developing negative mental states, such as depression, anxiety and stress [21], due to the nature of their work. Unlike depression, burnout is specific to an individual's relationship to his or her occupation and usually results from long-term exposure to occupational stress [22]. Burnout may lead to adverse outcomes, such as medical errors, suicide, depression and absenteeism [23,24]. It is known that stress and burnout are factors that can contribute to a decreased mental health [10,25]. The ICN [26] states that long and stressful shifts severely impact nurses' mental health, resulting in nurses leaving or planning to leave the profession. Stress and burnout were recognized internationally as work hazards for nurses even before the pandemic [27]. Some argue that burnout in itself is a form of mental illness. However, a more common assumption has been that burnout causes mental dysfunction, such as anxiety and depression [28]. Temporal, physical, emotional and mental workloads, as well as job stressors such as time pressure, have in previous studies been positively associated with negative stress and burnout symptoms [28,29]. Previous studies have stated that nurses' work environments contribute to high stress, job dissatisfaction and burnout [30,31]. Additionally, a previous study also stated that healthcare professionals (HCPs) in hospitals engage in many work-related tasks and experience relatively high levels of mental stress while caring for patients [32], while another study showed that workload and work pressure have an impact on job outcomes and quality of care [33]. Problems within the nurses' working environments are described as concerns over inadequate staffing, ability to provide safe care, working long hours with high levels of fatigue and a sense of not being valued or involved in decision-making processes concerning patients [34–36]. Mental ill health has, in previous studies, been associated with different factors, such as long hours worked, work overload and work pressure, lack of control over work, lack of participation in decision making, poor social support as well as poor support from managers and an unclear work role [10,28,37]. Repeated exposure to stressful patient-related situations makes nurses especially susceptible to stress-related outcomes, such as emotional exhaustion and post-traumatic stress disorder (PTSD) [38]. Stress-related outcomes in nurses can lead to grave consequences, including depression, lower job satisfaction, increased risk of medical errors, lower productivity and higher turnover intentions [28]. Ignoring the signs of anxiety and depression presented by nursing professionals could increase physical and emotional stress for the individual but could also result in low quality patient care and higher work burden on the organizations [18].

However, even though there are investigations into nurses' stress related to health and work environment, to our knowledge, there are no previous investigations on nurses´ total work situation, i.e., that investigates all areas of impact and determination for a sustainable working life, before and during the COVID-19 pandemic. It is, therefore, important to investigate what effect the COVID-19 pandemic had on healthcare organizations' impact and determinant areas associated with nurses´ work-related mental health diagnoses.

The objective of this present study is to investigate the association between work-related mental-health diagnoses and different factors in nurses' work situations before and during the COVID-19 pandemic. We want to test the hypothesis that there are no differences in nurses' work related mental-health diagnoses in 2017 and 2020. The specific research questions are:

- Is there a difference between 2017 and 2020 regarding nurses' work-related mental health?
- What associations are there between nurses' work-related mental health and their work situation in 2017?
- What associations are there between nurses' work-related mental health and their work situation in 2020, that is, during the COVID-19 pandemic?

This study also wants to increase knowledge and suggest measures against staff shortages and future challenges in healthcare.

2. Materials and Methods

2.1. Design

This longitudinal study is part of a greater research programme, "Sustainable working life for all ages" [19,39]. In the spring of 2017, a baseline survey was performed where links to an online survey were sent out to all healthcare staff in the Swedish Region of Skane via their work e-mail. The follow-up study was performed in the fall of 2020, where all healthcare staff who were employed in 2017 and that were still employed in 2020 were invited to partake in the online survey.

2.2. Study Population

A link to a web survey was sent out via work e-mail to all employees in the Healthcare sector in the Swedish region of Skane, that is to all physiotherapists, occupational therapists, doctors, psychologists, nurses (including specialties such as midwife, CRNA, O.R nurse), nurse aids, etc. In total, the link to the 2017 survey was sent out to 22,935 employees, out of which 11,902 completed the survey. In this study, we will look specifically at nurses. In 2017 there were 9219 nurses (including specialist nurses) employed in the region, out of which 4692 completed the survey (50.9%). Some of the reasons for not answering the survey were wrong e-mail address, absence from work, lack of time and concerns about the manager finding out what they wrote. In 2020, data was collected via web-survey from the same study group during the second Covid 19-pandemic wave in Sweden, i.e., from September to December. Again, all healthcare staff who were employed in 2017 and that were still employed in 2020 were invited by e-mail to partake in the study. The survey link was sent out to all 18,143 staff, out of which 7781 participants responded. The number of nurses completing the web survey in 2020 was 3107 (40.1%). Some of the reasons for not responding to the survey were the same as in 2017, but there were also many nurses who stated that they wanted to prioritize their work and some nurses that had left the region.

Of the 4692 participants in the 2017 survey, the median age of the participants was 48 (23–67) and among the 3107 participants in 2020 it was 52 (26–70). In 2017, 90.4% who answered the questionnaire were women and in 2020 that number was 90.5%. A large majority (54.1% vs. 59.4% respectively in 2017 and 2020) of participants had worked as nurses for more than 16 years.

2.3. Themes in the Analysis Model

The theoretical SwAge-model (sustainable working life for all ages) [17–19] was used as the theme areas in the analysis with the intention of investigating factors concerning the complexity of the nurses' work situations that could relate to their mental diagnoses caused by their work life and work environment. The SwAge-model consists of nine different impact and determinant areas that are important for a healthy and sustainable working life for all ages, and the four spheres of determination regarding employability. These four spheres and the nine impact and determinant areas are:

I. The health effects of the work environment, which include the following areas of determination:
   (1) Self-rated health, diagnoses and diverse physical and mental health functionality in work;
   (2) Physical work environment with unilateral movements, heavy lifting, risk of accidents, climate, chemical exposure and risk of contagion;
   (3) Mental work environment: stress and fatigue syndrome, threats and violence;
   (4) Working hours, work pace and possibility of recuperation during and between work shifts.

II. Financial incentives are associated with society's control of various financial motivations, such as through the social insurance system. Financial incentives include the following determinant area:
   (5) The personal financial situation's effects on individuals' needs and willingness to work. Issues with employability due to ill health and lack of support can jeopardize inclusion in working life and cause an inferior financial situation for the individual, e.g., through sick leave, unemployment and early retirement.

III. Relationships, social support and participation, i.e., attitudes in the social context in which the individual finds himself/herself, whether the individual feels included or excluded in the group and receives satisfactory social support from the environment when needed, which includes the following areas of determination:
   (6) The effects of the personal social environment with family, friends and in the leisure context;
   (7) The social work environment with leadership, discrimination and the significance of the employment relationship context for individuals' work.

IV. Performance of duties and activities relating to individual and instrumental support, which includes the following areas of determination:
   (8) Motivation, appreciation, satisfaction and stimulation when performing the work tasks;
   (9) Knowledge, skills, competence and competence development.

Seven out of the nine impact and determinate areas in the SwAge-model were used as independent variables in this investigation to analyze factors in the nurses' work situation associated with work-related mental health diagnoses. The Health (1) area was used as the outcome/dependent variable in the analysis, i.e., mental health diagnoses caused by the work situation. However, the Personal finances (5) area was excluded since there were no data on the nurses' private economic situation related to the work situation that could be used in the analysis.

2.4. Outcome Measures

The dependent variable was initially two individual statements: "I have a current diagnosis of exhaustion/stress" and "I have a current diagnosis of depression/anxiety". These individual statements were put together into one variable regarding their work-related mental-health diagnoses as an outcome measure. The self-reported doctor's diagnoses included in mental health were depression, anxiety, exhaustion and stress. The response options in the survey regarding diagnoses were taken from WHO's ICD-10 codes.

The independent variables used in the univariate estimates and multivariate models were calculated using a categorical variable of diagnoses caused by work, i.e., mental health, as the outcome measures in association with the seven determinate areas for a healthy and sustainable worklife and employability in the SwAge-model that have been used in previous studies investigating factors associated to a sustainable working life (see above).

2.5. Questionns and Statments

The questionnaires were written in Swedish and contained 158 questions based on the SwAge-model that has been used in different investigations since 2004 [19]. However, in the questionnaire that was sent out in the second pandemic wave in 2020, additional questions about the COVID-19 situation were added. Some questions were simple yes/no questions and some were open answer questions where the participants could write freely. Most questions were designed as statements, a validated Lickert scale was used, and the participants had four answer options ranging from fully agree (1–2, i.e., Fully agree, partly agree) to fully disagree (3–4, i.e., partly disagree, fully disagree). The sample data was collected and handled by researcher KN. In the present study, 24 statements sorted into seven of the determinate areas of the SwAge-model were used.

2.6. Statistical Analyses

Logistic regression analysis was used to test models to predict categorial outcomes and to assess how well a predictor variable associates with a categorial dependent variable [40]. The material was analyzed with the IBM SPSS software, version 27. Data are presented as odds ratios (ORs) with their 95% confidence intervals (CIs). Questions with four answer options were dichotomized for clear distinction of the participants' experiences. A multivariate analysis of variance (MANOVA) was performed comparing and testing the statistical significance of the multivariate sample mean differences to see which statements in the multivariate model saw the most increase between 2017 and 2020. Mental health was the dependent variable and the 24 statements in the seven impact and determinate areas were the independent variables. As with the logistic regression analysis, the MANOVA was analyzed with the IBM SPSS software, version 27.

2.6.1. Analyses within Each of the Seven Determinate Areas in the SwAge Analysis Model

Univariate logistic regression analysis was the first step to building multivariate models in each determinate area as well as for all determinate areas together. The univariate logistic regression analysis estimated for all statements within each of the seven determinate areas of the SwAge-model to investigate the association between the independent and the dependent variables. Initially, the associations for each statement were evaluated and the statements with p-values < 0.05, considered as the statistically significant level, were evaluated with other statements from the same determinate area. After this, the statements that continued to have a p-value < 0.05 were tested against the remaining statements one at a time. This continued for as long as the p-values for all included statements were <0.05.

2.6.2. Analyses including the Seven Determinate Areas in the SwAge Analysis Model

After the initial univariate analysis, a modulation was made for each determinate area in the SwAge-model. All the selected statements from the seven included determinate areas of the SwAge-model were analyzed in a logistical regression model. Thereafter, the analysis moved to step 2, where the statistically significantly statements (p-values < 0.05) from each determinate area was added, one determinate area at a time. These statements were tested to form the final model. In step 3, the out-sorted statements from step 2 and from each of the seven determinate areas were added one at a time to test the robustness of the model [41]. The multivariate models were tested for collinearity.

2.7. Ethical Considerations

The study was performed in accordance with the Helsinki declaration [42] and Swedish laws [43]. The benefits the knowledge this study would generate was considered to outweigh the potential risks that the study could bring. Rules for the handling and storage of data was and will be followed in accordance with university policies as well as guidelines for handling sensitive data according to GDPR [44]. The study was approved by the Swedish Ethical Review Agency (number 2016/867 and 2020-01897).

3. Results

3.1. Findings

There was an increase in diagnosis for both examined areas, i.e., exhaustion/stress and depression/anxiety between 2017 and 2020 (see Table 1). Of note, 128 nurses that previously reported no mental health diagnosis stated that they had been diagnosed with exhaustion/stress and/or depression/anxiety in 2020. In the logistic regression analysis, these diagnoses were combined into one variable: "mental health diagnoses".

Table 1. Percentage of nurses diagnosed with exhaustion/stress and/or depression/anxiety in 2017 and 2020.

Diagnosis	2017	2020
Exhaustion/stress	8.1%	26.4%
Depression/anxiety	5.3%	10.2%

3.2. Univariate Estimates and Multivariate Models for Work-Related Mental Health Diagnoses and Each of the Statements in the Analysed Areas

A logistic regression analysis was used to investigate which of the areas of importance for a healthy and sustainable work situation had the highest association with nurses' work-related mental health diagnoses in 2017 and in the second wave of COVID-19 in 2020. The statements in each impact and determinant area were analyzed by area. There were seven impact and determinant areas included in the study, which were physical work environment (2); mental work environment (3); work pace, work time, recuperation (4); private social environment (6); work social environment, organization, leadership (7); motivation and satisfaction of and to work tasks (8); knowledge and competency (9).

In the impact and determinant area "physical work environment", both included statements had a statistical association with nurses´ mental health diagnoses caused by their work for both 2017 and 2020 in the univariate estimates and in the multivariate model in 2017. However, the statement "For the most part I cannot cope with the physical work demands" also showed an association in the 2020 multivariate model.

All five statements in the impact and determinant area "Mental work environment" were statistically significant in the univariate estimates. In the 2017 multivariate model three statements were significant, which were "My work involves many psychologically heavy work tasks" (OR 1.78), "My work tasks usually clump together to the extent that I get frustrated" (OR 1.78) and "I wish for more opportunities to determine how to perform my work" (OR 1.60). In 2020, "My work tasks usually clump together to the extent that a lack of healthcare workers prior to the pandemic and many nurses are considering leaving the profession [10]. There is a serious nursing shortage in most European countries, which is insufficient to meet current healthcare demands [11,12]. Due to an ageing population, healthcare demands are predicted to increase, resulting in an estimated worldwide shortage of almost 6 million nurses by 2035 [7]. The ageing segment of the population is rapidly expanding and, thus, consuming more health services. Unfortunately, fewer new nurses are entering the work force; therefore, providing a healthy work environment to retain nurses in their workplace is essential for sustaining the profession [13].

Being able to work has a significant positive impact on people's health, and healthy workplaces are beneficial not only for employees but also for organizations and for society [14]. Decent work is one of the UN Global Goals for sustainable society development [15]. A sustainable work situation for employees is significant for a healthy organization that attracts people to work as well as promoting better health for employees, thus, also giving a better possibility for employability to an increased age [16–19]. Working in a hospital can be complicated due to the interaction between patients, nurses and the organization. This can, under normal circumstances, cause problematic work situations, but during the pandemic this was likely even more of a factor. It is, therefore, important to detect problems and shortcomings in the work situation in order to improve and support healthy and sustainable employability and understand what measures need to be taken. Areas of employability, and whether individuals can and want to work or not, has been stated as nine impact and determinant areas connected to sustainable healthy working life in the SwAge-model [6,16–19], i.e., (1) the employees self-rated health and diagnoses; (2) factors in the physical work environment; (3) factors in the mental work environment; (4) having time for recuperation within the employees' working hours, breaks and work pace; (5) the personal financial situation; (6) the employees' personal social environment outside of work; (7) the work social environment at the workplace, with leadership, colleagues, etcetera; (8) factors related to whether the employee experiences stimulation and motivation within work tasks and appreciation from the organization/work place regarding their performed tasks; (9) if the employees' have the right competence, skills and possibility for knowledge development in work.

As earlier mentioned, nurses play a key role in delivering care to patients [11]. How the nurses perform in their work environment is influenced by a number of human and environmental factors, including the type of information available, work experience, ambiguity, unpredictability, conflicting goals and time pressure [20]. Nurses face a higher risk of developing negative mental states, such as depression, anxiety and stress [21], due to the nature of their work. Unlike depression, burnout is specific to an individual's relationship to his or her occupation and usually results from long-term exposure to occupational stress [22]. Burnout may lead to adverse outcomes, such as medical errors, suicide, depression and absenteeism [23,24]. It is known that stress and burnout are factors that can contribute to a decreased mental health [10,25]. The ICN [26] states that long and stressful shifts severely impact nurses' mental health, resulting in nurses leaving or planning to leave the profession. Stress and burnout were recognized internationally as work hazards for nurses even before the pandemic [27]. Some argue that burnout in itself is a form of mental illness. However, a more common assumption has been that burnout causes mental dysfunction, such as anxiety and depression [28]. Temporal, physical, emotional and mental workloads, as well as job stressors such as time pressure, have in previous studies been positively associated with negative stress and burnout symptoms [28,29]. Previous studies have stated that nurses' work environments contribute to high stress, job dissatisfaction and burnout [30,31]. Additionally, a previous study also stated that healthcare professionals (HCPs) in hospitals engage in many work-related tasks and experience relatively high levels of mental stress while caring for patients [32], while another study showed that workload and work pressure have an impact on job outcomes and quality of care [33]. Problems within the nurses' working environments are described as concerns over inadequate staffing, ability to provide safe care, working long hours with high levels

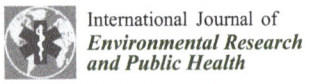

Article

Nurses' Work-Related Mental Health in 2017 and 2020—A Comparative Follow-Up Study before and during the COVID-19 Pandemic

Cicilia Nagel [1,2,*] and Kerstin Nilsson [1,2]

1. Division of Occupational and Environmental Medicine, Department of Laboratory Medicine, Lund University, 22184 Lund, Sweden
2. Division of Public Health, Kristianstad University, 29128 Kristianstad, Sweden
* Correspondence: cicilia.nagel@hkr.se; Tel.: +46-402-503-623

Abstract: The COVID-19 pandemic put a lot of strain on healthcare organizations. Nurses account for over 50% of healthcare staff, and how nurses perform in their work is influenced by a number of human and work environmental factors. However, to our knowledge, there has not been a previous study with the intention to look at all areas that affect a sustainable working life and how these impact nurses' mental well-being. The aim of this study is to investigate the association between, and the effect of, different factors in nurses' work situations associated with nurses' work-related mental-health diagnoses, before and during the COVID-19 pandemic. A questionnaire was sent out to all 9219 nurses in the Swedish county of Skane in the spring of 2017 and during wave two of the COVID-19 pandemic in the fall of 2020. The data were analyzed through logistic regression analysis. The results showed that lack of joy in the daily work, an increased workload and lack of support from co-workers had an increased association with work-related mental-health diagnoses. Future research regarding the long-term impact of COVID-19 on all areas of nurses' professional and personal lives is needed.

Keywords: work-related; mental-health diagnoses; work situation; work environment; nurses

1. Introduction

Healthcare workers around the world, primarily the nurses, were on the frontline of the Coronavirus pandemic that started in 2019 [1]. The second wave of the pandemic in Sweden occurred during the fall/winter 2020, the most serious wave of the pandemic regarding the burden on the healthcare sector. The pandemic has been described as a gigantic strain experiment on healthcare organizations, especially on healthcare staff due to exposure to hazards, such as psychological distress, fatigue, and trauma [1–5]. Healthcare workers had to perform their duties and face higher risks to their own health, such as the risk of infection [1]. Many nurses were afraid to become ill and die of COVID-19, which was incredibly stressful [6].

Nurses comprise half of the global health workforce [7,8]; however, for much of the general public, it is not fully understood what nurses do. Being a nurse includes promoting health, preventing illness as well as caring for people who are ill, disabled and dying. Advocating patients' rights, promoting a safe environment, conducting and/or taking part in research and education are also key nursing roles [9]. Nurses are often the first healthcare staff that the patient encounters. Their roles may vary depending on workplace, but often include triage, early recognition of life-threatening conditions, administration of medications, performance of life-saving procedures and initiation of early referral [7]. Despite nurses being a common profession in healthcare, there is an increasing demand for nurses worldwide [8]. According to the World Health Organization (WHO) [7], one out of six of the world's nurses are expected to retire in the next 10 years. Several countries experienced

37. Ryan, R.M.; Deci, E.L. Self-determination theory and the facilitation of intrinsic motivation, social development, and well-being. *Am. Psychol.* **2000**, *55*, 68–78. [CrossRef]
38. Nilsson, P.; Andersson, H.I.; Ejlertsson, G.; Blomqvist, K. How to make a workplace health promotion questionnaire process applicable, meaningful, and sustainable. *J. Nurs. Manag.* **2011**, *19*, 906–914. [CrossRef]
39. Bakker, A.B.; Demerouti, E. The Job Demands-Resources model: State of the art. *J. Manag. Psychol.* **2007**, *22*, 309–328. [CrossRef]
40. Graneheim, U.H.; Lundman, B. Qualitative content analysis in nursing research: Concepts, procedures and measures to achieve trustworthiness. *Nurse Educ. Today* **2004**, *24*, 105–112. [CrossRef]
41. Krueger, R.; Casey, M. *Focus Groups A Practical Guide for Applied Research*; Sage Publications: Thousand Oaks, CA, USA, 2009.

6. Antonovsky, A. The salutogenic model as a theory to guide health promotion. *Health Promot. Int.* **1996**, *11*, 11–18. [CrossRef]
7. Bauer, G.; Davies, J.K.; Pelikan, J. The EUHPID Health development model for the classification of public health indicators. *Health Promot. Int.* **2006**, *21*, 153–159. [CrossRef] [PubMed]
8. Clausen, T.; Tufte, P.; Borg, V. Why are they leaving? Causes of actual turnover in the Danish eldercare services. *J. Nurs. Manag.* **2014**, *22*, 583–592. [CrossRef] [PubMed]
9. Heinen, M.M.; van Achterberg, T.; Schwendimann, R.; Zander, B.; Matthews, A.; Kózka, M.; Ensio, A.; Sjetne, I.S.; Casbas, T.M.; Ball, J.; et al. Nurses' intention to leave their profession: A cross sectional observational study in 10 European countries. *Int. J. Nurs. Stud.* **2013**, *50*, 174–184. [CrossRef]
10. Kouvonen, A.; Oksanen, T.; Vahtera, J.; Stafford, M.; Wilkinson, R.; Schneider, J.; Väänänen, A.; Virtanen, M.; Cox, S.J.; Pentti, J.; et al. Low workplace social capital as a predictor of depression: The Finnish public sector study. *Am. J. Epidemiol.* **2008**, *167*, 1143–1151. [CrossRef]
11. Schaufeli, W.B.; Bakker, A.B.; Salanova, M. The measurement of work engagement with a short questionnaire. A cross-national study. *Educ. Psychol. Meas.* **2006**, *66*, 701–716. [CrossRef]
12. Jenny, G.J.; Bauer, G.F.; Vinje, H.F.; Vogt, K.; Torp, S. The Application of Salutogenesis to Work. In *The Handbook of Salutogenesis*; Mittelmark, M.B., Sagy, S., Eriksson, M., Bauer, G.F., Pelikan, J.M., Lindström, B., Espnes, G.A., Eds.; Springer: Cham, Switzerland, 2017; pp. 197–210.
13. Nilsson, K. A sustainable working life for all ages—The swAge-model. *Appl. Ergon.* **2020**, *86*, 103082. [CrossRef] [PubMed]
14. Persson, S.S.; Nilsson Lindström, P.; Pettersson, P.; Andersson, I.; Blomqvist, K. Relationships between healthcare employees and managers as a resource for well-being at work. *Soc. Health Vulnerability* **2018**, *9*, 1547035. [CrossRef]
15. Persson, S.S.; Nilsson Lindström, P.; Pettersson, P.; Nilsson, M.; Blomqvist, K. Resources for work-related well-being: A qualitative study about healthcare employees' experiences of relationships at work. *J. Clin. Nurs.* **2018**, *27*, 4302–4310. [CrossRef]
16. Dutton, J.E.; Ragins, B.R. *Exploring Positive Relationships at Work: Building a Theoretical and Research Foundation*; Psychology Press: Hove, UK, 2007.
17. Rousseau, D.M.; Ling, K. Commentary: Following the resources in positive organizational relationships. In *Exploring Positive Relationships at Work: Building a Theoretical and Research Foundation*; Dutton, J.E., Ragins, B.R., Eds.; Lawrence Erlbaum and Associates: Mahwah, NJ, USA, 2007; pp. 373–384.
18. Gharaveis, A.; Hamilton, D.K.; Pati, D. The impact of environmental design on teamwork and communication in healthcare facilities: A systematic literature review. *HERD* **2018**, *11*, 119–137. [CrossRef] [PubMed]
19. Orrung-Wallin, A.; Jakobsson, U.; Edberg, A.-K. Job satisfaction and associated variables among nurse assistants working in residential care. *Int. Psychogeriatr.* **2012**, *24*, 1904–1918. [CrossRef]
20. Feeney, B.C.; Collins, N.L. A new look at social support: A theoretical perspective on thriving through relationships. *Personal. Soc. Psychol. Rev.* **2014**, *19*, 113–147. [CrossRef]
21. Nappo, N. Job stress and interpersonal relationships cross country evidence from the EU15. A correlation analysis. *BMC Public Health* **2020**, *20*. [CrossRef] [PubMed]
22. Tourangeau, A.; Cranley, L.; Laschinger, H.K.S.; Pachis, J. Relationships among leadership practices, work environments, staff communication and outcomes in long-term care. *J. Nurs. Manag.* **2010**, *18*, 1060–1072. [CrossRef]
23. Keyes, C.L.M. Promoting and protecting mental health as flourishing. *Am. Psychol.* **2007**, *62*, 95–108. [CrossRef]
24. Seligman, M.E. *Flourish: A Visionary New Understanding of Happiness and Well-Being*; Free Press: New York, NY, USA, 2012.
25. McCormack, B.; Titchen, A. No beginning, no end: An ecology of human flourishing. *Int. Pract. Dev. J.* **2014**, *4*, 2. [CrossRef]
26. Gaffney, M. *Flourishing: How to Achieve a Deeper Sense of Well-Being, Meaning and Purpose—Even When Facing Adversity*; Penguin: London, UK, 2015.
27. Colbert, A.E.; Bono, J.E.; Purvanova, R.K. Flourishing via workplace relationships: Moving beyond instrumental support. *Acad. Manag. J.* **2016**, *59*, 1199–1223. [CrossRef]
28. Dewing, J.; McCormack, B. Creating flourishing workplaces. In *Person-Centred Practice in Nursing and Health Care: Theory and Practice*, 2nd ed.; McCormack, B., McCance, T., Eds.; John Wiley & Sons, Ltd.: Hoboken, NJ, USA, 2017; pp. 150–161.
29. Swedish Association of Local Authorities and Regions. *Öppna Jämförelser 2020. Vård Och Omsorg Om Äldre*; Socialstyrelsen: Stockholm, Sweden, 2021. (In Swedish)
30. Socialstyrelsen. *Tillståndet Och Utvecklingen Inom Hälso- Och Sjukvård Och Socialtjänst: Lägesrapport 2015*; Socialstyrelsen: Stockholm, Sweden, 2015. (In Swedish)
31. Stringer, E.; Genat, W. *Action Research in Health*; Merrill Prentice Hall: Hoboken, NJ, USA, 2004.
32. Hummelvoll, J.K. The multistage focus group interview: A relevant and fruitful method in action research based on a co-operative inquiry perspective. *Nor. Tidsskr. Sykepl.* **2008**, *10*, 3–14.
33. Elo, S.; Kyngäs, H. The qualitative content analysis process. *J. Adv. Nurs.* **2008**, *62*, 107–115. [CrossRef] [PubMed]
34. Sias, P.M. *Organizing Relationships: Traditional and Emerging Perspectives on Workplace Relationships*; Sage Publications Inc.: Thousand Oaks, CA, USA, 2009.
35. Cohen, S.; Gottlieb, B.; Underwood, L. Social relationships and health. In *Measuring and Intervening in Social Support*; Cohen, S., Underwood, L., Gottlieb, B., Eds.; Oxford University Press: Oxford, UK, 2000; pp. 3–25.
36. Hobfoll, S.E. Social and psychological resources and adaptation. *Rev. Gen. Psychol.* **2002**, *6*, 307–324. [CrossRef]

study with a participatory approach, the weakest part is perhaps the lack of follow-up of whether the participants' suggestions for changes were introduced and how they turned out. This weakness was due to limited time for the project.

The researchers have nursing and public health backgrounds, which strengthens the credibility as it enhanced the possibility to see things from different perspectives. The fact that all researchers participated in the analysis and that there was high agreement between them also strengthens the study's credibility. Similar issues were discussed in the four focus groups, which demonstrates dependability. The transferability of the results is enhanced by descriptions of the study context, the participants, and the procedure and analysis process [40].

5. Conclusions

In view of the increased rationalization in society, in which meetings are minimized and are required to be strictly effective and production-oriented, our results regarding the importance of informal and formal meetings and work relationships need to be taken into account if we aim to create sustainable health-promoting workplaces. This study contributes to workplace health promotion research with its salutogenic and participatory approach and represents a new opportunity to explore and understand workplace relationships as a resource by strengthening, or maintaining, positive activities and processes. It is therefore vital to develop dialogues about relationship processes, and raise awareness of the importance of different relationships for improving the work situation and healthcare. The study also shows that the components of flourishing could be used to create a model for such dialogues. Taking the employees' own experiences into account in group dialogues seems to improve employee engagement and could be a fruitful way to conduct workplace health promotion interventions. However, further studies are required to explore the utility of our results in intervention studies, in various workplace settings, between night and day shifts, and among different occupational groups.

Author Contributions: Conceptualization, S.S.P., K.B. and P.N.L.; methodology, S.S.P., K.B. and P.N.L.; formal analysis, S.S.P., K.B. and P.N.L.; writing—original draft preparation, S.S.P.; writing—review and editing, K.B. and P.N.L.; supervision, K.B. and P.N.L. All authors have read and agreed to the published version of the manuscript.

Funding: This research received no external funding.

Institutional Review Board Statement: The study was conducted according to the guidelines of the Declaration of Helsinki, and approved by the Ethical Review Board of Lund, Sweden (dnr: 2015/565).

Informed Consent Statement: Informed consent was obtained from all subjects involved in the study.

Data Availability Statement: Not applicable.

Acknowledgments: We would like to thank all the healthcare staff who participated in this study. We would also like to thank the research platform Collaboration for Health at Kristianstad University, Kristianstad, Sweden, for financial support.

Conflicts of Interest: The authors declare no conflict of interest.

References

1. Lindmark, U.; Wagman, P.; Wåhlin, C.; Rolander, B. Workplace health in dental care—A salutogenic approach. *Int. J. Dent. Hyg.* **2016**, *16*, 103–113. [CrossRef]
2. Nilsson, P.; Andersson, I.; Ejlertsson, G.; Troein, M. Workplace health resources based on sense of coherence theory. *Int. J. Work. Health Manag.* **2012**, *5*, 156–167. [CrossRef]
3. Persson, S.S.; Lindström, P.N.; Pettersson, P.; Andersson, I. Workplace relationships impact self-rated health: A survey among Swedish municipal healthcare employees. *WORK J.Prev. Assess. Rehabil.* **2017**, *60*, 85–94. [CrossRef]
4. Bringsén, Å.; Andersson, I.; Ejlertsson, G.; Troein, M. Exploring workplace related health resources from a salutogenic perspective. *WORK J.Prev. Assess. Rehabil.* **2012**, *42*, 403–414.
5. Häusser, J.A.; Mojzisch, A.; Niesel, M. Ten years on: A review of recent research on the Job Demand-Control (-Support) model and psychological well-being. *Work Stress* **2010**, *24*, 1–35. [CrossRef]

A practical implication is to use meetings, both formal and informal, as a means to enhance relationships in everyday practice. Conditions for meetings provide the opportunity for people to share experiences and get to know each other in the work group, which in itself contributes to a health-promoting workplace [14,15,38]. Using the concept of flourishing both in the planning of work tasks and in issues concerning the psychosocial work environment, could contribute to a flourishing and sustainable workplace. Using the four components in formal meetings enables the creation of a clear model to show what challenges and suggestions have emerged, and thus makes it possible to develop connectivity, autonomy, and use of competence in an optimal way. The identified challenges and suggestions for improvements can, for instance, undergo process evaluation at the staff meetings, in order to make the relationships a resource for the flourishing of individuals and the organization alike. It is advantageous to base dialogues on the four flourishing components to highlight both the salutogenic aspects and the challenges to creating a sustainable workplace that causes the individual workers to flourish. Previous research about using dialogue as a tool has shown that a structured dialogue model makes it easier to notice what is happening in daily work relations and provides the possibility to work in a promoting way [38].

Furthermore, a practical implication of informal meetings is to create conditions for things such as joint breaks. Conditions for informal meetings contribute to the opportunity for the staff to share their thoughts and feelings about different work situations. This promotes social relationships and the opportunity to give each other more support in everyday practice. Relationships can function as a job resource that helps employees to manage strain and job demands [39]. Especially in human-related work, such as healthcare, work tasks are often challenging and energy-draining, on the one hand, and energy-giving through daily human meetings, on the other [34].

Regardless of the subject, dialogue is essential in research with a salutogenic and participatory approach. In this study the dialogues in the multi-stage focus groups developed during the study process and had the effect that all groups decided to proceed with the suggestions and try to put them into action. Our interpretation is that the groups themselves, based on the participatory approach, were an enhancing action for the workplace relationships among the healthcare staff. This further justifies dialogue as useful in improvement work to achieve a health-promoting workplace. This should be taken into account in public health and workplace health promotion, considering society's rationalisation efforts, according to which, meetings should be minimized and must be effective and production-oriented.

4.2. Limitations and Trustworthiness

The methodological aspects of credibility, dependability, and transferability need to be considered for a study to be seen as trustworthy [40]. From a credibility perspective, multi-stage focus groups were considered appropriate for this study, as it was hoped they would create a reflective environment for the participants, be emancipatory, and yield detailed data. Although a situation where the participants know each other very well can lead to a lack of discussion, a sense of security within the group facilitates a trustful discussion where participants feel free to share their feelings, thoughts, and perceptions [41]. If the study is to be repeated in the future, the focus group method may need to be modified according to any current pandemic restrictions, for example, by offering digital participation or smaller group sizes. Results obtained using a deductive analysis approach can be questioned from a credibility point of view [40], as the deductive analysis brings a risk that unexpected results may be neglected. However, the participants' reflections and suggestions were often unexpected. Among the unexpected results was the large gap in the relationship between night and day staff. We were also surprised that the relationship with care recipients was hardly discussed. At the meetings, the participants instead focused on the relationship with their colleagues since a good relationship with their colleagues and the manager was a prerequisite for good care and a positive relationship with their care recipients. Being a it is important to build a work structure based on positive relationships [13,27,34,35]. To achieve this, well-thought-out strategies for informal and formal meetings in the workplace are required.

Strong relationships with colleagues and managers and positive relationships with care recipients are closely linked. Our results showed that positive informal and formal meetings seemed to have a dual purpose. They made the staff themselves flourish at their workplace, but they were also a prerequisite for providing good care and having positive relationships with care recipients, which was also central to their own well-being. In the focus groups, the caring staff rarely talked about relationships with care recipients. Instead, they spoke about relationships with colleagues, professionals from other occupations, and managers. The caring staff chose to talk about their workplace relationships, not primarily to improve their own well-being but to achieve improved relationships with care recipients as a way of providing better care, which ultimately improved their own well-being. In human care professions, when employees are faced with high emotional demands [34], awareness of types of work relationships and why they function as a resource and as a prerequisite for flourishing is valuable.

A salutogenic approach to workplace health needs to emphasise positive relationships based on respect, security, and reciprocity. One interpretation of our study results is that there existed more of a "we-feeling" between caring colleagues working the same shift and more of an "us-and them feeling" between people from different shifts and representing different care professions. The we-feeling contributed to togetherness among the caring staff and created flow and confidence at informal meetings. This "we-feeling" of togetherness also contributed to good formal meetings because of respect, security, and strong reciprocity. Such a sense of belonging and security has also been shown in previous research [3] to contribute to well-being as well as recognition of self-worth. On the other hand, the results in this study also showed more of an "us-and-them feeling" in the relationships with caring staff from other shifts, the manager, and other occupational care groups. Hence, a major part of the challenge of turning the relationships with the manager and other occupational care groups into a resource seemed to lie with the organizational structure, as physical meetings in daily situations were sometimes considered inadequate. If an organization relies on interactions between people, relationships should be emphasized as more important to the organization than, for instance, organizational principles and structures [36]. By using the relationships as a tool for the development of the organization and by having a less hierarchical structure—a structure that is based on a democratic mindset between different professions—everyone's competence can be anchored in the overall organization and everyone can work towards the same goal [35]. This salutogenic approach may in turn benefit the flourishing of the individuals, and the organization [27,28].

4.1. Practical and Theoretical Implications

In this study with a salutogenic and a participatory design, practical and theoretical implications where deeply intertwined. A theoretical implication is that the concept of flourishing, and its four specific components, can be used in practice to identify, interpret, and explain positive relationships, and situations and elements of a workplace that affect employee health. The components of flourishing have links to the three components of motivational needs in Ryan and Deci's Self-Determination Theory (2000): autonomy, competence, and belongingness [37]. These three components create inner motivation for the individual to act in situations or in relationships that are important for health experience and well-being. There is also a connection between the concept flourishing and the model of person-centredness [28]. Person-centredness is usually discussed in relation to care, but an organization can also work in a person-centred manner with its employees and in the organization of work. Different dimensions of relationships at work become important to understand and improve, as relationships are vital for flourishing. Healthful relationships among employees may thereby also contribute to a person-centredness culture.

I get frustrated" (OR 2.05), "My work involves many psychologically heavy work tasks" (OR 1.76) and "I wish for greater control over my work (OR 1.75) showed significance.

All three of the investigated statements in the impact and determinant area "Work pace, work time, recuperation" showed an association in both the univariate estimates and the multivariate model for a healthy and sustainable working life.

In the impact and determinant area "Private social environment", both statements were statistically significant in the univariate estimates of 2017. The statement "I need to work more at home/care for relatives and will probably therefore work less in the future" showed an association in the multivariate model of 2017, whereas the statement "I want to spend more time enjoying leisure activities and will therefore work less in the future" showed an association in both the univariate estimates and multivariate model of 2020.

The area "Work social environment, organization, leadership" consisted of six statements that all indicated an association in the univariate estimates of 2017 and 2020. In 2017, three statements showed significance, which were "Not having enough staff means that I cannot perform my work in the way I want" (OR 2.04), "Big changes in my work situation causes me to want to leave" (OR 1.41) and "The social community at my workplace does not make me want to stay" (OR 1.33). In 2020, only two statements showed significance, including "I do not feel I have enough support from my co-workers" (OR 3.14) and "Big changes in my work situation causes me to want to leave" (OR 1.73).

Similar to the previous determinant area, all statements in the impact and determinate area "Motivation and satisfaction of and to work tasks" indicated an association in the univariate estimates of both 2017 and 2020. However, only two statements showed association in the 2017 and 2020 multivariate models: "I do not experience joy in my daily work" and "I do not experience satisfaction in my daily work".

The impact and determinant area "Knowledge and Competency" consisted of two statements that were both found to be statistically significant in the univariate estimates of 2017 and 2020, but only the statement "I do not feel like my competencies are being utilized in a satisfactory way" showed association with nurses' work-related mental health diagnoses in the 2017 and 2020 multivariate model (Table 2).

Table 2. Univariate and multivariate variables 2017 and 2020. Univariate estimates and multivariate models in each of the analyzed areas between the statements (agree vs. disagree) and work-related mental health diagnoses and other factors. OR = Odds ratio; CI = Confidence interval. * The variable shows no statistical significance in the multivariate modelling and is, therefore, not included in the final multivariate model shown in this column.

Area	Statement	Univariate Estimates for Each Variable in 2017		Multivariate Model in Each Area in 2017		Univariate Estimates for Each Variable in 2020		Multivariate Model in Each Area in 2020	
		OR	CI 95%	OR	CI 95%	OR	CI 95%	OR	CI 95%
Physical work environment	For the most part I cannot cope with the physical work demands	1.74	1.22–2.48	1.67	1.17–2.40	2.01	1.17–3.46	2.01	1.17–3.46
	My current work is too physically straining for my health	1.37	1.08–1.73	1.32	1.04–1.68	1.44	0.99–2.08	*	*
Mental work environment	My work involves many psychologically heavy work tasks	2.21	1.75–2.78	1.78	1.40–2.26	2.17	1.60–2.95	1.76	1.28–2.41
	I wish for more opportunities to determine how to perform my work	2.00	1.63–2.45	1.60	1.29–1.98	1.81	1.37–2.40	*	*
	I wish for greater control over my work	1.89	1.55–2.31	*	*	2.24	1.69–2.97	1.75	1.30–2.36
	At my workplace there are not enough possibilities to be re-allocated to less demanding work tasks for those who need it	1.36	1.10–1.68	*	*	1.29	0.96–1.72	*	*
	My work tasks usually clump together to the extent that I get frustrated	2.32	1.89–2.84	1.78	1.45–2.23	2.63	1.98–3.49	2.05	1.51–2.78

Table 2. Cont.

Area	Statement	Univariate Estimates for Each Variable in 2017		Multivariate Model in Each Area in 2017		Univariate Estimates for Each Variable in 2020		Multivariate Model in Each Area in 2020	
		OR	CI 95%	OR	CI 95%	OR	CI 95%	OR	CI 95%
Work pace, work time, recuperation	I do not feel like I get enough rest/recuperation between work shifts	1.83	1.50–2.23	1.44	1.17–1.78	2.23	1.68–2.97	1.73	1.27–2.35
	I do not have time to perform the work duties I have planned for the day	1.74	1.42–2.14	1.312	1.06–1.63	2.50	1.84–3.39	1.79	1.27–2.53
	The work pace in my daily work is too high	2.27	1.85–2.78	1.88	1.51–2.34	2.22	1.67–2.96	1.55	1.12–2.15
Private social environment	I want to spend more time enjoying leisure activities and will therefore work less in the future	1.33	1.02–1.74	*	*	1.51	1.04–2.19	1.51	1.04–2.19
	I need to work more at home/care for relatives, and will probably therefore work less in the future	1.46	1.17–1.81	1.42	1.14–1.77	1.02	0.72–1.43	*	*
Worksocial environment, organization, leadership	The social community at my workplace does not make me want to stay	1.50	1.20–1.88	1.33	1.06–1.68	1.47	1.06–2.04	*	*
	Big changes in my work situation causes me to want to leave	1.81	1.45–2.26	1.41	1.12–1.78	2.15	1.53–3.02	1.73	1.21–2.47
	I do not feel I have enough support from my closest manager	1.24	1.01–1.52	*	*	1.56	1.16–2.08	*	*
	I do not feel I have enough support from my co-workers	1.36	1.00–1.84	*	*	3.53	2.41–5.17	3.14	2.11–4.67
	I feel bullied or shut out from the community at my work place	1.91	1.21–3.02	*	*	2.35	1.26–4.39	*	*
	Not having enough staff mean that I cannot perform my work in the way I want	2.26	1.83–2.79	2.04	1.64–2.54	1.44	1.08–1.91	*	*
Motivation and satisfaction of and to work tasks	I do not feel like my daily work is meaningful	2.22	1.63–3.01	*	*	2.35	1.47–3.76	*	*
	I do not feel like my work is stimulating	2.14	1.67–2.73	*	*	1.99	1.36–2.90	*	*
	I do not experience joy in my daily work	2.73	2.20–3.39	2.02	1.45–2.82	3.45	2.53–4.70	2.39	1.48–3.84
	I do not experience satisfaction in my daily work	2.48	2.01–3.08	1.49	1.07–2.07	3.10	2.26–4.24	1.64	1.01–2.66
Knowledge and Competency	I do not get enough opportunities at work to utilise my skills and knowledge	1.74	1.36–2.23	*	*	1.70	1.17–2.46	*	*
	I do not feel like my competencies are being utilised in a satisfactory way	1.82	1.46–2.28	1.64	1.21–2.22	2.10	1.53–2.90	2.17	1.42–3.32

A multivariate analysis of variance (MANOVA) was performed in the multivariate model in order to see which of the 24 statements showed the most increase between 2017 and 2020. MANOVA was used since it does not affect the Type I error rate to the same extent as other independent tests. The results of the MANOVA mirrored the logistic regression analysis and the four statements that saw the most increase were "I do not have the time to perform the work duties I have planned for the day", "I want to spend more time enjoying leisure activities and will therefore work less in the future", "I do not feel I have enough support from co-workers" and "I do not experience joy in my daily work". Results of the MANOVA showed that there was a statistical difference between the combined dependent variables. Wilks´ Λ = 0.09, $F(40,1582)$ = 4.200, $p < 0.001$, partial η^2 = 0.096, observed power = 1.00. Based on the low Wilks´ Λ, we want to be careful rejecting the null hypothesis. The observed power was 1.00, indicating that there was a 100% chance that the results could have been significant.

3.3. Multivariate Model of all Impact and Determinant Areas in the Work Situation in Association with Nurses' Mental Health Diagnoses Caused by the Work Situation in 2017 and in 2020

In real life, nurses are not only affected by one of the impact and determinant areas from the SwAge-model, there is impact from all nine areas. Therefore, in the next step of the analysis we aimed to make a collected analysis of the seven relevant impact and determinate areas in this study. Hence, all the statements from the seven deteminant and impact areas for a sustainable healthy working life (the swAge-model) included in this investigation were modelled into a single multivariate model for each year, i.e., 2017 and for the second wave of COVID-19 in 2020. The variables that were statistically significant (p-value < 0.05) from each area were used in the modelling, and each of the eliminated statements (i.e., the variables not statistic significant in the earlier analysis of each area) were added once more one at a time to test the robustness of the model.

In the 2017 multivariate model, six statements showed significance: "I do not experience joy in my daily work" (OR 1.97), "My work involves many psychologically heavy work tasks" (OR 1.66), "The work pace in my daily work is too high" (OR 1.37), "I wish for more opportunities to determine how to perform my work" (OR 1.37), "My work tasks usually clump together to the extent that I get frustrated" (OR 1.34) and "I need to work more at home/care for relatives and will probably therefore work less in the future" (OR 1.27). In 2020, five statements showed significance: "I do not experience joy in my daily work" (OR 2.17), "I do not feel enough support from my co-workers" (OR 2.00), "My work tasks usually clump together to the extent that I get frustrated" (OR 1.81), "My work involves many psychologically heavy work tasks" (OR 1.69) and "I do not get enough rest/recuperation between work shifts (OR 1.41). There were no statistically significant statements in 2017 or in 2020 from the area "physical work environment" and "knowledge and competency" in the final total multivariate model, including all relevant impact and determinant areas for a healthy and sustainable working life (Table 3).

Table 3. The final multivariate model for all areas and statement together for 2017 and for 2020. Statistically significant variables in relation to nurses' work-related mental health diagnosis in 2017 and 2020. OR = Odds ratio; CI = Confidence intervl. Nagelkerke R square 0.073. * The variable shows no statistical significance in the multivariate modelling and is, therefore, not included in the final multivariate model shown in this column.

Area	Statement	2017 OR	2017 CI 95%	2020 OR	2020 CI 95%
Mental work environment	My work involves many psychologically heavy work tasks	1.66	1.29–2.13	1.69	1.22–2.34
	I wish for more opportunities to determine how to perform my work	1.37	1.10–1.72	*	*
	My work tasks usually clump together to the extent that I get frustrated	1.34	1.06–1.71	1.81	1.33–2.48
Work time, work pace, recuperation	I do not feel that I get enough rest/recuperation between work shifts	*	*	1.41	1.03–1.93
	The work pace in my daily work is too high	1.37	1.07–1.74	*	*
Private social environment	I need to work more at home/care for relatives, and will probably therefore work less in the future	1.27	1.02–1.56	*	*
Work social environment, organization, leadership	I do not feel enough support from my co-workers	*	*	2.00	1.31–3.08
Motivation and satisfaction of and to work tasks	I do not experience joy in my daily work	1.97	1.56–2.48	2.17	1.52–3.09

3.4. Multivariate Model of the Work Situation in the Second Wave of COVID-19 in Association with Nurses' Mental Diagnoses Caused by the Work Situation, including COVID-19-Specific Questions

COVID-19 had a significant impact on the healthcare systems in Sweden, particularly during the fall/winter of 2020. COVID-19-specific questions were, therefore, added to the investigation during the second wave of COVID-19 in 2020. Therefore, 25 COVID-19-specific variables in the seven impact and determinant areas were included in the next step of the analysis of the multivariate model regarding the second wave of COVID-19 in 2020 to see whether there were particular areas that affected the nurses. The statements in each impact and determinant area were analyzed within that particular determinant area. All statements showed significance in the univariate model. Sixteen statements remained significant in the multivariate model; out of these, five showed a slightly higher OR, which were "I do not feel enough support from my co-workers" (OR 2.86), "I do not experience joy in my daily work" (OR 2.46), "My workload has been higher during COVID-19 compared to my average workload" (OR 2.33), "My work tasks usually clump together to the extent that I get frustrated" (OR 2.07) and "I do not feel like my competencies are being utilized in a satisfactory way" (OR 2.02) (Table 4).

Table 4. Univariate estimates and the total multivariate model including all seven investigated areas in 2020 with COVID-19-specific questions. Statistically significant variables in relation to work-related mental health diagnoses in 2020. OR = Odds ratio; CI = Confidence interval. Nagelkerke R square 0.115. * The variable shows no statistical significance in the multivariate modelling and is, therefore, not included in the final multivariate model shown in this column.

Area	Statement	Univariate Estimates OR	CI 95 %	Multivariate Model OR	CI 95%
Physical work environment	For the most part I cannot cope with the physical work demands	2.01	1.17–3.46	1.93	1.10–3.38
	My current work is too physically straining for my health	1.44	1.00–2.08	*	*
	The hygiene routines in my daily work are not enough to protect me from serious risk of being infected by COVID-19	1.50	1.05–2.15	*	*
	I do not experience the personal protective equipment (PPE) as satisfactory from an infection protection point of view	1.48	1.03–2.12	*	*
	The accessibility to proper PPE has not been enough to perform my work duties safely	1.17	0.83–1.65	*	*
	The PPE is designed in a way that makes it difficult to perform my work duties safely	1.12	0.77–1.61	*	*
	In my daily work there are obstacles that prevent employees from fully compling with COVID-19 safety procedures	1.22	0.90–1.65	*	*
	The PPE prevents me from performing my work duties in a (for me) comfortable and satisfactory way	1.18	0.89–1.57	*	*
	The measures for preventing ill health and disease among the staff during the COVID-19 pandemic are not good enough at my workplace	1.22	0.88–1.68	*	*
	I feel that there have been significant risks of being infected by COVID-19 in my workplace	1.51	1.13–2.01	1.50	1.13–2.00
	My work situation during COVID-19 has not contained more physical load when compared to normal circumstances	1.13	0.81–1.58	*	*

Table 4. Cont.

Area	Statement	Univariate Estimates		Multivariate Model	
		OR	CI 95 %	OR	CI 95%
Mental work environment	My work tasks usually clump together to the extent that I get frustrated	2.63	1.98–3.49	2.07	1.51–2.83
	My work involves many psychologically heavy work tasks	2.17	1.60–2.95	1.81	1.31–2.51
	I wish for more opportunities to determine how to perform my work	1.81	1.37–2.40	*	*
	I wish for greater control over my work	2.24	1.69–2.97	1.73	1.18–2.54
	My work situation during COVID-19 has been more stressful in comparison to normal circumstances	1.63	1.22–2.18	*	*
	I have had anxiety over myself being severely ill with COVID-19	1.53	1.16–2.03	*	*
	I have had anxiety over dying due to COVID-19	1.44	1.06–1.97	*	*
Work time, work pace, recuperation	My workload has been higher during COVID-19 compared to my average workload	1.38	1.04–1.83	2.33	1.19–4.56
	I do not have time to perform the work duties I have planned for the day	2.50	1.84–3.39	1.70	1.20–2.42
	I do not feel that I get enough rest/recuperation between work shifts	2.23	1.68–2.97	1.68	1.22–2.30
	The work pace in my daily work is too high	2.22	1.67–2.96	1.56	1.13–2.17
	My work situation during COVID-19 has had a negative impact on my ability to recuperate during work shifts due to reduced possibilities to take breaks, etc.	1.60	1.18–2.16	*	*
	My work situation during COVID-19 has had a negative impact on my ability to recuperate between work shifts	1.86	1.38–2.52	*	*
	I have not been able to take my vacation the way I had planned due to COVID-19	1.21	0.77–1.90	*	*
Private social environment	I want to spend more time enjoying leisure activities and will therefore work less in the future	1.51	1.04–2.19	*	*
	I need to work more at home/care for relatives, and will probably therefore work less in the future	1.02	0.72–1.43	*	*
	I feel that I have risked getting infected by COVID-19 in my leisure time (in the store, trip to/from work, etc.)	1.32	0.99–1.75	*	*
	My work situation during COVID-19 has had a negative impact on my private life (my family, partner, etc.)	1.70	1.28–2.25	1.42	1.05–1.92
	I have felt concern about a close relative being or getting severely ill by COVID-19	1.74	1.29–2.36	*	*
	I am/have been concerned that I will bring the COVID-19 virus home from work, which will infect family/friends, etc.	1.72	1.29–2.28	*	*
	I am/have been concerned that I will bring the COVID-19 virus from my private life and infect people and risk groups at my work	1.41	1.06–1.88	*	*
Work social environment, organization, leadership	The social community at my workplace does not make me want to stay	1.47	1.06–2.04	*	*
	Big changes in my work situation causes me to want to leave	2.15	1.53–3.02	1.64	1.11–2.42
	I do not feel enough support from my co-workers	3.53	2.41–5.17	2.86	1.84–4.44
	I do not feel I have enough support from my closest manager	1.56	1.16–2.08	*	*
	I feel bullied or shut out from the community at my workplace	2.35	1.26–4.39	*	*
	Not having enough staff means that I cannot perform my work in the way I want	1.44	1.08–1.91	*	*
	My closest manager has not given me enough support during the COVID-19 pandemic	1.62	1.20–2.18	*	*
	I have not received enough information/knowledge from management to perform my work duties in a satisfactory way during the COVID-19 pandemic	1.35	0.96–1.89	*	*

Table 4. Cont.

Area	Statement	Univariate Estimates		Multivariate Model	
		OR	CI 95 %	OR	CI 95%
Motivation and satisfaction of and to work tasks	I do not experience joy in my daily work	3.45	2.53–4.70	2.46	1.50–4.04
	I do not feel like my daily work is meaningful	2.35	1.47–3.76	*	*
	I do not feel like my work is stimulating	1.99	1.36–2.90	*	*
	I do not experience satisfaction in my daily work	3.10	2.26–4.24	1.69	1.03–2.78
	The COVID-19 pandemic has not increased my motivation for my work tasks	1.43	0.98–2.10	*	*
	At my workplace there are not enough possibilities to be re-allocated to less demanding work tasks for those who need it	1.29	0.97–1.72	*	*
Knowledge and Competency	I do not get enough opportunities at work to utilise my skills and knowledge	1.70	1.17–2.46	*	*
	I do not feel like my competencies are being utilised in a satisfactory way	2.10	1.53–2.90	2.02	1.31–3.10
	I have not received enough information, knowledge, and competence development at work in order to feel safe performing my work tasks during the COVID-19 pandemic	1.65	1.22–2.24	1.49	1.09–2.03

3.5. Final Multivariate Model with COVID-19-Specific Variables of the Work Situation in Association with Nurses' Mental Health Diagnoses Caused by the Work Situation

We wanted to see which of the variables were most likely to impact nurses' mental health and, therefore, be chosen for a final multivariate model. All statistically significant variables from Table 4 were added one at a time to form a multivariate model. The discarded statements were then added to the model one at a time to test the robustness of the model. In the end, the model consisted of eight statements that showed a connection with nurses' mental health diagnoses (Table 5).

Table 5. Final multivariate model with COVID-19-specific variables. Statistically significant variables in relation to work-related mental health diagnoses in 2020. OR = Odds ratio; CI = Confidence interval. Cox and Snell R Square 0.058; Nagelkerke R square 0.121.

Area	Statement	Multivariate Model	
		OR	CI 95%
Mental work environment	I wish for greater control over my work	1.45	1.04–2.01
	My work involves many psychologically heavy work tasks	1.72	1.23–2.40
	I have had anxiety over myself being severely ill with COVID-19	1.40	1.03–1.89
	My work tasks usually clump together to the extent that I get frustrated	1.91	1.36–2.68
Work time, work pace, recuperation	I do not feel that I get enough rest/recuperation between work shifts	1.41	1.01–1.95
Work social environment, organization, and leadership	I do not feel enough support from my co-workers	1.96	1.27–3.01
	Not having enough staff means that I cannot perform my work in the way I want	1.53	1.08–2.16
Motivation and satisfaction of and to work tasks	I do not experience joy in my daily work	2.14	1.49–3.09

4. Discussion

Nurses are one of the biggest workgroups within the healthcare sector, and nursing is an important social security profession [7,8]. Unfortunately, many nurses are currently on short- or long-term sick leave, and too many nurses choose to leave the profession in the beginning of their educational training or a short time after their entry into the profession [10]. During the COVID-19 pandemic, nurses' work situations were tested to the limit [1–5]. The aim of the study was, therefore, to investigate the association between work-related mental health diagnoses and nurses' work situations in 2017 and 2020, i.e., before and during the second wave of the COVID-19 pandemic. With the intention of investigating the complexity of the nurses' work situations, the swAge-model was used as the theme model in the analysis. In the results, we could see that the percentage of nurses having a diagnosis for exhaustion/stress had tripled between 2017 and 2020, and the percentage of nurses with a diagnosis of depression/anxiety had doubled. These are alarming numbers, and the fact that so many nurses suffer from work-related mental health issues is something that needs to be addressed and dealt with.

4.1. Impact and Determinant Areas Important for Nurses' Mental Health Diagnoses Caused by Their Work

The seven different impact and determinant areas of importance for a healthy and sustainable working life were analyzed one at a time before multivariate modelling to understand the wider complexity of the nurses´ work situations in relation to mental health diagnoses caused by their work. Earlier studies stated the importance of investigating the total complexity of the work situation and not only one or two areas of importance for a sustainable working life if the intention is to develop practically important knowledge for measured activities [16–21]. The result of this investigation showed that all seven of the impact and determinant areas appeared to have an association with nurses' mental health diagnoses caused by work.

According to the result of the univariate estimates, the nurses felt unable to cope with the physical work demands in both 2017 and in 2020. A too demanding physical work environment is problematic for a sustainable working life [16–18]. A lot of nurses' physical activity is spent standing and/or walking [45–47]; however, depending on where you work, the physical activity can also consist of working in strenuous work postures or moving patients from bed to wheelchair or on/off operating tables [48–51]. A physically demanding work environment could contribute to stress since people tend to get more tired from a physically demanding work environment, and if you are tired, you tend to not keep up with the work pace and be more sensitive to stressful situations, thus, increasing a vulnerability to mental health diagnoses, such as burnout [19,20].

The mental work environment was earlier described as a very important area for employees' mental health [16–18,52]. In the nurses´ mental work environment area, all five statements were statistically significant in 2017 with "psychologically heavy work task" having a strong connection; in 2020, this statement was still significant but the "I wish for more opportunities to determine how to perform my work" statement showed a slightly higher association. Having a perceived sense of control is identified as important for the well-being and mental health of nurses [53]. Previous studies state that the more nurses are exposed to stressful situations, the more likely it is that it will drain their psychological resources and they will experience stress-related outcomes, i.e., their job demands exceed their job resources and the result can be poor mental health [54,55].

Rest and recuperation are important to the individual's health and vital in a sustainable working life [16–18]. In the "work pace, work time, recuperation area" in the analysis, it was a "lack of time to perform work duties" that showed a high association in 2017 and it was still significant in the regression analysis in 2020; however, in 2020, it was the "accumulation of work tasks" that seemed to have a stronger association. Not having enough time for work tasks or feeling like the work tasks are piling up can cause frustration and ultimately lead to certain work tasks not being carried out and a wish to leave the profession [16–18]. A recent study found a strong negative association between high work time demands and emotional exhaustion [56]. A worst-case scenario is that lack of time can affect quality of care and/or affect nurses' health [57,58]. A British survey [59] showed that, in some cases, this time constraint can result in malpractice and the neglect of patients.

Recuperation between work shifts is important for all aspects of an individual's well-being. Recovery is necessary for the body to reverse changes in the psychobiological system (such as increased heartrate from stressful work situations) [60].

In the impact and determinant area of "private social environment for a sustainable working life", it was interesting that it was the "need to work more from home/care for relatives" that was statistically significant in 2017, whereas "wanting to spend more time enjoying leisure activities" showed as not being significant; however, in 2020, the roles were reversed. The balance between the work and the private social situation is important for employees' sustainable working life [16–18]. Sweden, as a country, did not enforce lock-down during the COVID-19 pandemic. There were restrictions as to how and when you could go to gyms, for example, and a lot of activities were held on-line instead of in person. However, could the fact that there were restrictions in place influence the respondents' feelings? A recent study showed that nurses felt it was important to leave all their experiences from working during the pandemic behind at work and when at home to focus on being at home cooking and cleaning as well as practicing self-care by exercising, walking, or spending time in nature [61].

Concerning the social environment at work, the organization and leadership are very important factors for a healthy and sustainable working life. In our study, the data from 2017 showed that lack of support from managers and co-workers seemed to have the least connection with nurses' work-related mental health diagnoses. However, in 2020, lack of support from co-workers had one of the highest connections. Our study did not show any statistical significance regarding lack of support from managers in 2017 or in 2020. It is interesting that lack of support from co-workers changed from a low connection to having one of the highest connections with work-related mental health diagnoses. Is this due to the fact that nurses relied on support from colleagues more during the COVID-19 pandemic or has the pandemic simply put the spotlight on what was always there? Previous studies have shown that collegial support affects communication, organizational commitment, teamwork, stress, negative interaction, human relations, job satisfaction and the hierarchy in the workplace [16–18,62]. Positive social relations at work can ease the burden of emotional demands and work time demands [16–18,63].

Motivation and satisfaction regarding work tasks are important in order to have a healthy and sustainable working life. Our results show that in 2017, both lack of joy in the daily work as well as having no job satisfaction seemed to have high associations with mental health and work-related diagnoses. Lack of joy in the daily work continues to have increased association with work-related diagnoses both in the 2017 and the 2020 multivariate model. According to a study [64], experiencing joy at work is important both for the nurse and for healthcare in general. Several studies [65–67] show that job satisfaction is a vital component in nursing and that it is strongly related to factors such as job stress [16–18,67], intention to leave [16–18,65,67,68], quality of care [69] and patient satisfaction [67]. Studies have shown that nurses reported higher levels of job satisfaction when they felt high levels of support from their manager [17,70].

When it came to the impact and determinant area "knowledge and competency", only the feeling of not having their competencies utilized showed to be statistically significant to nurses´ work-related mental health diagnoses. An earlier study [71] showed that good interaction between colleagues was a resource for high quality of care, which allowed everyone to use their competence well. Additionally, not being able to use their skills could most likely affect nurses' willingness to stay in their workplace.

4.2. Multivariate Analysis of the Total Complexity in the Nurses' Work Situation in Association with Work-Related Mental Diagnoses in 2017 and in 2020

In reality, each impact and determinant area is not operated separately. Therefore, all impact and determinant areas involved in this investigation were analyzed together in a total multivariate model to investigate the association between nurses' work situations and nurses´ mental health diagnoses. Out of the original seven included impact and determinant areas, only five remained statistically significant and were, therefore, included in the final multivariate models for 2017 and 2020. The included areas were "mental work environment", "work time, work pace, recuperation", "private social environment", "work social environment, organization, leadership" and "motivation and satisfaction of and to work tasks". Only three statements showed an association with nurses' work-related mental health diagnoses in both 2017 and 2020, they were "My work involves many psychologically heavy work tasks", "My work tasks usually clump together to the extent that I get frustrated" and "I do not experience joy in my daily work". Two additional statements showed significance in the 2020 model, which were "I do not feel that I get enough rest/recuperation between work shifts" and "I do not feel enough support from my co-workers". Feeling that you are unable to provide proper care to patients can lead to ethical and moral stress among nurses, which, in turn, can affect their health and psychological well-being [72,73] and cause job dissatisfaction [73]. Nurses and other healthcare workers' mental health diagnoses have been shown to threaten the quality of care and patient safety [74–76]; this adds further importance to the fact that healthcare organizations must take the nurses' work situation very seriously.

4.3. The COVID-19 Pandemics Effect on Nurses' Work Situation

Several studies have shown that many healthcare workers have experienced anxiety, depression [77–79] and burnout [79] during the COVID-19 pandemic. The final multivariate model showed that anxiety over being seriously ill can be associated with nurses' work-related mental health diagnosis. The COVID-19 pandemic had a huge impact on the healthcare organizations, with many millions of people, including nurses, becoming infected by the virus, thus, causing an increased workload for nurses [1–5]. Being at risk of being infected by COVID-19, becoming seriously ill, dying or infecting others has been cited as a major risk for work-related mental illness for healthcare workers during the COVID-19 pandemic. In this investigation, some of the variables have not shown a change between 2017 and 2020, most likely indicating that the COVID-19 pandemic did not impact these particular variables. The result in the final multivariate model did show that the nurses' increased risk of being infected by COVID-19 in their workplace was associated with work-related mental health illness. However, issues related to personal protective equipment was not statistically significant. Instead, the result showed that especially lack of support from co-workers, lack of joy in their daily work as well as an increased workload and the accumulation of work tasks showed increased associations with nurses' work-related mental health diagnoses during the COVID-19 pandemic. A previous systematic review stated that the COVID-19 pandemic forced nurses to have a greater workload, but also that many nurses had trouble falling asleep and/or not getting enough sleep, which they attributed to lack of time to decompress mentally between work shifts [10]. Additionally, nurses felt like their competencies were not utilized in a satisfactory way. Not being given the opportunity to use their skills or feeling that the organization does not utilize or appreciate the skills and knowledge that the employees possess has, in previous studies, been associated with a lack of job satisfaction and motivation and could lead to employees not wanting to continue working at the workplace [16–18].

The pandemic put the spotlight on nurses' work situations, but is the spotlight pointing in the right place? Many healthcare organizations had problems in their work environment prior to the pandemic (including lack of staff and the work situation). Have certain aspects of the nurses' work situation become more important during the COVID-19 pandemic or has the pandemic simply shown cracks in the façade? Perhaps only the future can tell since we are still living with the pandemic.

4.4. Limitations

One limitation of the study is that we had a large percentage of non-responders, the answer rate was 50.1% and 40.1% in 2017 and 2020, respectively. However, considering that it was a survey, the low response rate was expected, and we are very grateful to those nurses who took the time and answered the survey, especially in 2020 when there was an on-going pandemic. Another limitation is that when you use dichotomization, there is always a risk of losing valuable information. The dichotomization was made by an experienced researcher who thoroughly made considerations in which response choice dichotomization was used. The fifth impact and determinate area, i.e., "personal finances" was not included in the study since there was no data on the nurses' private economic situation related to the work situation that could be used in the analysis. However, this area could have an impact on the results, for instance, if nurses went to work despite being sick due to not being able to afford the loss in pay. This, in turn, could contribute an added stress. In this study, we have used the respondents' self-reported doctors' diagnoses that they felt were caused by their work. One opportunity could have been to use registers with reported work-related illnesses. However, in these registers there are only those diagnoses that have been deemed as work injuries and, therefore, the diagnoses in our study would probably not have been reported. It is also well known that the number of reported work-related illnesses is underreported [80]. Therefore, we found it more valuable to ask the nurses about which of their diagnoses they felt had been caused by their work. One limitation is the possibility of responders misunderstanding the questions regarding their current mental health diagnoses since no specific timeframe was given, i.e., "I was diagnosed with exhaustion/stress or depression/anxiety within the last six months". Another limitation is the low score on Wilks´ Λ, which would mean that we cannot rule out the possibility of other factors influencing nurses' work-related mental health other than those we have presented.

5. Conclusions

Based on the results of this survey, there were some differences in what was associated with the nurses' work-related mental health diagnoses in 2017 and in 2020. The COVID-19 pandemic put nurses' working situations to a severe test. The result from this comparative analysis, where we examined the work situations and work-related mental health diagnoses before and during the second wave of the COVID-19 pandemic, showed that increased workload and experiencing a lack of joy in the nurses´ daily work as well as experiencing a perceived lack support from their co-workers had the strongest association with nurses' work-related mental health diagnoses in 2020. It is hard to get around the fact that nurses will continue to face psychologically and physically heavy work tasks, but it is important for organizations to have an open climate so that nurses can talk about their experiences. For nurses to have more opportunities to determine how to perform their work tasks, it is important that they feel like they have a safe work environment and that they have adequate staff and resources and feel involved in decision-making. This study's analysis model is based on theories about factors that influence a healthy and sustainable working life, and the results are consistent with what the SwAge-model has previously shown [16–18].

Nurses and other healthcare workers' mental health diagnoses have been shown to threaten the quality of care and patient safety [74,75]. Therefore, the result from this study investigating nurses' work-related mental health diagnoses could be important knowledge for the future development of healthcare organizations. The results from this study could also be used by hospitals and ministries of health, etc. as a template to improve the working conditions and quality of life at work for nurses. If these two things improve, perhaps nurses would be more inclined to remain in their current workplace/profession. Future research regarding the long-term impact from COVID-19 on all areas of nurses' professional and personal lives is needed.

Author Contributions: Conceptualization, C.N. and K.N.; methodology, C.N. and K.N.; software, C.N.; formal analysis, C.N.; writing—original draft preparation, C.N.; writing—review and editing, All authors; supervision, K.N.; project administration, K.N.; funding acquisition, K.N. All authors have read and agreed to the published version of the manuscript.

Funding: This research was funded by Interreg (European Regional Development Fund, EU), grant number NYPS20303383; FORTE FORMAS, grant number 2020-02746 and the Research Platform for Collaboration for Health, Kristianstad University, Sweden, funding number 9/2021.

Institutional Review Board Statement: The study was conducted in accordance with the Declaration of Helsinki and approved by the Swedish Ethical Review Agency (2016/867 approved 07 December 2016 and 2020-01897 approved 29 April 2020).

Informed Consent Statement: Informed consent was obtained from all subjects involved in the study.

Data Availability Statement: Not applicable.

Acknowledgments: The authors wish to acknowledge the valuable input given to us by Lars Rylander, Jens Peter Ellekilde Bonde, Sandra Sögaard Töttenborg, Esben Meulengracht Flachs, Kajsa Kirstine Ugelvig Petersen and Christel Nielsen.

Conflicts of Interest: The authors declare no conflict of interest. The funders had no role in the design of the study; in the collection, analyses, or interpretation of data; in the writing of the manuscript, or in the decision to publish the results.

References

1. World Health Organization (WHO). Available online: https://www.who.int/emergencies/diseases/novel-coronavirus-2019 (accessed on 27 June 2022).
2. WHO. *Protecting Workers' Health*; Word Health Organization: Geneva, Switzerland, 2019.
3. WHO. *Healthy Workplaces: A Model for Action for Employers, Workers, Policymakers, and Practitioners*; World Health Organization: Geneva, Switzerland, 2019.
4. WHO. *Mental Disorders*; World Health Organization: Geneva, Switzerland, 2019.
5. Shone, E. More Than 850 Health and Social Care Workers Have Died of COVID in England and Wales Since the Pandemic Began. *The Scotsman*, 27 January 2021. Available online: https://www.yorkshireeveningpost.co.uk/health/coronavirus/more-than-850-health-and-social-care-workers-have-died-of-covid-in-england-and-wales-since-the-pandemic-began-3114202 (accessed on 20 September 2022).
6. Nilsson, K. Situationen under COVID-19 pandemin för 7 781 hälso- och sjukvårdsanställda: Enkätsvar vid uppföljningsstudien Hållbart arbetsliv inom hälso- och sjukvården 2020. *Lund Arbets- Och Miljömedicin Syd.* **2020**, *14*, 1–45.
7. WHO. State of the World's Nursing 2020, Investing in Education, Jobs and Leadership. 2020. Available online: https://www.who.int/publications/i/item/9789240003279 (accessed on 3 August 2022).
8. Drennan, V.M.; Ross, F. Global nurse shortages—The facts, the impact and action for change. *Br. Med. Bull.* **2019**, *130*, 25–37. [CrossRef] [PubMed]
9. ICN Nursing Definitions. Nursing Definitions | ICN—International Council of Nurses. Available online: https://www.icn.ch/nursing-policy/nursing-definitions (accessed on 3 August 2022).
10. Nagel, C.; Westergren, A.; Persson, S.S.; Lindström, P.N.; Bringsén, Å.; Nilsson, K. Nurses' Work Environment during the COVID-19 Pandemic in a Person-Centred Practice—A Systematic Review. *Sustainability* **2022**, *14*, 5785. [CrossRef]
11. Zander, B.; Busse, R.; Rafferty, A.M.; Sermeus, W.; Bruyned, L. Nursing in the European Union. *EuroHealth* **2016**, *22*, 3–6.
12. McCarthy, G.; Lehane, E. Intention to 'leave' or 'stay' in nursing. *J. Nurs. Manag.* **2007**, *15*, 248–255. [CrossRef] [PubMed]
13. Nunstedt, H.; Eriksson, M.; Obeid, A.; Hillstrom, L.; Truong, A.; Pennbrant, S. Salutary factors and hospital work environments: A qualitative descriptive study of nurses in Sweden. *BMC Nurs.* **2020**, *19*, 125. [CrossRef]
14. European Network for Workplace Health Promotion. The Case for WHP. 2018. Available online: https://www.enwhp.org/?i=portal.en.the-case-for-whp (accessed on 27 June 2022).
15. UN Global Goals for Sustainable Society Development. Available online: https://www.un.org/sustainabledevelopment/ (accessed on 27 June 2022).
16. Nilsson, K. A sustainable working life for all ages—The swAge-model. *Appl. Ergon.* **2020**, *103082*, 1–27. [CrossRef] [PubMed]
17. Nilsson, K.; Nilsson, E. Organizational Measures and Strategies for a Healthy and Sustainable Extended Working Life and Employability—A Deductive Content Analysis with Data Including Employees, First Line Managers, Trade Union Representatives and HR-Practitioners. *Int. J. Environ. Res. Public Health* **2021**, *18*, 5626. [CrossRef]
18. Nilsson, K. *Attraktivt och Hållbart Arbetsliv på MäNniskors Villkor—Arbete, Hälsa och Ledarskap med SwAge-modellen i Teori och Praktik*; Studentlitteratur: Lund, Sweden, 2021; pp. 1–420.
19. SwAge-Model. Available online: www.swage.org/en.html (accessed on 27 June 2022).
20. Aiken, L.H. Hospital nurse staffing and patient mortality, nurse burnout, and job dissatisfaction. *J. Am. Med. Assoc.* **2002**, *288*, 1987–1993. [CrossRef] [PubMed]
21. Maharaj, S.; Lees, T.; Lal, S. Prevalence and Risk Factors of Depression, Anxiety, and Stress in a Cohort of Australian Nurses. *Int. J. Environ. Res. Public Health* **2019**, *16*, 61. [CrossRef]

22. Ruotsalainen, J.H.; Verbeek, J.H.; Mariné, A.; Serra, C. Preventing occupational stress in healthcare workers. *Sao Paulo Med. J.* **2016**, *134*, 92. [CrossRef] [PubMed]
23. Dimou, F.M.; Eckelbarger, D.; Riall, T.S. Surgeon burnout: A systematic review. *J. Am. Coll. Surg.* **2016**, *222*, 1230–1239. [CrossRef] [PubMed]
24. Portero de la Cruz, S.; Cebrino, J.; Herruzo, J.; Vaquero-Abellán, M. A Multicenter Study into Burnout, Perceived Stress, Job Satisfaction, Coping Strategies, and General Health among Emergency Department Nursing Staff. *J. Clin. Med.* **2020**, *9*, 1007. [CrossRef] [PubMed]
25. Van der Heijden, B.; Brown Mahoney, C.; Xu, Y. Impact of Job Demands and Resources on Nurses' Burnout and Occupational Turnover Intention Towards an Age-Moderated Mediation Model for the Nursing Profession. *Int. J. Environ. Res. Public Health* **2019**, *16*, 2011. [CrossRef]
26. ICN. Available online: https://www.icn.ch/news/rapid-development-covid-resources-usa (accessed on 2 August 2022).
27. Adriaenssens, J.; de Gucht, V.; Maes, S. The impact of traumatic events on emergency room nurses: Findings from a questionnaire survey. *Int. J. Nurs. Stud.* **2012**, *49*, 1411–1422. [CrossRef]
28. Michie, S.; Williams, S. Reducing work related psychological ill health and sickness absence: A systematic literature review. *Occup. Environ. Med.* **2003**, *60*, 3–9. [CrossRef]
29. Pérez-Fuentes, M.M.; Gázques-Linares, J.J.; Simón-Marquez, M.M. Analysis of burnout predictors in nursing: Risk and protective psychological factors. *Eur. J. Psychol. Appl. Leg.* **2018**, *11*, 33–40. [CrossRef]
30. Broetje, S.; Jenny, G.J.; Bauer, G.F. The key job demands and resources of nursing staff: An integrative review of reviews. *Front. Psychol.* **2020**, *11*, 84. [CrossRef]
31. Khamisa, N.; Peltzer, K.; Oldenburg, B. Burnout in relation to specific contributing factors and health outcomes among nurses: A systematic review. *Int. J. Environ. Res. Public Heath* **2013**, *10*, 2214–2240. [CrossRef]
32. Van Bogaert, P.; Timmermans, O.; Weeks, S.M.; van Heusden, D.; Wouters, K.; Franck, E. Nursing unit teams matter: Impact of unit-level nurse practice environment, nurse work characteristics, and burnout on nurse reported job outcomes, and quality of care, and patient adverse events—A cross-sectional survey. *Int. J. Nurs. Stud.* **2014**, *51*, 1123–1134. [CrossRef] [PubMed]
33. Hämmig, O. Explaining burnout and the intention to leave the profession among health professionals—A cross-sectional study in a hospital setting in Switzerland. *BMC Health Serv. Res.* **2018**, *18*, 785. [CrossRef]
34. Burmeister, E.A.; Kalisch, B.J.; Xie, B.; Doumit, M.A.A.; Lee, E.; Ferraresion, A.; Terzioglu, F.; Bragadóttir, H. Determinants of nurse absenteeism and intent to leave: An international study. *J. Nurs. Manag.* **2019**, *27*, 143–153. [CrossRef]
35. Hinshaw, A.S. Navigating the perfect storm. Balancing a culture of safety with workforce challenges. *Nurs. Res.* **2008**, *57*, S4–S10. [CrossRef] [PubMed]
36. Sasso, L.; Bagnasco, A.; Catania, G.; Zanini, M.; Aleo, G.; Watson, R.; RN4CAST@IT Working Group. Push and pull factors of nurses' intention to leave. *J. Nurs. Manag.* **2019**, *27*, 946–954. [CrossRef]
37. Lin, K.-C.; Huang, C.-C.; Wu, C.-C. Association between stress at work and primary headache among nursing staff in Taiwan. *Headache* **2007**, *47*, 576–584. [CrossRef]
38. Li, H.; Cheng, B.; Zhu, X.P. Quantification of burnout in emergency nurses: A systematic review and meta-analysis. *Int. Emerg. Nurs.* **2018**, *39*, 46–54. [CrossRef] [PubMed]
39. Nilsson, K. *Hållbart Arbetsliv Inom Hälso- och Sjukvården—Enkätsvar om Hur 11902 Medarbetare Upplever Sin Arbetssituation*; Lund University: Lund, Sweden, 2017; Rapport nr 13/2017.
40. Pallant, J. SPSS Survival manual. In *A Step by Step Guide to Data Analysis Using IBM SPSS*, 7th ed.; Open University Press: London, UK, 2020; pp. 1–361.
41. Norman, G.F.; Streiner, D.L. Biostatistics. In *The Bare Essentials*, 4th ed.; People's Medical Publishing House: Shelton, CT, USA, 2014; pp. 1–422.
42. WMA. Declaration of Helsinki: Ethical Principles for Medical Research Involving Human Subjects. World Medical Association. 64th WMA General Assembly, Brazil. 2008. Available online: https://www.wma.net/policies-post/wma-declaration-of-helsinki-ethical-principles-for-medical-research-involving-human-subjects/ (accessed on 20 June 2022).
43. SFS. Lag om Etikprövning. 2003, 460. Available online: https://www.riksdagen.se/sv/dokument-lagar/dokument/svensk-forfattningssamling/lag2003460-om-etikprovning-av-forskning-som_sfs-2003-460 (accessed on 20 June 2022).
44. Dataskyddsförordning (2016). Förordning (EU) 2016/679. Available online: https://www.imy.se/verksamhet/dataskydd/det-har-galler-enligt-gdpr/introduktion-till-gdpr/dataskyddsforordningen-i-fulltext/ (accessed on 20 June 2022).
45. Chappel, S.E.; Verswijweren, S.J.J.M.; Aisbett, B.; Considine, J.; Ridgers, N.D. Nurses' occupational physical activity levels: A systematic review. *Int. J. Nurs. Stud.* **2017**, *73*, 52–62. [CrossRef] [PubMed]
46. Yu, F.; Narayanan, A.; Mackay, L.; Ward, K.; King, A.; Smith, M. Describing objectively measured intensive care nurses' physical work activity behavioural patterns during a 12-hr shift. *J. Clin. Nurs.* **2020**, *29*, 4331–4342. [CrossRef] [PubMed]
47. Dutra, C.K.d.R.; Guirardello, E.d.B. Nurse work environment and its impact on reasons for missed care, safety climate, and job satisfaction: A cross-sectional study. *J. Adv. Nurs.* **2021**, *77*, 2398–2406. [CrossRef] [PubMed]
48. Gustafsson, K.; Marklund, S.; Aronsson, G.; Leineweber, C. Physical work environment factors affecting risk for disability pension due to mental or musculoskeletal diagnoses among nursing professionals, care assistants and other occupations: A prospective, population-based cohort study. *BMJ Open* **2019**, *9*, e026491. [CrossRef]

49. da Costa, B.R.; Vieira, E.R. Risk factors for work-related musculoskeletal disorders: A systematic review of recent longitudinal studies. *Am. J. Ind. Med.* **2010**, *53*, 285–323. [CrossRef] [PubMed]
50. Koppelaar, E.; Knibbe, H.J.J.; Miedema, H.S.; Burdorf, A. The influence of ergonomic devices on mechanical load during patient handling activities in nursing homes. *Ann. Occup. Hyg.* **2012**, *56*, 708–718. [PubMed]
51. Warming, S.; Precht, D.H.; Suadicani, P.; Ebbehoj, N.E. Musculoskeletal complaints among nurses related to patient handling tasks and psychosocial factors—Based on logbook registrations. *Appl. Ergon.* **2009**, *40*, 569–576. [CrossRef] [PubMed]
52. Karasek, R.; Theorell, T. *Healthy Work. Stress, Productivity, and the Reconstruction of Working life*; Basic Books: New York, NY, USA, 1992.
53. Sin, S.S.; Huak, C.Y. Psychological impact of the SARS outbreak on a Singaporean rehabilitation department. *Int. J. Ther. Rehabil.* **2004**, *11*, 417–424. [CrossRef]
54. Van den Broeck, A.; De Cuyper, N.; De Witte, H.; Vansteenkiste, M. Not all job demands are equal: Differentiating job hindrances and job challenges in the Job-Demands-Resources model. *Eur. J. Work. Organ. Psychol.* **2010**, *19*, 735–759. [CrossRef]
55. de Wijn, A.N.; van der Doef, M.P. Patient related stressful situations and stress-related outcomes in emergency nurses: A cross-sectional study on the role of work factors and recovery during leisure time. *Int. J. Nurs. Stud.* **2020**, *107*, 103579. [CrossRef]
56. Riell, E.M.; Thomas, J. The moderating role of work pressure on the relationships between emotional demands and tension, exhaustion, and work engagement: An experience samplibg study among nurses. *Eur. J. Work. Organ. Psychol.* **2019**, *28*, 414–429.
57. Ericson-Lidman, E.; Åhlin, J. Assessments of stress of conscience, perceptions of conscience, burnout, and social support before and after implementation of a participatory action-research-based intervention. *Clin. Nurs. Res.* **2017**, *26*, 205–223. [CrossRef]
58. Richards, K. Work/life balance: The disease of 'busyness'. *Nurs. Econ.* **2015**, *33*, 117–119.
59. Borland, S. Three in Four Nurses Say They Are Too Busy to Talk to Patients. 2011. Available online: https://www.dailymail.co.uk/health/article-2048933/Three-nurses-say-busy-talk-patients.html (accessed on 3 August 2022).
60. Meijman, T.F.; Mulder, G. Psychological aspects of workload. In *Handbook of Work and Organizational Psychology*; Drenth, P.J.D., Thierry, H., Eds.; Psychology Press: Hove, UK, 1998; pp. 5–33.
61. Maben, J.; Conolly, A.; Abrams, R.; Rowland, E.; Harris, R.; Kelly, D.; Kent, B.; Couper, K. 'You can't walk through water without getting wet' UK nurses' distress and psychological health needs during the COVID-19 pandemic: A longitudinal interview study. *Int. J. Nurs. Stud.* **2022**, *131*, 104242. [CrossRef]
62. Kılıç, E.; Altuntaş, S. The effect of collegial solidarity among nurses on the organizational climate. *Int. Nurs. Rev.* **2019**, *66*, 356–365. [CrossRef] [PubMed]
63. Schneider, A.; Weigl, M. Associations between psychosocial work factors and provider mental well-being in emergency departments: A systematic review. *PLoS ONE* **2018**, *13*, e0197375. [CrossRef] [PubMed]
64. Sampaio, F.; Sequeira, C.; Teixeira, L. Nurses' mental health during the COVID-19 outbreak: A cross-sectional study. *J. Occup. Environ. Med.* **2020**, *62*, 783–787. [CrossRef] [PubMed]
65. De Simone, S.; Planta, A.; Cicotto, G. The role of job satisfaction, work engagement, self-efficacy and agentic capacities on nurses' turnover intention and patient satisfaction. *Appl. Nurs. Res.* **2018**, *39*, 130–140. [CrossRef] [PubMed]
66. Puah, L.N.; Ong, L.D.; Chong, W.Y. The effects of perceived organizational support, perceived supervisor support and perceived co-worker support on safety and health compliance. *Int. J. Occup. Saf. Ergon.* **2016**, *22*, 333–339. [CrossRef]
67. Sharif, S.P.; Ahadzadeh, A.S.; Nia, H.S. Mediating role of psychological well-being in the relationship between organizational support and nurses' outcomes: A cross-sectional study. *J. Adv. Nurs.* **2018**, *74*, 887–899. [CrossRef]
68. Lu, H.; Zhao, Y.; While, A. Job satisfaction among hospital nurses: A literature review. *Int. J. Nurs. Stud.* **2019**, *94*, 21–31. [CrossRef]
69. Halcomb, E.; Bird, S. Job satisfaction and career intention of Australian General Practice nurses: A cross-sectional survey. *J. Nurs. Scholarsh.* **2020**, *52*, 270–280. [CrossRef]
70. Gillet, N.; Fouquereau, E.; Coillot, H.; Cougot, B.; Moret, L.; Dupont, S.; Bonnetain, F.; Colombat, P. The effects of work factors on nurses' job satisfaction, quality of care and turnover intentions in oncology. *J. Adv. Nurs.* **2018**, *74*, 1208–1219. [CrossRef]
71. Persson, S.S.; Blomqvist, K.; Nilsson Lindström, P. Meetings are an Important Prerequisite for Flourishing Workplace Relationships. *Int. J. Environ. Res. Public Health* **2021**, *18*, 8092. [CrossRef]
72. Bergman, L.; Falk, A.-C.; Wolf, A. Registered nurses' experiences of working in the intensive care unit during the COVID-19 pandemic. *Nurs. Crit. Care* **2021**, *26*, 467–475. [CrossRef] [PubMed]
73. Da Rosa, P.; Brown, R.; Pravecek, B.; Carotta, C.; Garcia, A.S.; Carson, P.; Callies, D.; Vukovich, M. Factors associated with nurses emotional distress during the COVID-19 pandemic. *Appl. Nurs. Res.* **2021**, *62*, 151502. [CrossRef] [PubMed]
74. Cheng, H.; Yang, H.; Ding, Y.; Wang, B. Nurses' mental health and patient safety: An extension of the job demands-resources model. *J. Nurs. Manag.* **2020**, *28*, 653–663. [CrossRef] [PubMed]
75. Teoh, K.R.H.; Hassard, J.; Cox, T. Doctors' working conditions, wellbeing and hospital quality of care: A multilevel analysis. *Saf. Sci.* **2020**, *135*, 105–115. [CrossRef]
76. Nagel, C.; Rylander, L.; Ellekilde Bonde, J.P.; Sögaard Töttenborg, S.; Meulengracht Flachs, E.; Ugelvig Petersen, K.K.; Nielsen, C.; Nilsson, K. Predictors of nurses' work-related mental health during the COVID-19 pandemic. (Unpublished work).
77. Pappa, S.; Ntella, V.; Giannakas, T.; Giannakoulis, V.G.; Papoutsi, E.; Katsaounou, P. Prevalence of depression, anxiety and insomnia among healthcare workers during the COVID-19 pandemic: A systematic review and meta-analysis. *Brain Behav. Immun.* **2020**, *88*, 901–907. [CrossRef]

78. Shechter, A.; Diaz, F.; Moise, N.; Anstey, D.E.; Ye, S.; Agarwal, S.; Abdalla, M. Psychological distress, coping behaviors, and preferences for support among New York healthcare workers during the COVID-19 pandemic. *Gen. Hosp. Psychiatry* **2020**, *66*, 1–8. [CrossRef]
79. Sanghera, J.; Pattani, N.; Hashmi, Y.; Varley, K.F.; Cherevu, M.S.; Bradley, A.; Burke, J.R. The impact of SARS-CoV-2 on the mental health of healthcare workers in a hospital setting—A systematic review. *J. Occup. Health* **2020**, *62*, e12175. [CrossRef]
80. Swedish Work Environment Authority. Work-Related Disorders 2020. Workenvironment Statistic Report 2021, 3. Arbetsmiljöverket. Arbetsorsakade besvär 2020. Arbetsmiljö statistik Rapport 2021, 3. 2021. Available online: https://www.av.se/globalassets/filer/statistik/arbetsorsakade-besvar-2020/rapport-arbetsorsakade-besvar-2020.pdf?hl=Arbetsorsakade%20besv%C3%A4r%202020.%20Arbetsmilj%C3%B6%20statistik%20Rapport%202021,%203 (accessed on 8 September 2022).

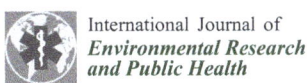

Article

Perceived Work Ability during Enforced Working from Home Due to the COVID-19 Pandemic among Finnish Higher Educational Staff

Saila Kyrönlahti [1,*], Subas Neupane [1], Clas-Håkan Nygård [1], Jodi Oakman [2], Soile Juutinen [3] and Anne Mäkikangas [3]

1 Faculty of Social Sciences, Unit of Health Sciences, Tampere University, 33014 Tampere, Finland; subas.neupane@tuni.fi (S.N.); clas-hakan.nygard@tuni.fi (C.-H.N.)
2 Centre for Ergonomics and Human Factors, School of Psychology and Public Health, La Trobe University, Melbourne, VIC 3086, Australia; j.oakman@latrobe.edu.au
3 Work Research Centre, Faculty of Social Sciences, Tampere University, 33014 Tampere, Finland; soile.juutinen@tuni.fi (S.J.); anne.makikangas@tuni.fi (A.M.)
* Correspondence: saila.kyronlahti@tuni.fi; Tel.: +358-503182275

Abstract: **Background:** Due to COVID-19 pandemic, many employees were forced to suddenly shift to working from home (WFH). How this disruption of work affected employees' work ability is not known. In this study, we investigated the developmental profiles of work ability among Finnish higher education employees in a one-year follow-up during the enforced WFH. Secondly, we investigated demographic, organizational, and ergonomic factors associated with the developmental profiles. **Methods:** A longitudinal web-survey was conducted with four measurement points (April 2020–February 2021). Employees of a Finnish university who answered the questionnaire at baseline and at least at two follow-up surveys (n = 678) were included (71% women, 45% teachers/research staff, 44% supporting staff, 11% hired students). Perceived work ability was measured on a scale of 1–5 in all timepoints. Latent class growth curve analysis was used to identify profiles of work ability. Multinomial logistic regression was used to determine the associations of demographic factors, perceived stress, musculoskeletal pain, functionality of home for work, and organizational support with the work ability profiles. **Results:** Six distinct work ability profiles were identified. For most (75%), work ability remained stable during the follow-up. A total of 17% had a favourable trend (very good-stable or increasing) of work ability, and 8% had non-favourable (poor-stable or decreasing). Poor ergonomics at home, low organizational support, high stress, and musculoskeletal pain were associated with non-favourable development of work ability. **Conclusions:** Heterogeneity in development of work ability during forced WFH was found. Several factors were identified through which work ability can be supported.

Keywords: ergonomics; stress; musculoskeletal pain

1. Introduction

In response to the outbreak of COVID-19 disease in spring 2020, national policies on social distancing were placed in most countries, including Finland. The social distancing policies mandated an abrupt shift to working from home (WFH), which has had a profound impact mainly on white-collar workers. Although the prevalence of WFH was increasing, for many, it was not routinely undertaken [1]. According to EU Labour Force Survey, in 2019, before the current pandemic, less than 5% of the EU labour force regularly worked from home [2]. In response to the COVID-19 public health measures, mandatory WFH was instigated across much of the world. On average, WFH was reported by 37% in EU after the pandemic and lockdowns started [3]. The figures for some countries, including Finland, have been much higher (50–60%) [3].

The sudden disruption of work meant very little time for formal measures to be instigated by individual workers and their organizations and the subsequent impact on employee well-being. Prior research has identified that the WFH enables flexibility and an improved work–life interface [4,5]. However, recent studies have also shown negative consequences of mandatory WFH to workers' well-being. The closure of schools and childcare had a negative impact on those with caring responsibilities [6]. Work–life conflict emerged especially for families with young children, impacting women to a greater extent than men [3,6]. Technostress and work strain increased due to an expansion in the use of digital working tools, especially among workers not accustomed to digital technologies and remote working [7]. Furthermore, for many, the home offices were inadequately equipped for WFH, with poor physical, cognitive, and organizational ergonomic factors, such as inadequate workspace and equipment for work and social isolation from work community, potentially impacting work ability. For example, consequences of poor physical ergonomics may have impacted work ability through musculoskeletal pain [8].

Despite increasing evidence on the impacts of WFH during the COVID-19 pandemic, the impact on employees' work ability is yet to be studied. Work ability is a comprehensive indicator that describes a worker's ability to meet the demands of work given the individual's resources [9]. The individual resources cover a broad and holistic range of factors from a worker's health and functional ability to competencies, values, and attitudes towards work. Work demands, on the other hand, cover the actual content and demands of work but also the physical and social work environment, community, organization, and management of the work [9]. The different domains of work ability were significantly affected by the mandatory shift to WFH.

The starting points for individual employees vary greatly, with some employees more accustomed and prepared than others to shift to WFH; therefore, a person-centred estimation strategy that considers the possible heterogeneity in the development of work ability during mandatory WFH is warranted. The aim of this study is to investigate the developmental profiles of work ability among Finnish higher education staff during the mandatory WFH from April 2020 to February 2021. The second aim is to study how demographic factors, stress, musculoskeletal pain, the functionality of home for work, and organizational support predict membership in the different work ability profiles.

2. Methods

2.1. Study Population

The data used in this study were collected as a part of the Well-being 2020 research project, which aimed to explore working at home and its impact on well-being among the staff of Tampere Universities during the coronavirus crisis. The longitudinal study was conducted with four measurement points: in April 2020 (T1), June 2020 (T2), October 2020 (T3), and February 2021 (T4). Data were collected through a web-based questionnaire created with the LimeSurvey.

The study flowchart is presented in Figure 1. At T1, all members of the university community were invited via email to participate in the survey with one reminder. Of the 6929 university employees, 2661 employees responded (response rate 38%). The baseline respondents who were willing to continue their participation in the study received the first follow-up survey with one reminder at T2, resulting in 909 responses. Invitations to participate in the second follow-up survey (T3), with two reminders, were sent to those who had responded to both earlier surveys and agreed to continue their participation. At T3, 692 employees responded. The third follow-up survey (T4) was sent with two reminders to employees who had participated in all earlier surveys and agreed to continue their participation. At T4, 535 employees responded.

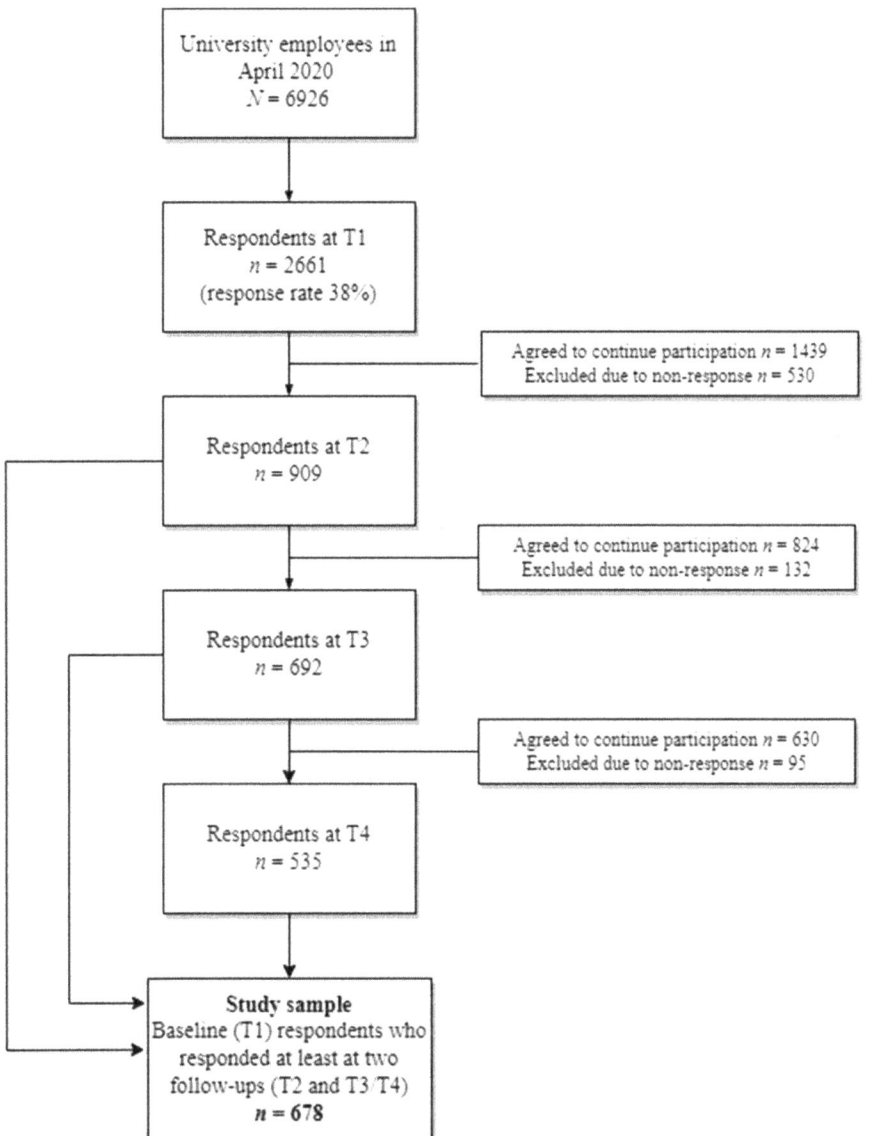

Figure 1. Flowchart of university employees included in the study of work ability profiles during COVID-19 lockdown. T1–T4 are data collection points: T1, April 2020; T2, June 2020; T3, October 2020; T4, March 2021.

The current study uses data from respondents who answered the questionnaire at baseline and at least at two of the three follow-up surveys ($n = 678$). The mean age of participants was 44.3 years (SD = 11.2) at baseline. Educational attainment was most commonly a Master's degree (48%). As regards the participants' primary position, 45% were teaching and research staff, 44% were support staff, 8% were doctoral/licentiate students, and 3% were BSc/MSc students at T1.

2.2. Measures

2.2.1. Work Ability

To assess work ability the respondents were asked: *"How would you describe your work ability or your ability to make progress towards your degree in the past two weeks?"* (modified from [10]). The respondents were asked to evaluate their work ability on a 5-point Likert-scale from 1 (very poor) to 5 (very good). The same question with same answer options was asked in each of the follow-up rounds but with the following recall periods: *"during past two months"* (T2), *"during autumn 2020"* (T3), and *"in early 2021"* (T4).

2.2.2. Predictor Variables

Baseline characteristics included demographic factors (age, gender, primary position at university, relationship status, current housing situation, number of under-school-aged and school-aged children), ergonomic and organizational factors (functionality of respondents' home for work, organizational support), and musculoskeletal pain and stress.

The functionality of respondents' home for work was assessed at baseline with five items ("I have adequate space at home for remote working; "I have the necessary equipment at home for remote working"; "I can find enough peace at home for working"; "I can maintain a healthy work-life balance when working from home"; "My home internet connection works well enough"). Each item was measured on a scale from 1 (strongly disagree) to 5 (strongly agree). Using principal component analyses (PCA), the original items were reduced to one factor (Table S1), for which the standardized factor score values ranged from −3.7 to 1.4. The factor score was used as a continuous variable in the analyses.

Organizational support was assessed with six items developed for the current study. Four related to university management and support (*"The top management of the university have communicated clearly about the current exceptional circumstances"*; *"My practical questions have been answered quickly enough"*; *"I have received enough instructions for performing my tasks and duties from home"*; *"I have received support for my work when I have encountered difficulties"*). Two items related to the operation of information systems and teleworking tools (*"I have received enough instructions for using the electronic systems and tools such as Teams, Zoom, Panopto, Moodle"*; *"The electronic systems and tools have worked well technically"*). Respondents indicated their agreement with the statements from 1 (strongly disagree) to 5 (strongly agree). The original items were reduced to one factor (Table S1), for which the standardized factor score values ranged from −4.4 to 1.4. The factor score was used as a continuous variable in the analyses. Details on the PCA to create the composite variables is described in the Supplementary Materials (Table S1).

Musculoskeletal pain was assessed at baseline by the question: *"Have you experienced pains, aches or other discomfort in your back, neck, or arms during the past two weeks?"* (modified from [11]). The answer options ranged from 1 (never) to 5 (always) and were recategorized into three classes: low (comprising answer options "never" and "rarely"), moderate ("sometimes"), and high ("often" and "always"). Stress was assessed at baseline by the question *"Stress means you feel tense, restless, nervous of anxious or are unable to sleep because your mind is troubled. Have you been feeling stressed in the last two weeks?"* [12]. The response scale ranged from 1 (not at all) to 5 (very much) and recategorized into low, moderate, and high.

3. Statistical Analyses

3.1. Trajectory Analyses

Latent class growth curve analysis (LCGA) was used to examine heterogeneity in the development of work ability during the follow-up and to classify individuals into distinct profiles based on their response patterns to the questions about work ability at four timepoints. Work ability at each timepoint was treated as ordinal variables ranging from 1 to 5, with equally spaced levels. Assuming homogeneity of variance within the profiles, the posterior probabilities of belonging to each profile were obtained for each respondent, and they were allocated to the profile for which the probability was the highest [13,14]. The best fit model was chosen based on the interpretation of the identified profiles as well as several statistical model fit criteria (Table S2) [15]. Models with one to seven classes with a linear and quadratic shape trajectories were examined.

A six-profile solution best fitted the data based on the model fit indices (Table S2). The six-class solution excluding the quadratic terms was supported by the LMR likelihood ratio test ($p = 0.030$); it ranked best in terms of the highest entropy value (0.79) and the lowest sample-size-adjusted BIC. Although some of the profiles were rather small, they were important in terms of the content. The minimum class size was above 1%, which can be considered adequate [16]. The average posterior probabilities were likewise reasonably high (>0.70) for all profiles. The models were rerun with different starting values to ensure the optimal solution was found. LCGA were run with Mplus software V.7.2 (Mplus, Los Angeles, CA, US). The class assignment information was exported to SPSS v. 26 (IBM), which was used for the explanatory analyses.

Baseline characteristics by the derived work ability profiles are reported as mean and standard deviation (SD) for continuous variables and proportions for categorical variables. Differences between profiles were examined with chi-square test for categorical variables and analysis of variance for continuous variables.

3.2. Multinomial Regression Modelling

We used multinomial logistic regression to determine the associations between baseline demographic and ergonomic factors, organizational support, stress, and musculoskeletal pain with the work ability profiles. Odds ratios (OR) with 95% confidence intervals (CIs) were determined for each model. First, each predictor variable was individually examined in univariate regression models using profile membership as a categorical dependent variable. Then, a forward stepwise multinomial regression was used to test which factors significantly ($\alpha = 0.10$) predicted participants' work ability when all other variables were mutually adjusted. The variables that survived the selection were simultaneously added into the final model. Multicollinearity was checked using variance inflation factor. Model fit was estimated from Pearson's goodness-of-fit test. The proportion of variance explained was determined from Nagelkerke's pseudo R^2.

Those who did not give information on gender ($n = 21$) were excluded from the explanatory analysis. Furthermore, due to too-small class size (<1%), those who reported their gender as other ($n = 7$) were excluded.

4. Results

4.1. Work Ability Trajectories

Figure 2 depicts the profiles of work ability. The majority of respondents (52%) belonged to "good-stable" profile, in which work ability remained at a good level across the follow-up. Approximately one-fourth (23%) of respondents were categorized into the "moderate-stable" profile, characterized by stable, moderate level of work ability. "Very good-stable" profile (13% of respondents) reported initially very good work ability, which slightly decreased after T2; yet, the change was not statistically significant ($p = 0.06$ for slope). Our analysis also revealed two rather small work ability profiles in which the slope of change in work ability during follow-up was statistically significant ($p < 0.05$). These small profiles were named "very good-decreasing" (2% of participants), in which participants initially reported very good work ability that decreased to a poor level during follow-up, and "good-increasing" (4% of participants), in which participants reported good work ability at T1, which improved to very good level during follow-up. Finally, a "poor-stable" profile emerged (6% of respondents), in which those reporting poor work ability remained at a poor level across the follow-up.

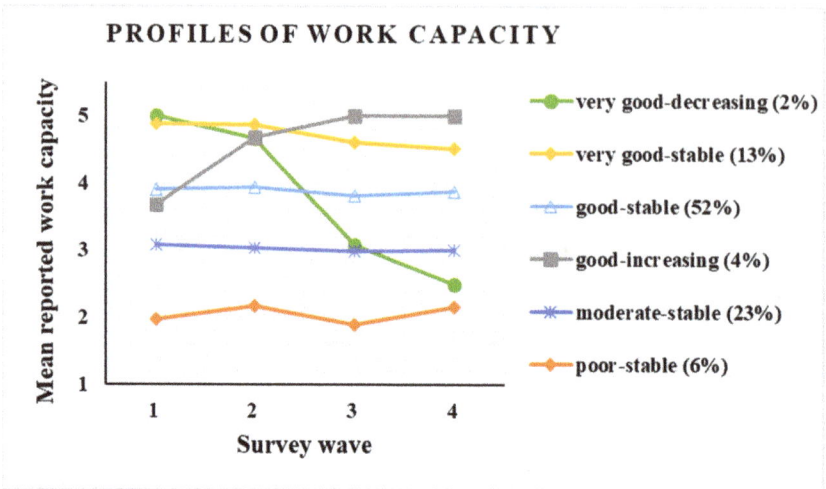

Figure 2. Profiles of work ability during COVID-19 lockdown among university employees (number of participants in each profile: high-decreasing = 12, high = 87, good = 375, good-increasing = 26, moderate = 157, poor = 39). T1–T4 are data collection points: T1, April 2020; T2, June 2020; T3, October 2020; T4, March 2021.

Because some of the derived work ability profiles were too small to yield reliable results in regression models, we combined some of them into bigger classes. The two profiles showing the most optimal development of work ability ("very good-stable" and "good-increasing") were combined. Similarly, the profiles showing the least optimal ("poor-stable" and "decreasing") development of work ability were merged into one class. The "good-stable" profile was chosen as the reference category because it was the most common class.

4.2. Baseline Characteristics

The derived profiles of work ability differed in almost all studied factors (Table 1). Those in the less optimal work ability profiles were younger and more often men and teaching/research staff than those in "good-stable" and "very good-stable and good-increasing" profiles. A clear gradient was observed in the two factor-variables (functionality of home for work and organizational support) such that those in the most optimal scored higher than those in the less favourable profiles. Stress and musculoskeletal pain were more prevalent in the less optimal work ability profiles.

4.3. Regression Analyses

Table 2 shows the univariate associations of the predictor variables with a membership of the "very good-stable and good-increasing", "moderate-stable", and "poor-stable and decreasing" work ability profiles, with the "good-stable" profile as a reference. Age was conversely associated with "moderate-stable" and "poor-stable and decreasing" profiles, while male gender was associated with "poor-stable and decreasing" profile. Having children under school-age was associated with "moderate-stable" profile. Support staff were less likely to belong to "moderate-stable" and "poor-stable and decreasing" profiles as compared to other staff groups. Further, those living in flat or in terraced/semi-detached house were more likely to belong to "moderate-stable" profile than those living in a single-family detached house.

Table 1. Baseline characteristic of the study population and each of the derived work ability profiles among university staff (n = 678).

	All (n = 678)	Very Good-Stable and Good-Increasing (n = 113)	Good-Stable (n = 357)	Moderate-Stable (n = 157)	Poor-Stable and Decreasing (n = 51)	p for Difference
Demographic factors						
Age, years, mean (SD)	44.3 (11.2)	46.6 (11.0)	45.4 (11.3)	41.2 (10.4)	40.7 (11.3)	<0.001
Gender, %						0.031
Women	75	76	74	65	55	
Men	21	22	22	30	41	
Other/prefer not to say	4	2	4	5	4	
Primary position, %						<0.001
Teaching/research staff	45	37	42	56	53	
Support staff	44	57	49	30	22	
Doctoral/licentiate student	8	5	7	10	22	
BSc/MSc student	3	2	3	5	4	
Relationship status, %						0.056
Single	17	13	15	22	26	
In a relationship	83	87	85	78	74	
School-aged children (yes %)	29	31	28	32	24	0.669
Children under school-age (yes %)	18	12	17	25	14	0.033
Current housing						0.016
Single-family detached house	34	42	36	24	25	
Flat	44	36	42	49	57	
Terraced/semi-detached house	23	22	22	27	18	
Ergonomic and organizational factors						
Functionality of home as workplace, mean (SD) [a]	0.0 (1.0)	0.69 (0.71)	0.06 (0.89)	−0.43 (0.98)	−0.60 (1.28)	<0.001
Organizational support [b], mean (SD)	0.0 (1.0)	0.50 (0.83)	0.11 (0.91)	−0.35 (0.91)	−0.82 (1.35)	<0.001
Musculoskeletal pain, %						<0.001
Low	49	71	50	35	39	
Moderate	19	18	19	16	24	
High	32	11	31	49	37	
Work-related stress, %						<0.001
Low	51	81	54	27	31	
Moderate	22	10	25	30	8	
High	27	9	21	43	61	

Note. SD, standard deviation. Summary statistics calculated among participants with non-missing data. Missing values included: age n = 5, gender n = 2, primary position n = 2, relationship status n = 22, current housing n = 3, under-school-aged children n = 5, and school-aged children n = 5. [a] Standardized factor score, range from −3.7 to 1.4. [b] Standardized factor score, range from −4.4 to 1.

Table 2. Univariate associations between profiles of work ability among university staff during COVID-19 lockdown with baseline predictors. Multinomial logistic regression analysis odds ratios (OR) and 95% confidence intervals (CI).

	Very Good-Stable and Good-Increasing vs. Good-Stable	Moderate-Stable vs. Good-Stable	Poor-Stable and Decreasing vs. Good-Stable
	OR (95% CI)	OR (95% CI)	OR (95% CI)
Demographic factors			
Age	1.01 (0.99–1.03)	**0.97 (0.95–0.98)**	**0.97 (0.94–0.99)**
Gender			
Women	ref.	ref.	ref.
Men	0.93 (0.55–1.56)	1.52 (0.99–2.32)	**2.47 (1.33–4.58)**
Primary position			
Teaching/research staff	ref.	ref.	ref.
Support staff	1.29 (0.82–2.03)	**0.51 (0.33–0.77)**	**0.37 (0.18–0.78)**
Doctoral/licentiate student	0.73 (0.26–2.04)	1.13 (0.56–2.27)	2.31 (0.99–5.39)
BSc/MSc student	0.64 (0.14–3.00)	1.15 (0.43–3.07)	1.01 (0.21–4.81)
School-aged children			
No	ref.	ref.	ref.
Yes (one or more)	1.05 (0.65–1.68)	1.06 (0.70–1.62)	0.78 (0.39–1.56)
Children under school-age			
No	ref.	ref.	ref.
Yes (one or more)	0.58 (0.30–1.12)	**1.63 (1.03–2.59)**	0.78 (0.34–1.82)
Relationship status			
Single	ref.	ref.	ref.
In relationship	1.22 (0.65–2.30)	0.64 (0.39–1.04)	**0.50 (0.25–0.99)**
Current housing			
Single-family detached house	ref.	ref.	ref.
Flat	0.74 (0.46–1.21)	**1.96 (1.22–3.16)**	1.82 (0.90–3.67)
Terraced/semi-detached house	0.86 (0.48–1.54)	**2.14 (1.25–3.69)**	1.20 (0.49–2.93)
Ergonomic and organizational factors			
Functionality of home as workplace	**2.94 (2.11–4.10)**	**0.63 (0.51–0.77)**	**0.53 (0.39–0.71)**
Organizational support	**1.76 (1.33–2.32)**	**0.61 (0.45–0.74)**	**0.41 (0.31–0.55)**
Work-related stress			
Low	ref.	ref.	ref.
Moderate	**0.24 (0.12–0.49)**	**2.29 (1.40–3.75)**	0.58 (0.19–1.81)
High	**0.27 (0.13–0.57)**	**4.09 (2.53–6.59)**	**5.45 (2.77–10.75)**
Musculoskeletal pain			
Low	ref.	ref.	ref.
Moderate	0.61 (0.34–1.08)	1.11 (0.63–1.93)	1.44 (0.65–3.18)
High	**0.25 (0.13–0.47)**	**2.10 (1.37–3.22)**	1.60 (0.81–3.15)

Note: ref. indicates the reference group.

The score for the functionality of home for work was positively associated with membership in "very good-stable and good increasing" profiles and conversely associated with membership in "moderate-stable" and "poor-stable and decreasing" profiles. Organizational support was similarly associated with work ability profiles: the higher the score, the more likely a respondent was to belong to the more optimal work ability profiles. The odds of belonging to "poor-stable and decreasing" or "moderate-stable" profiles were higher for those who reported high work-related stress. High musculoskeletal pain predicted a membership in "moderate-stable" profile, while those reporting high musculoskeletal pain were unlikely to belong to the most optimal work ability profiles.

In the multivariate model (Table 3), increasing age increased the probability of belonging to "moderate-stable" profile. Men were more likely than women to belong to the poorer work ability profiles.

Table 3. Multivariate associations between profiles of work ability among university staff during COVID-19 lockdown with baseline predictors. Multinomial logistic regression analysis OR and 95% confidence intervals (CI).

Predictor	Very Good-Stable and Good-Increasing vs. Good-Stable	Moderate-Stable vs. Good-Stable	Poor-Stable and Decreasing vs. Good-Stable
	OR (95% CI)	OR (95% CI)	OR (95% CI)
Individual/background factors			
Age	0.98 (0.96–1.00)	**0.97 (0.95–0.99)**	0.98 (0.94–1.02)
Gender			
Women	ref.	ref.	ref.
Men	0.78 (0.42–1.42)	**1.73 (1.05–2.84)**	**2.53 (1.23–5.21)**
Primary position			
Teaching/research staff	ref.	ref.	ref.
Support staff	0.98 (0.58–1.66)	0.60 (0.15–1.96)	0.98 (0.16–6.05)
Doctoral/licentiate student	0.99 (0.58–1.66)	**0.60 (0.37–0.96)**	0.59 (0.26–1.31)
BSc/MSc student	0.35 (0.11–1.14)	0.91 (0.39–2.12)	2.84 (0.96–8.44)
Ergonomic and organizational factors			
Functionality of home as workplace	**2.60 (1.80–3.75)**	0.80 (0.63–1.00)	**0.70 (0.50–0.97)**
Satisfied with the activities of Tampere University	**1.46 (1.09–1.97)**	**0.69 (0.55–0.87)**	**0.50 (0.35–0.70)**
Work-related stress			
Low	ref.	ref.	ref.
Moderate	**0.28 (0.13–0.60)**	**2.17 (1.26–3.71)**	0.51 (0.15–1.65)
High	0.50 (0.23–1.12)	**2.98 (1.74–5.12)**	**3.57 (1.63–7.79)**
Musculoskeletal pain			
Low	ref.	ref.	ref.
Moderate	0.86 (0.46–1.63)	1.00 (0.55–1.84)	1.59 (0.66–3.88)
High	**0.38 (0.18–0.77)**	**1.82 (1.11–2.98)**	1.35 (0.61–2.99)

Note: Stepwise forward variable selection. α = 0.10. Chi-square p-value for model fit < 0.001 (273.847 with 33 degrees of freedom). Nagelkerke value 0.391; ref. indicates the reference group.

All ergonomic and organizational factors significantly predicted membership of the work ability profiles. One SD increase on functionality of home for work score was associated with OR of 2.60 (95% CI 1.80–3.75) of belonging to "very good-stable and good-increasing" profiles, whereas it decreased the probability of belonging to (the least optimal profiles) "moderate-stable" (OR 0.80; 95% CI 0.63–1.00) and "poor-stable and decreasing" profiles (OR 0.70; 95% CI 0.50–0.97). Similarly, one SD increase on organizational support score was associated with higher probability of belonging to "very good-stable and good-increasing" profiles (OR 1.46; 95% CI 1.09–1.97), whereas it decreased the probability of belonging to "moderate-stable" (OR 0.69; 95% CI 0.55–0.87) and "poor-stable and decreasing" profiles (OR 0.50; 95% CI 0.35–0.70).

High stress predicted membership in "moderate-stable" profile and in "poor-stable and decreasing" profiles. Moderate stress level decreased the odds of belonging to "very good-stable and good-increasing" profiles. Finally, those reporting high musculoskeletal pain had lower odds of belonging to the optimal profiles. Instead, musculoskeletal pain increased the risk of belonging to the "moderate-stable" profile.

Model fitting information showed that the observed and the estimated values did not differ significantly ($p = 0.17$). Chi-square test showed that the fitted model significantly improved the intercept-only model ($p < 0.001$). Approximately 39% of the variation in profiles was explained by the variables included in the final model.

An attrition analysis was conducted to examine baseline differences between the study population and those who were dropped out ($n = 1658$). The results show that women (71% of the study population and 57% of the attrition group $\chi^2(3) = 37.06, p < 0.001$) and support staff (44% of study and 34% attrition group, $\chi^2(3) = 28.38, p < 0.001$) were overrepresented in the study population. The study population reported a higher mean work ability (3.74 vs. 3.59, $p < 0.001$) than the attrition group. The groups did not differ in age, $t(1327.35) = 1.96$, $p = 0.05$.

5. Discussion

The present longitudinal study used repeated questionnaires to identify developmental pathways of work ability among white-collar workers during exceptional circumstances that required the employees to suddenly shift to WFH. We found that among approximately half of the university staff, work ability remained at a good-stable level throughout the one-year follow-up, whereas near to one-fourth (23%) of the respondents reported a stable moderate level of work ability. Two small profiles with less optimal work ability profiles were also found: one that showed a steep decline of work ability from very good to a poor level and another for whom work ability remained at a stable poor level. Despite the exceptional situation, for 4% of the respondents, work ability improved during the follow-up period.

The longitudinal design and the use of the person-centred method in analysing the development of work ability is a major strength of our study. A traditional variable-centred approach could not have captured the individual variability in the development of work ability. Our results contribute to an understanding of how employees' work ability is affected by sudden changes in their work demands and resources. The results indicate that job-related well-being experiences during enforced remote work diverge significantly, and for some employees, remote working has been difficult. Recent evidence is in accordance with our results, which demonstrated heterogeneity in the development of work well-being during the enforced remote work among white-collar workers [17,18].

We also identified factors that predicted membership in the different work ability profiles. Of the demographic factors, younger age was associated with the least optimal work ability profiles. This contradicts some of the earlier findings, which, overall, have shown that age is reversely associated with work ability [19]. On the other hand, recent evidence has shown that younger people report lower levels of well-being during the pandemic, with lower overall levels of life satisfaction and optimism and a greater risk of depression as compared with older people [3]. Our results also showed that male gender predicted less optimal work ability profiles. Previous studies suggest that the sociopsychological consequences of the COVID-19 mandated lockdown affected women's psychological health more strongly than men's [3,20] owing partly to increasing caring responsibilities during the lockdown, which has given rise to increasing work–life conflicts [3,4,19,21]. In our data, most respondents did not have children, which may explain the difference in results.

It was less surprising that a higher level of stress and musculoskeletal pain predicted poorer work ability. The adverse effects of stress on workers' health are well-documented (e.g., [22,23]) but according to our knowledge, the effects on work ability in a WFH context have not been studied before. Similarly, previous evidence has shown that musculoskeletal pain is associated with reduced work ability [24,25] and that the prevalence of musculoskeletal pain increased after switching to WFH during the COVID-19 pandemic [26,27]. In line, our results show that the prevention of stress and musculoskeletal pain are key to maintaining and promoting work ability. The suitability of one's home for WFH is a key resource for safe and productive working. Increased musculoskeletal pain during a COVID-19 pandemic may, in part, signal poor physical working arrangements at home. Further, telecommunication connections and software suitable for teleworking are essential preconditions for effective teleworking. In our study, a high score on the variable encompassing a range of factors important for WFH ergonomics was associated with increased likelihood of belonging to the "very good-increasing" work ability profile. Lower scores, on the other hand, significantly increased the risk for less favourable work ability profiles.

Employees' experience of the support provided by the organization is a significant work resource that promotes commitment and work performance [28,29]. In line, our results showed that respondents' experiences of organizational support provided during the forced WFH was associated with work ability. Sufficient support increased the likelihood of belonging to the most optimal work ability profiles, while perceived insufficient support predicted non-optimal work ability profiles.

Limitations

Selection bias may have affected the results of our trajectory analyses, as the attrition analyses revealed that those who continued participating in the study after baseline survey had better work ability at baseline as compared to those who dropped out. The baseline situation strongly predicted the development of work ability; therefore, the proportion of participants in the least optimal work ability profiles may be underestimated.

Another limitation is that data collection commenced during the COVID-19 lockdown in April 2020, and we did not adjust our analyses for any pre-pandemic factors. In particular, the fact that some of the employees may have been more accustomed and therefore better prepared to WFH than others may have affected the work ability profiles found as well as the observed associations. The majority of the sample (65%), however, did not have previous remote work experience prior to the COVID-19 pandemic, as approximately one-third of the participants had not worked remotely at all, and 40% had worked remotely less than one day per week. [18] Moreover, the COVID-19 pandemic situation itself gave rise to health concerns and mandated social isolation, which undoubtedly affected the respondents' work ability.

The COVID-19 situation mandated WFH, but it has been previously suggested that a tailored WFH organizational policy, in which employees' needs and preferences for WFH are considered, is an optimal approach to facilitate employees' well-being [30]. The results of our exploratory analyses provide insights on the factors that are important in promoting good work ability when working from home. Future studies are warranted to investigate the mechanisms through which the identified predictors of work ability operate.

6. Conclusions

To our knowledge, this was the first study to investigate the development of work ability and its predictors among white-collar workers during the WFH mandated by the COVID-19 public health restrictions. For most employees, work ability was maintained across the follow-up, but heterogeneity in the development of work ability indicates that individual starting points for WFH should be considered. Functionality of employees' home for work with adequate physical, cognitive, and organizational ergonomics are important in maintaining work ability while working from home. The results can advise organizations to optimize multi-location work conditions in the future. Means to provide workers with a functional work environment and adequate organizational support while working from home in order to promote white-collar workers' work ability should be considered.

Supplementary Materials: The following supporting information can be downloaded at: https://www.mdpi.com/article/10.3390/ijerph19106230/s1, see Refs. [31,32] Table S1: Principal component analysis of items describing university employees' adequacy of home as workplace (i) and organizational support (ii) during COVID-19 lockdown; Table S2: Model fit indices of latent class growth analysis: profiles of work ability during COVID-19 lockdown among university employees (*n* = 678).

Author Contributions: Conceptualization, S.K.; statistical analysis, S.K.; writing—original draft preparation, S.K.; data acquisition, A.M. and C.-H.N.; data curation, A.M. and S.J.; writing—review and editing, S.K., S.N., C.-H.N., J.O., S.J. and A.M. All authors have read and agreed to the published version of the manuscript.

Funding: This research was partly funded by the Finnish Work Environment Fund (grant number 200392) (A.M.).

Institutional Review Board Statement: This study was conducted according to the guidelines of the Declaration of Helsinki. Ethical review and approval were waived for this study, due to further approvals were not required after the chairman of the Ethics Committee reviewed the research privacy notice and questionnaire after which the study was approved by the University Rector's Office, Human Resources Directors and the executive board.

Informed Consent Statement: Informed consent was obtained from all subjects involved in the study.

Data Availability Statement: The data are available from A.M. upon reasonable request.

Acknowledgments: The data of the study are part of a larger research project funded by the Finnish Work Environment Fund (number 200392; Principal Investigator Anne Mäkikangas).

Conflicts of Interest: The authors declare no conflict of interest.

References

1. Sostero, M.; Milasi, S.; Hurley, J.; Fernandez Macias, E.; Bisello, M. *Teleworkability and the COVID-19 Crisis: A New Digital Divide?* JRC121193; European Commission: Seville, Spain, 2020.
2. Eurostat. EU-Labour Force Survey Database. Employed Persons Working from Home as a Percentage of the Total Employment in 2019. Available online: https://ec.europa.eu/eurostat/web/main/data/database (accessed on 31 January 2021).
3. Eurofound. *Living, Working and COVID-19*; COVID-19 Series; Publications Office of the European Union: Luxembourg, 2020.
4. Allen, T.D.; Johnson, R.C.; Kiburz, K.M.; Shockley, K.M. Work–family conflict and flexible work arrangements: Deconstructing flexibility. *Person. Psychol.* **2013**, *66*, 345–376. [CrossRef]
5. Nijp, H.H.; Beckers, D.G.J.; Geurts, S.A.E.; Tucker, P.; Kompier, M.A.J. Systematic review on the association between employee worktime control and work–non-work balance, health and well-being, and job-related outcomes. *Scand. J. Work. Environ. Health* **2012**, *38*, 299–313. [CrossRef]
6. Graham, M.; Weale, V.; Lambert, K.A.; Kinsman, N.; Stuckey, R.; Oakman, J. Working at home: The impacts of COVID 19 on health, family-work-life conflict, gender, and parental responsibilities. *J. Occup. Environ. Med.* **2021**, *63*, 938–943. [CrossRef]
7. Oksanen, A.; Oksa, R.; Savela, N.; Mantere, E.; Savolainen, I.; Kaakinen, M. COVID-19 Crisis and Digital Stressors at Work: A Longitudinal Study on the Finnish Working Population. *Comput. Hum. Behav.* **2021**, *122*, 106853. [CrossRef]
8. Bayattork, M.; Jakobsen, M.D.; Sundstrup, E.; Seidi, F.; Bay, H.; Andersen, L.L. Musculoskeletal pain in multiple body sites and work ability in the general working population: Cross-sectional study among 10,000 wage earners. *Scand. J. Pain* **2018**, *19*, 131–137. [CrossRef]
9. Ilmarinen, J. Work ability—A comprehensive concept for occupational health research and prevention. *Scand. J. Work. Environ. Health* **2009**, *35*, 1–5. [CrossRef]
10. Ilmarinen, J.; Tuomi, K.; Klockars, M. Changes in the work ability of active employees over an 11-year period. *Scand. J. Work. Environ. Health* **1997**, *23* (Suppl. S1), 49–57. [PubMed]
11. Kuorinka, I.; Jonsson, B.; Kilbom, A.; Vinterberg, H.; Biering-Sørensen, F.; Andersson, G.; Jørgensen, K. Standardised Nordic questionnaires for the analysis of musculoskeletal symptoms. *Appl. Ergon.* **1987**, *18*, 233–237. [CrossRef]
12. Elo, A.-L.; Leppänen, A.; Jahkola, A. Validity of a single-item measure of stress symptoms. *Scand. J. Work. Environ. Health* **2003**, *29*, 444–451. [CrossRef] [PubMed]
13. Muthén, B. Latent variable analysis: Growth mixture modeling and related techniques for longitudinal data. In *Handbook of Quantitative Methodology for the Social Sciences*; Kaplan, D., Ed.; Sage Publications: Newbury Park, CA, USA, 2004.
14. Berlin, K.S.; Parra, G.R.; Williams, N.A. An Introduction to Latent Variable Mixture Modeling (Part 2): Longitudinal Latent Class Growth Analysis and Growth Mixture Models. *J. Pediatr. Psychol.* **2014**, *39*, 188–203. [CrossRef]
15. Nylund, K.L.; Asparouhov, T.; Muthén, B.O. Deciding on the Number of Classes in Latent Class Analysis and Growth Mixture Modeling: A Monte Carlo Simulation Study. *Struct. Equ. Model. A Multidiscip. J.* **2007**, *14*, 535–569. [CrossRef]
16. Jung, T.; Wickrama, K.A.S. An Introduction to Latent Class Growth Analysis and Growth Mixture Modeling. *Soc. Pers. Psychol. Compass* **2007**, *2*, 302–317. [CrossRef]
17. Oakman, J.; Lambert, K.; Neupane, S.; Kyrönlahti, S.; Nygård, C.-H. Musculoskeletal pain trajectories of employees working from home during the COVID-19 pandemic. *Int. Arch. Occup. Environ. Health*, 2022; in press.
18. Mäkikangas, A.; Juutinen, S.; Mäkiniemi, J.-P.; Sjöblom, K.; Oksanen, A. Work Engagement and Its Antecedents in Remote Work: A Person-Centered View. *Work Stress*, 2022; in press.
19. Van den Berg, T.I.J.; Elders, L.A.M.; De Zwart, B.C.H.; Burdorf, A. The effects of work-related and individual factors on the Work Ability Index: A systematic review. *Occup. Environ. Med.* **2009**, *66*, 211–220. [CrossRef]
20. Meyer, B.; Zill, A.; Dilba, D.; Gerlach, R.; Schumann, S. Employee psychological well-being during the COVID-19 pandemic in Germany: A longitudinal study of demands, resources, and exhaustion. *Int. J. Psychol.* **2021**, *56*, 532–550. [CrossRef]
21. Palumbo, R. Let me go to the office! An investigation into the side effects of working from home on work-life balance. *Int. J. Public Sect. Manag.* **2020**, *33*, 771–790. [CrossRef]
22. Blackmore, E.R.; Stansfeld, S.A.; Weller, I.; Munce, S.; Zagorski, B.M.; Stewart, D.E. Major Depressive Episodes and Work Stress: Results From a National Population Survey. *Am. J. Public Health* **2007**, *97*, 2088–2093. [CrossRef] [PubMed]
23. Kivimäki, M.; Kawachi, I. Work Stress as a Risk Factor for Cardiovascular Disease. *Curr. Cardiol. Rep.* **2015**, *17*, 630. [CrossRef] [PubMed]

24. Kapteyn, A.; Smith, J.P.; van Soest, A. Dynamics of work disability and pain. *J. Health Econ.* **2008**, *27*, 496–509. [CrossRef] [PubMed]
25. Miranda, H.; Kaila-Kangas, L.; Heliövaara, M.; Leino-Arjas, P.; Haukka, E.; Liira, J.; Viikari-Juntura, E. Musculoskeletal pain at multiple sites and its effects on work ability in a general working population. *Occup. Environ. Med.* **2010**, *67*, 449–455. [CrossRef]
26. Moretti, A.; Menna, F.; Aulicino, M.; Paoletta, M.; Liguori, S.; Iolascon, G. Characterization of Home Working Population during COVID-19 Emergency: A Cross-Sectional Analysis. *Int. J. Environ. Res. Public Health* **2020**, *17*, 6284. [CrossRef]
27. Oakman, J.; Kinsman, N.; Stuckey, R.; Graham, M.; Weale, V. A rapid review of mental and physical health effects of working at home: How do we optimise health? *BMC Public Health* **2020**, *20*, 1825. [CrossRef]
28. Rhoades, L.; Eisenberger, R. Perceived organizational support: A review of the literature. *J. Appl. Psychol.* **2002**, *87*, 698–714. [CrossRef]
29. Mäkiniemi, J.-P.; Oksanen, A.; Mäkikangas, A. Loneliness and Well-Being during the COVID-19 Pandemic: The Moderating Roles of Personal, Social and Organizational Resources on Perceived Stress and Exhaustion among Finnish University Employees. *Int. J. Environ. Res. Public Health* **2021**, *18*, 7146. [CrossRef]
30. Astrid, D.W.; Beckers, D.G.; Nijp, H.H.; Hooftman, W.; de Boer, A.G.; Geurts, S.A. Working from home: Mismatch between access and need in relation to work–home interference and fatigue. *Scand. J. Work. Environ. Health* **2021**, *47*, 619–627. [CrossRef]
31. Sharma, S. *Applied Multivariate Techniques*; John Wiley & Sons, Inc.: New York, NY, USA, 1996; p. 493.
32. Pallant, J. *SPSS Survival Manual*, 5th ed.; Allen & Unwin: Crows Nest, NSW, Australia, 2013; pp. 97–101.

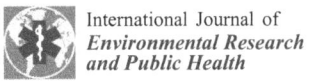

International Journal of *Environmental Research and Public Health*

Article

Sustainable Working Life in a Swedish Twin Cohort—A Definition Paper with Sample Overview

Annina Ropponen [1,2,*], Mo Wang [1], Jurgita Narusyte [1,3], Karri Silventoinen [1,4], Petri Böckerman [5,6,7] and Pia Svedberg [1]

1. Division of Insurance Medicine, Department of Clinical Neuroscience, Karolinska Institutet, SE-171 77 Stockholm, Sweden; mo.wang@ki.se (M.W.); jurgita.narusyte@ki.se (J.N.); karri.silventoinen@helsinki.fi (K.S.); Pia.Svedberg@ki.se (P.S.)
2. Finnish Institute of Occupational Health, 00032 Työterveyslaitos, Finland
3. Center of Epidemiology and Community Medicine, Stockholm County Council, 104 31 Stockholm, Sweden
4. Population Research Unit, Faculty of Social Sciences, University of Helsinki, 00014 Helsinki, Finland
5. School of Business and Economics, University of Jyväskylä, 40014 Jyväskylä, Finland; petri.bockerman@labour.fi
6. Labour Institute for Economic Research, 00100 Helsinki, Finland
7. IZA Institute of Labor Economics, 53113 Bonn, Germany
* Correspondence: annina.ropponen@ki.se

Citation: Ropponen, A.; Wang, M.; Narusyte, J.; Silventoinen, K.; Böckerman, P.; Svedberg, P. Sustainable Working Life in a Swedish Twin Cohort—A Definition Paper with Sample Overview. *IJERPH* 2021, *18*, 5817. https://doi.org/10.3390/ijerph18115817

Academic Editor: Paul B. Tchounwou

Received: 13 April 2021
Accepted: 26 May 2021
Published: 28 May 2021

Publisher's Note: MDPI stays neutral with regard to jurisdictional claims in published maps and institutional affiliations.

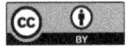

Copyright: © 2021 by the authors. Licensee MDPI, Basel, Switzerland. This article is an open access article distributed under the terms and conditions of the Creative Commons Attribution (CC BY) license (https://creativecommons.org/licenses/by/4.0/).

Abstract: *Background*: A unified or consensus definition of "sustainable working life" remains lacking, although studies investigating risk factors for labour market exit are numerous. In this study, we aimed (1) to update the information and to explore a definition of "sustainable working life" via a systematic literature review and (2) to describe the working life trajectories via the prevalence of sickness absence (SA), disability pension (DP), and unemployment in a Swedish twin cohort to provide a sample overview in our Sustainable Working Life-project. *Methods*: A systematic literature review was conducted to explore the studies with the search phrase "sustainable working life" in PubMed, PsycInfo, and the Web of Science Database of Social Sciences in January 2021, resulting in a total of 51 references. A qualitative synthesis was performed for the definitions and the measures of "sustainable working life." Based on the Swedish Twin project Of Disability pension and Sickness absence (STODS), the current dataset to address sustainable working life includes 108 280 twin individuals born between 1925 and 1990. Comprehensive register data until 2016 for unemployment, SA and DP were linked to all individuals. Using STODS, we analysed the annual prevalence of SA, DP, and unemployment as working life trajectories over time across education and age groups. *Results*: The reviewed 16 full articles described several distinct definitions for sustainable working life between 2007 and 2020 from various perspectives, i.e., considering workplaces or employees, the individual, organizational or enterprise level, and the society level. The definition of "sustainable working life" appearing most often was the swAge-model including a broad range of factors, e.g., health, physical/mental/psychosocial work environment, work motivation/satisfaction, and family situation and leisure activities. Our dataset comprised of 81%–94% of individuals who did not meet SA, DP, or unemployment during the follow-up in 1994–2016, being indicative for "sustainable working life." The annual prevalence across years had a decreasing trend of unemployment over time, whereas the prevalence of SA had more variation, with DP being rather stable. Both unemployment and DP had the highest prevalence among those with a lower level of education, whereas in SA, the differences in prevalence between education levels were minor. Unemployment was highest across the years in the youngest age group (18–27 years), the age group differences for SA were minor, and for DP, the oldest age group (58–65 years) had the highest prevalence. *Conclusions*: No consensus exists for a "sustainable working life," hence meriting further studies, and we intend to contribute by utilising the STODS database for the Sustainable Working Life project. In the upcoming studies, the existing knowledge of available definitions and frameworks will be utilised. The dataset containing both register data and self-reports enables detailed follow-up for labour market participation for sustainable working life.

Keywords: systematic literature review; sustainable working life; labour market; prevalence; sick leave; unemployment

1. Introduction

A "sustainable working life" can be defined as the absence of disruptions and interruptions of working careers due to various reasons, including unemployment, rehabilitation, sickness absence (SA), and disability pension (DP) [1]. Furthermore, sustainable work refers to working and living conditions that support people in engaging and remaining in paid work throughout an extended working life [2]. Reducing the extent of work incapacity in terms of SA and DP is highly prioritised in the public policy of Nordic countries [3]. The SA and DP have increased in the industrialised world during the recent decades even when health conditions have generally improved at the same time, as seen, for example, in the increasing healthy life expectancy [4–6]. Another major concern is the overall inclusiveness of the working-age population in the labour market, which is emphasised by the Europe 2020 strategy for smart, sustainable, and inclusive economic growth [7].

The consequences of being absent from the labour market are severe; for example, SA/DP are linked to a number of negative health-related consequences, such as disease (the same disease for which SA/DP has been granted, or another disease), well-being, economy, career development, social integration, and premature death [8]. Even when substantial efforts have already been invested in investigating the risk factors for individuals' absence from the labour market (i.e., SA/DP), there is still a gap in studies analysing factors that promote a "sustainable working life." Furthermore, to the best of our knowledge, no consensus definition of "sustainable working life" exists, although many have approached this topic [1,2].

The Nordic countries provide excellent opportunities to investigate "sustainable working life" because their national registries are representative of their populations. Further, twin cohorts including comprehensive survey data with decades of follow-up have been collected in the Nordic countries, thus enabling the investigation of the role of both genetic factors and childhood environment in the association of predictive factors for "sustainable working life." Using genetically informative data is important since the variation in complex phenotypes is caused by a combination of genetic and environmental factors and their mutual interactions [9]. The possibility to take into account genetic contributions to variation in "sustainable working life" is also important in order to show possible causality between various factors of interest and sustainable work-life participation. To the best of our knowledge, such studies have primarily focused on the associations between risk factors and interruptions, e.g., SA/DP or unemployment [10–15]. However, these earlier studies in which researchers of this article have been involved have shown that the heritability varies based on diagnosis groups for DP [16–18].

In this study, we utilised as the starting point the feasibility study of measuring "sustainable working life," in which a systematic literature review was conducted for the period 2010–2017 [1]. This earlier review utilised "sustainable work" as a search term but found only a few relevant studies. Hence in order to identify more studies, the researchers included additional terms (i.e., NEET, work-life balance, and life course). Having this as the background, we designed a systematic literature review to update the information on "sustainable working life" and to explore a definition. Another aim was to describe the working life trajectories via the annual prevalence of SA, DP, and unemployment in a Swedish twin cohort to provide a sample overview in our Sustainable Working Life project. As an example of factors of interest for "sustainable working life," we focused on SA, DP, and unemployment as they are the most common reasons for exit from the labour market.

2. Materials and Methods

2.1. Literature Review

We conducted systematic literature searches in late January 2021 to explore the studies of "sustainable working life" published in English. Having the earlier review [1] as the starting point, we did not limit the time period of searches but utilised the search phrase "sustainable working life." First, a literature search was conducted in PubMed (n = 36 references), PsycInfo (n = 2), and the Web of Science database of Social Sciences (n = 13) that resulted in 51 references in total (Figure 1). Then, all references were evaluated as full texts by 2 evaluators (AR and MW) who performed the evaluations separately and blinded [19]. The evaluation criterion applied was that the articles included a definition for "sustainable working life." All types of articles and designs were considered. In 2 cases of discrepancy between evaluators, a third author (PS) made the tie-breaking decision regarding inclusion/exclusion. Due to wide variation in the designs, definitions, and measures of the included studies, we did not make formal comparisons or conduct a meta-analysis of these articles. Instead, we conducted a qualitative synthesis that provided the basis to collect the definitions of "sustainable working life" and the measures of "sustainable working life" utilised in the articles. After the removal of 2 duplicates, the main reasons for excluding the articles (n = 34) were no definition of "sustainable working life" or that the article was identified due to "department of sustainable working life" in one university (i.e., the search phrase existed in affiliations, not in the text of the article).

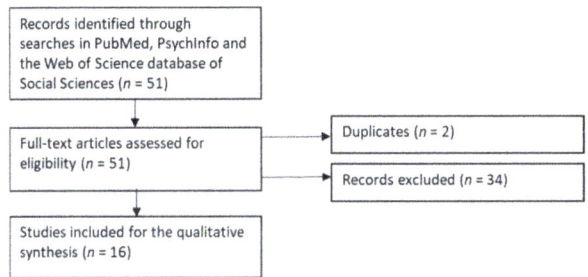

Figure 1. Flow diagram for systematic literature searches [20].

2.2. The Swedish Twin Project of Disability Pension and Sickness Absence

The Swedish Twin project Of Disability pension and Sickness absence (STODS) forms a national resource for genetic epidemiological studies regarding SA and DP but also for other labour market outcomes such as unemployment. STODS includes the twins identified in the Swedish Twin Registry (STR) who were born between 1925 and 1990, i.e., 119 907 twin individuals (approximately 1/3 are monozygotic [MZ], 1/3 same-sexed dizygotic [DZ], and 1/3 opposite-sexed DZ). Extensive survey data linked with the data obtained from national registers are already available. The survey data were collected through telephone interviews during the time period 1998–2002 (available for twins born 1925–1958) and through a Web-based questionnaire in 2005 (twins born 1959–1986) by STR. These data include background information (zygosity, age, and sex) and information on socioeconomic position (e.g., education), work-related factors (e.g., work history, work load, shift work, job insecurity, and Job demand-control-support (JDC-S) [21]), health (e.g., pain, musculoskeletal and mental disorders and common diseases), and health behaviour (e.g., physical activity, tobacco use, and alcohol consumption) [22,23]. Register data currently available for the time period 1994–2018 on DP (date, type, grade, and ICD diagnoses) and SA (grade and date of when each SA spell began and ended) and SA diagnoses for the time period 2005–2018 were collected from the Swedish Social Insurance Agency database MiDAS. Data on income, socioeconomic status, occupation, unemployment, old age pension, emigration, and rehabilitation currently available for the time period 1990–2016 were collected from Statistic Sweden (SCB) LISA database [24] and from other SCB databases that include corresponding information for other years not covered by LISA. The mortality data (date of death and diagnoses) were collected from the national death register, and data on non-fatal disease outcomes were collected from the inpatient and specialised outpatient registers held by the National Board of Health and Welfare. Register data for the STODS cohort are regularly updated.

As a data-based part for the sample overview of the data included in this Sustainable Work Life project, we described the annual prevalence (%) of the full sample without SA, DP, and unemployment for the time period 1994 to 2016 (n = 108 280, Supplemental Table S1), and we analysed the prevalence of SA, DP, and unemployment as working life trajectories until 2016. We also estimated differences in prevalence over time across education (measured as years of education and categorised as <10 years, 10–12 years, and >12 years) and age groups (categorised based on the distribution into 18–27 years, 28–37 years, 38–47 years, 48–57 years, and 58–65 years).

3. Results

3.1. Literature Review

The reviewed 16 full articles described several distinct definitions for "sustainable working life" (Table 1). Out of the articles, four were reviews, and six were qualitative studies complicating the evaluation of measures for "sustainable working life" (Table 2). The timeline of published studies indicated that "sustainable working life" is a relatively new concept since the earliest article with this specific phrase was published in 2007, and most were published in 2019 and 2020. Another aspect is region: six studies involving employees were conducted in Sweden as well as four of the reviews, whereas single studies were available from Australia, Italy, Netherlands, and the UK.

"Sustainable working life" seems to be defined from various perspectives, i.e., considering workplaces or employees, although some studies also suggested considering the individual level, the organizational and enterprise level, and the society level (Table 1). The definition of "sustainable working life" appearing most often was the swAge-model. This model defines "sustainable working life" to include health, physical work environment, mental/psychosocial work environment, working time and work pace, knowledge and competence, work motivation and work satisfaction, the attitude of managers and the organization/enterprise towards older workers, and the family situation and leisure activities (Table 1). In the swAge-model, the measures of "sustainable working life" would be:

1. Health effects of the work environment (and associations with biological age)
   - Function variation, diagnoses, and self-rated health
   - Physical working environment: Load, vibration, wear, dangerous substances, climate, access to tools, etc.
   - Mental work environment: Stress, demands, control, threats, violence, etc.
   - Working time, working rate, recovery: schedule, shifts, breaks, etc.
2. Finance (and associations with chronological age)
   - Economy: Personal financial situation, security, employability, insurance, etc.
3. Support and community (and associations with social age)
   - Private social environment: Private life, family life, and leisure in relation to work
   - Work social environment: Social support, discrimination, participation, attitudes, and leadership
4. Execution of task (and associations with cognitive age)
   - Work tasks, activity: Stimulation, motivation, and job satisfaction
   - Competence, knowledgeability, employability, and development in relation to the task

To sum up, the literature review indicated that definition and measures of "sustainable working life" vary to a large extent; therefore, no consensus on a definition exists.

Table 1. Comparative analysis of the definitions for "sustainable working life" in terms of target population and theoretical model or related measure.

Year	Author(s) (Ref)	Definition	Comparative Features	Number of Citation	Time-Span of Citations
2007	Kaneklin and Gorli [25]	Sustainable working life is the capacity for organizations to create and regenerate value through the application of participative policies and practices to promote both organizational performances and people's well-being. Relief of social dimension that inhabits organizational changes and maintain it close to the functional and strategic organizational changes, since the structural and functional dimensions of an organization must come together with the social and cultural dimensions for a sustainable working life.	Population: Healthcare sector organizations in Italy. Design: Action research.	2	2007–2020
2013	Hansen et al. [26]	Personal- and practice-based, professional, and systemic themes containing a number of sub-themes representing the experiences (i.e., ability to work part-time, achieve a healthy work-life balance, etc.), initiatives (e.g., alternatives to ownership of practice or develop teams with multidisciplinary support), or conditions (e.g., payment systems supportive of continued involvement in teaching or educational opportunities) that promote a long and sustainable working life in rural general practice.	Population: Australian rural general practitioners >45 years on age. Design: Semi-structured qualitative interview.	0	-
2013	Koolhaas et al. [27]	The increase in problems due to ageing and health-related problems from the age of 45 years onwards implies the importance of attention to obstacles and retention factors for maintaining or enhancing a sustainable working life.	Population: Workers aged ≥45 years in nine different companies in Netherlands. Design: A cross-sectional in-depth survey.	13	2013–2020
2015	Leider et al. [28]	Sustainable working life consists of parameters: work ability, productivity, vitality, and/or work role functioning.	Population: - Design: Systematic literature review utilizing Web of Science, Medline/PubMed and Embase to identify papers published in peer-reviewed journals between 1997 and 2013.	42	2015–2020
2015	Vänje [29]	Sustainable working life includes the perspectives of crafting employees' individual resources as well as collaboration between employees and their managers in order to create organizational development.	Population: - Design: Literature review using the Royal Institute of Technology's (KTH's) library search engine KTHB Primo, EndNote and the Social Sciences Citation Index at Web of Science (ISI), the Swedish search engines LIBRIS (http://libris.kb.se/) and KVINNSAM (http://www.ub.gu.se/kvinn/kvinnsam/) from the mid-1980s until 2014.	5	2015–2019

Table 1. *Cont.*

Year	Author(s) (Ref)	Definition	Comparative Features	Number of Citation	Time-Span of Citations
2016	Nilsson [30]	Four different concepts of ageing; the nine factors of importance for working life; and their relation to older workers' decision to extend their working life or retire. Employees' biological ageing is important due to individual health and well-being in association with their work situation (work pace, time, and environment); employees' chronological ageing involves statutory retirement age, social insurance, policies and economic incentives in working life and society. Adequate personal finances, i.e., providing for a living, food, and essential factors, but also motivation factors (e.g., the possibility for social inclusion/participation in an inspiring work situation and for motivating and stimulating activities and tasks based on the individuals' knowledge) are important.	Population: - Design: Literature review in Medline, PubMed, Scopus, Science Direct, Web of Knowledge, Cochrane Library and Google Scholar, in addition Swedish library database LIBrIS and Lund University library database, and also the Organisation for economic Co-operation and Development (OECD), the World Health Organisation (WHO), the World economic Forum (WeF), and the European Union (EU) in 2003–2015.	7	2016–2020
2017	Eriksson et al. [31]	Sustainable workplaces as work environments that embrace factors that contribute to employee health and well-being, as well as organizational efficiency. By integrating human and economic values, sustainable workplaces can even impact societal effectiveness.	Population: - Design: Scoping review in Web of Science, Scopus, Pubmed, Cinahl, Academic Search Premier, PsycInfo, and Embase for 2009–2014.	3	2019–2020
2018	Forslin et al. [32]	A well-functioning balance between a working and private life is important for a sustainable working life over time.	Population: Those with a definite MS diagnosis and an outpatient appointment with a neurologist in Sweden and alive, of working age at the 10-year follow-up (<55 years of age at baseline). Design: A 10-year longitudinal observational study.	5	2019–2020
2018	Wälinder et al. [33]	Social support and low strain (JCD-model) are linked with workers' well-being and a sustainable working life in the health-care sector.	Population: Hospital workers in university hospitals in Sweden Design: Cross-sectional survey study	0	-

Table 1. *Cont.*

Year	Author(s) (Ref)	Definition	Comparative Features	Number of Citation	Time-Span of Citations
2019	Gyllensten et al. [34]	Sustainable working life according to swAge-model depends on health, physical work environment, mental/psycho-social work environment, working time and work pace, knowledge and competence, work motivation and work satisfaction, the attitude of managers and the organisation/enterprise towards older workers, the family situation, and leisure activities.	Population: Employees of health and elderly care homes in Sweden Design: Focus group interviews	1	2019
2019	Thompson et al. [35]	The concept of sustainable working life includes organizations devising career paths that support staff to retain their health (physical and mental), productivity, and motivation over an extended period of employment. Vulnerable employees may cycle between the more- and the less-adaptive poles of each chrontope, and even between chrontopes, given that people with chronic illness are known to draw on a range of self-management strategies over time.	Population: Multiplesclerosis patients in UK. Design: Dialogical analysis of focus group interviews.	0	-
2020	Blomé et al. [36]	The swAge-model: the individual motives and considerations for continuing to work and the older workers' retirement decisions are based on: (a) their health in relation to the work situation and work environment versus health in retirement; (b) their personal economic situation in employment versus in retirement; (c) their opportunities for social inclusion in working life situations versus in retirement; (d) their opportunities for meaningful and self-crediting activities in working life versus in retirement	Population: Focus group interviews of 3–7 older workers, managers, trade union representatives, and human resource personnel from public organizations, large private companies and from private small-to-medium-sized enterprises in Sweden. Design: Secondary analysis of age management with the theoretical swAge-model.	3	2020

Table 1. *Cont.*

Year	Author(s) (Ref)	Definition	Comparative Features	Number of Citation	Time-Span of Citations
2020	Gyllensten et al. [37]	Continuing to work at an older age is determined by "push factors," i.e., chronic diseases, physical demands, and poor working conditions, and "'pull factors," such as one's spouse not working, care-taking of relatives, and leisure time expectations. Additionally, norms about working and retiring, economic incentives, attitudes at the workplace, work satisfaction, and social relationships at work and home are important factors for extended working life.	Population: All individuals employed at one car manufacturer in Sweden during 2005–2015. Design: A case-control study for 10-year follow-up.	0	-
2020	Lindmark et al. [38]	Focus on the prevention of ill health, health-promoting factors (e.g., occupational balance, emotional intelligence, social interaction/teamwork) for improvement of people's capacity to develop abilities and resources to feel good and cope with different situations in a healthy way are essential for health and sustainable working life.	Population: Students of higher education programs in the healthcare and social work sectors in Sweden. Design: Baseline results of a multicentre longitudinal study.	0	-
2020	Nilsson [39]	The swAge-model describes three influence levels of importance for work-life participation and to a sustainable, extended working life: the individual level, micro level; the organizational and enterprise level, meso level; and the society level, macro level.	Population: - Design: Descriptive for swAge-model which will be developed based on grounded theory using qualitative and quantitative studies, intervention projects, and literature reviews.	1	2020
2020	Nunstedt [40]	A reduced workload, varied tasks, individual schedules, clear leadership, and cooperation between nurses and other professionals are factors that contribute to a good working climate, sense of coherence, and meaningfulness. Hence, these can be used for action programmes, which, in turn, can promote a sustainable working life.	Population: Nurses in a hospital in western Sweden. Design: Qualitative and descriptive in design including a literature review, interviews, a qualitative content analysis, and a deductive approach for theoretical discussion.	1	2021

Table 2. Suggested measures for "sustainable working life" in terms of source population or data.

Author(s) (Ref)	Measure	Source
Kaneklin and Gorli [25]	n.a.	n = 14 middle managers
Hansen, Pit, Honeyman, and Barclay [26]	• Encouragement and support at all stages of career, wishing to work part-time. • Try to achieve control over your working life by maintaining a healthy work-life balance through the implementation of mental and lifestyle strategies. • Eat healthily, be physically active, and recognise and respond to signs of stress and burnout. • Support and assistance to those wishing to sell their practice but remain at work • Work in a good team and promote good team communication through regularly scheduled meetings. • Have a gradual retirement plan. Promotion of practice structures enabling to retire gradually without being financially penalised. • Implement practice-based health promotion strategies. • Pursue a special professional interest. • Become involved in teaching and mentoring young workers. Implement legislation to make it financially viable for semi-retires to remain at work • Ensure that a good range of educational opportunities are available and easily accessible • Reduce the bureaucratic burden • Implement strategies to improve the status and recognition. • Build on and improve utilisation of the current local locum database.	n = 16
Koolhaas, van der Klink, Vervoort, de Boer, Brouwer, and Groothoff [27]	Workers' perspectives on problems, obstacles, retention factors, and needs due to ageing classified with the International Classification of Functioning, Disability and Health (ICF).	n = 3008 workers, response rate 36%
Leider, Boschman, Frings-Dresen, and van der Molen [28]	• Job rotation comprises rotating between tasks within jobs and/or between activities • Exposures related to musculoskeletal complaints • Sustainable working life: work ability, productivity, vitality, and/or work role functioning.	Search terms: job rotation, musculoskeletal complaints, terms for related exposures and terms for sustainable working life parameters. n = 16 included studies.
Vanje [29]	n.a.	Discourse analysis of documents was used in an integrative review including 128 articles.
Nilsson [30]	Health; economic incentives; family, leisure, and surrounding society; physical work environment; mental work environment; work pace and working hours; competence and skills; motivation and work satisfaction; and the attitude of managers and organisation to older workers.	
Eriksson, Orvik, Strandmark, Nordsteien, and Torp [31]	n.a.	In-depth analysis of 20 studies
Forslin, Fink, Hammar, von Koch, and Johansson [32]	Employment status at the 10-year follow-up categorised as full-time work, part-time work (working, but less than full time), and no work.	Baseline and follow-up surveys, n = 154

Table 2. *Cont.*

Author(s) (Ref)	Measure	Source
Wålinder, Runeson-Broberg, Arakelian, Nordqvist, Runeson, and Rask-Andersen [33]	Well-being at work Zest for work (i.e., emotions about work) Intention to stop working with health care	n = 1405 hospital employees
Gyllensten, Wentz, Håkansson, Hagberg, and Nilsson [34]	Organisational issues • High demands • Lack of staff • Lack of recovery at work Health-related problems • Tiredness and aches • Individually created solutions to cope with chronic health problems Private issues • Poor personal finances postpone retirement • Lack of private life Meaningfulness and appreciation • Meaningful job • Downgrading of competencies Social support • Belonging • Support from colleagues increases motivation for delaying pension	n = six focus groups with four to eight participants in each group
Thompson, Ford, Stroud, and Madill [35]	n.a.	Dialogical analysis of 20 workers
Blomé, Borell, Håkansson, and Nilsson [36]	• Contemporary policies and practice in the work environment • Social participation and attitudes • Experience and mentorship	Qualitative interviews, n = 16
Gyllensten, Torén, Hagberg, and Söderberg [37]	Employers' register for employment status: active at work, retired (either retired at the age 55–62 or working ≥63 years during the observation years)	n = 572 cases and 771 controls
Lindmark, Ahlstrand, Ekman, Berg, Hedén, Källstrand, Larsson, Nunstedt, Oxelmark, Pennbrant, Sundler, and Larsson [38]	Health-promoting dimensions: • Health-promoting resources (i.e., sense of coherence) • Occupational balance • Emotional intelligence • Health and welfare • Social interaction • Work and workplace experiences/perception	n = 2283 students

Table 2. *Cont.*

Author(s) (Ref)	Measure	Source
Nilsson [39]	1. Health effects of the work environment (and associations with biological age) • Function variation, diagnoses, and self-rated health • Physical working environment: Load, vibration, wear, dangerous substances, climate, access to tools, etc. • Mental work environment: Stress, demands, control, threats, violence, etc. • Working time, working rate, recovery: schedule, shifts, breaks, etc. 2. Finance (and associations with chronological age) Economy: Personal financial situation, security, employability, insurance, etc. 3. Support and Community (and associations with social age) • Private social environment: Private life, family life, and leisure in relation to work • Work social environment: Social support, discrimination, participation, attitudes, and leadership 4. Execution of task (and associations with cognitive age) • Work tasks, activity stimulation, motivation, and job satisfaction • Competence, knowledgeability, employability, and development in relation to the task	Grounded theory
Nunstedt [40]	1. Job satisfaction 2. Professional role 3. Job engagement 4. Belonging in the workplace 5. Working conditions and factors for remaining in the profession 6. Opportunities for learning and development in the workplace 7. The professional role in the future	$n = 12$

n.a. = not applicable.

3.2. Prevalence of Sickness Absence, Disability Pension and Unemployment as Working Life Trajectories

In our dataset of the full sample for those without unemployment, SA, or DP numbers varied between 82340 and 64189 from 1994 to 2016 and included 81%–94% of individuals who did not meet SA, DP, or unemployment during the follow-up (Supplemental Table S1). The annual prevalence across years is shown in Figure 2, indicating a decreasing trend of unemployment over time, whereas the prevalence of SA has had more variation and DP being rather stable.

Figures 3–5 show the prevalence of unemployment, SA, and DP across education categories. Both unemployment and DP have the highest prevalence among those with a lower level of education compared to the highest level of education with the lowest prevalence. For SA, the differences in prevalence between education levels were minor. The Supplemental Figures S1–S3 show age group differences in the prevalence of unemployment, SA, and DP, indicating unemployment being highest across the years in the youngest age group (18–27 years), whereas for SA, the age group differences were minor (although the youngest age group had the lowest prevalence), and for DP, the oldest age group (58–65 years) had the highest prevalence.

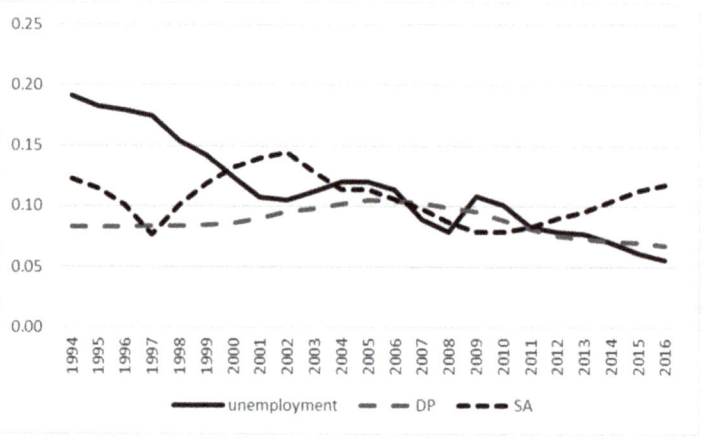

Figure 2. The annual prevalence of unemployment, disability pension (DP), and sickness absence (SA) from 1994 to 2016.

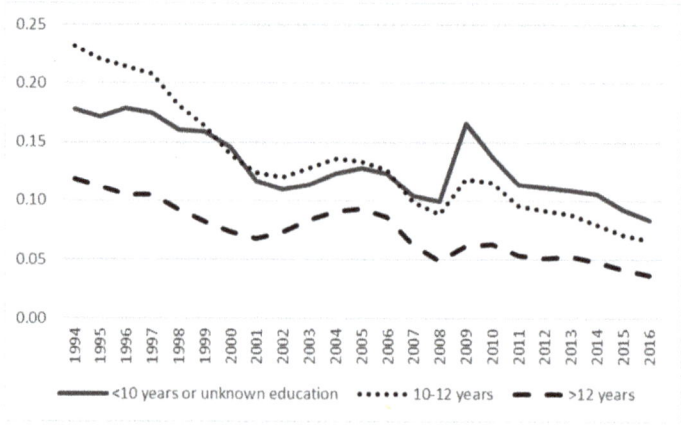

Figure 3. The prevalence of unemployment across categories of education.

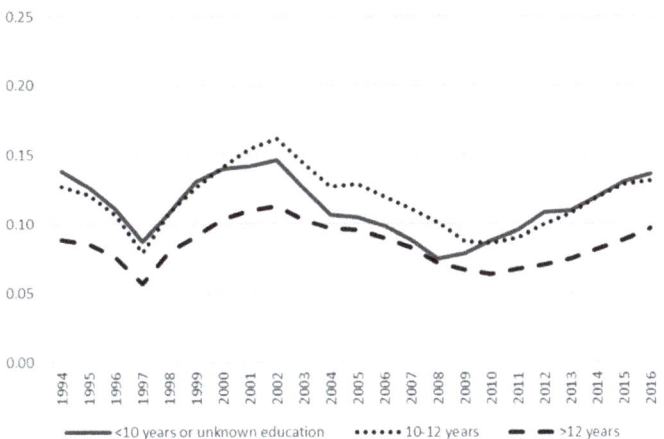

Figure 4. The prevalence of sickness absence across categories of education.

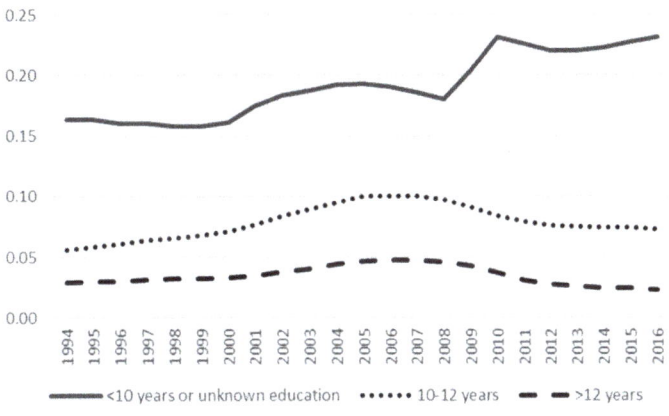

Figure 5. The prevalence of disability pension across categories of education.

4. Discussion

In this study, we conducted a systematic literature review to explore a definition and measures for "sustainable working life" and described the working life trajectories via the prevalence of SA, DP, and unemployment in a Swedish twin cohort as a cohort profile of our Sustainable Working Life project. In line with the feasibility study conducted in 2017 for measures of "sustainable working life" [1], the relevant studies were still few. In this study, we were not able to detect a unified definition of "sustainable working life," although the swAge-model has gained interest in recent years [30,39]. The sample overview part of this study in which we estimated the annual prevalence of SA, DP, and unemployment, indicated variation across years for the follow-up from 1994 to 2016, but also that our sample included most (81%–94%) of individuals without such exit from the labour market. As an example of factors of interest for "sustainable working life" along with the swAge-model [39], we tested the effects of education and age on the prevalence of unemployment: SA and DP indicated differences across categories and even across time. Hence, our sample will have ample power and longitudinal design for further investigations of influential factors of "sustainable working life."

Strengths and Limitations

STODS is based on the population-based STR with comprehensive survey data collected by STR but with the addition of register data from several authorities covering the years 1994–2018, for almost 120,000 twin individuals. The twin data enable analyses controlling for familial confounding, which is genetics and mainly childhood and shared environment, hence extending the knowledge based on other samples without such possibility. Furthermore, the register data available for follow-up are detailed, including the date for starting and ending times of a spell for "sustainable working life" outcomes as well as diagnoses to define the analyses. Hence, we expect that we can contribute to the knowledge of "sustainable working life" through studies with the longitudinal design of genetically informative twins but also controlling and/or investigating many other influential factors for "sustainable working life" as identified in the systematic literature review part of this study. Even the measures suggested by the swAge-model [39] could be tested.

A limitation in the systematic review part of our study was that no consensus exists for the definition of "sustainable working life." Although the topic has raised interest since 2010, many studies have created frameworks or lists of influential factors [1,37,39]. Another limitation is the regional emphasis: "sustainable working life" has raised particular interest in Sweden, limiting the generalisation and the applicability of the findings to Nordic countries only, where there are well-developed welfare systems, working life, and populations. The studies have also utilised various designs (i.e., from cross-sectional to longitudinal), methodologies (qualitative vs. quantitative), and samples (including studies with occupational groups, population-based samples or even students), whereas some studies were theoretical in nature. This further complicates the search for a definition or certain, commonly agreed on measures of "sustainable working life." However, the expectation is that in our Sustainable Working Life project, we can add to the existing knowledge via the utilisation of available definitions and frameworks since our survey data cover self-reported aspects comprehensively. Furthermore, the register data enable detailed follow-up for labour market participation in terms of "sustainable working life," as well as labour market non-participation in line with earlier studies based on STODS for SA, DP, and unemployment [10,41–45].

In conclusion, no consensus exists for the definition of "sustainable working life." Hence, "sustainable working life" merits further studies, and we intend to contribute by utilising the STODS database for our Sustainable Working Life project.

Supplementary Materials: The following are available online at https://www.mdpi.com/article/10.3390/ijerph18115817/s1, Table S1. The full sample, prevalence of those without unemployment, sickness absence or disability pension pre a year from 1994 to 2016, Figure S1. Prevalence of unemployment across age categories, Figure S2. Prevalence of sickness absence across age categories, Figure S3. Prevalence of disability pension across age categories.

Author Contributions: A.R., J.N., K.S., P.B., and P.S. were involved in the study conception and design. P.S. was responsible for the acquisition of data. A.R. and M.W. conducted the systematic literature review and A.R. the statistical analyses. A.R. drafted the manuscript, and A.R., M.W., J.N., K.S., P.B., and P.S. contributed to the interpretation of data and the critical revision of the manuscript. All authors have read and agreed to the published version of the manuscript.

Funding: This study was supported by Forte (2019-01284). The study utilised data from the Swedish Twin project Of Disability pension and Sickness absence (STODS), one cohort of the REWHARD consortium supported by the Swedish Research Council (grant no 2017-00624). The Swedish Twin Registry (STR) is managed by Karolinska Institutet and receives funding through the Swedish Research Council under grant no 2017-00641.

Institutional Review Board Statement: The study was conducted according to the guidelines of the Declaration of Helsinki, and approved by the Regional Ethical Review Board of Stockholm, Sweden (Dnr: 2007/524-31, 2010/1346-32/5, 2014/311-32, 2015/1809-32, 2017/128-32).

Informed Consent Statement: Not applicable.

Data Availability Statement: The data presented in this study are not publicly available. Readers may contact the last author regarding details. The data are not publicly available due to the legal restrictions set out in the General Data Protection Regulation, the Swedish law SFS 2018:218, the Swedish Data Protection Act, the Swedish Ethical Review Act, and the Public Access to Information and Secrecy Act. These types of sensitive data can only be made available after legal review, for researchers who meet the criteria for access to these types of sensitive and confidential data.

Conflicts of Interest: The authors declare no conflict of interest.

References

1. Eurofound. *Measuring Sustainable Work over the Life Course-Feasibility Study*; European Foundation for the Improvement of Living and Working Conditions (Eurofound): Dublin, Ireland, 2018.
2. Eurofound. *Sustainable Working over the Life Course: Concept Paper*; Publications Office of the European Union: Luxembourg, 2015.
3. Thorsen, S.; Friborg, C.; Lundstrøm, B.; Kausto, J.; Örnelius, K.; Sundell, T.; Kalstø, Å.M.; Thune, O.; Gross, B.O.; Petersen, H.; et al. *Sickness Absence in the Nordic Countries*; Nordic Social Statistical Committee: Copenhagen, Denmark, 2015.
4. ILO. *Disability Inclusion Strategy and Action Plan 2014-17 a Twin-Track Approach of Mainstreaming and Disability-Specific Actions*; International Labour Office: Geneva, Switzerland, 2015.
5. OECD. *Sickness, Disability and Work: Breaking the Barriers*; OECD Publishing: Paris, France, 2010.
6. Forouzanfar, M.H.; Afshin, A.; Alexander, L.T.; Anderson, H.R.; Bhutta, Z.A.; Biryukov, S.; Brauer, M.; Burnett, R.; Cercy, K.; Charlson, F.J.; et al. Global, regional, and national comparative risk assessment of 79 behavioural, environmental and occupational, and metabolic risks or clusters of risks, 1990–2015: A systematic analysis for the Global Burden of Disease Study 2015. *Lancet* **2016**, *388*, 1659–1724. [CrossRef]
7. European Commission. *A Strategy for Smart, Sustainable and Inclusive Growth 2010*; Communication from the Commission, Europe 2020; European Commission: Brussels, Belgium, 2020.
8. Kivimäki, M.; Head, J.; Ferrie, J.E.; Shipley, M.J.; Vahtera, J.; Marmot, M.G. Sickness absence as a global measure of health: Evidence from mortality in the Whitehall II prospective cohort study. *BMJ* **2003**, *327*, 364. [CrossRef]
9. Plomin, R.; Colledge, E. Genetics and Psychology: Beyond Heritability. *Eur. Psychol.* **2001**, *6*, 229–240. [CrossRef]
10. Narusyte, J.; Ropponen, A.; Alexanderson, K.; Svedberg, P. Internalizing and externalizing problems in childhood and adolescence as predictors of work incapacity in young adulthood. *Soc. Psychiatry Psychiatr. Epidemiol.* **2017**. [CrossRef]
11. Narusyte, J.; Ropponen, A.; Alexanderson, K.; Svedberg, P. Genetic and Environmental Influences on Disability Pension Due To Mental Diagnoses: Limited Importance of Major Depression, Generalized Anxiety, and Chronic Fatigue. *Twin Res. Hum. Genet.* **2016**, *19*, 10–16. [CrossRef] [PubMed]
12. Ropponen, A.; Svedberg, P. Single and additive effects of health behaviours on the risk for disability pensions among Swedish twins. *Eur. J. Public Health* **2014**, *24*, 643–648. [CrossRef] [PubMed]
13. Svedberg, P.; Ropponen, A.; Alexanderson, K.; Lichtenstein, P.; Narusyte, J. Genetic susceptibility to sickness absence is similar among women and men: Findings from a Swedish twin cohort. *Twin Res. Hum. Genet.* **2012**, *15*, 642–648. [CrossRef] [PubMed]
14. Amin, R.; Svedberg, P.; Narusyte, J. Associations between adolescent social phobia, sickness absence and unemployment: A prospective study of twins in Sweden. *Eur. J. Public Health* **2019**, *29*, 931–936. [CrossRef]
15. Böckerman, P.; Maczulskij, T. Unfit for work: Health and labour-market prospects. *Scand. J. Public Health* **2018**, *46*, 7–17. [CrossRef] [PubMed]
16. Narusyte, J.; Ropponen, A.; Silventoinen, K.; Alexanderson, K.; Kaprio, J.; Samuelsson, Å.; Svedberg, P. Genetic Liability to Disability Pension in Women and Men: A Prospective Population-Based Twin Study. *PLoS ONE* **2011**, *6*, e23143. [CrossRef] [PubMed]
17. Narusyte, J.; Ropponen, A.; Silventoinen, K.; Alexanderson, K.; Kaprio, J.; Samuelsson, Å.; Svedberg, P. The Genetic Liability to Disability Retirement: A 30-Year Follow-Up Study of 24,000 Finnish Twins. *PLoS ONE* **2008**, *3*, e3402. [CrossRef]
18. Gjerde, L.C.; Knudsen, G.P.; Czajkowski, N.; Gillespie, N.; Aggen, S.H.; Røysamb, E.; Reichborn-Kjennerud, T.; Tambs, K.; Kendler, K.S.; Orstavik, R.E. Genetic and environmental contributions to long-term sick leave and disability pension: A population-based study of young adult Norwegian twins. *Twin Res. Hum. Genet.* **2013**, *16*, 759–766. [CrossRef] [PubMed]
19. Xiao, Y.; Watson, M. Guidance on Conducting a Systematic Literature Review. *J. Plan. Educ. Res.* **2019**, *39*, 93–112. [CrossRef]
20. Moher, D.; Liberati, A.; Tetzlaff, J.; Altman, D.G. Preferred Reporting Items for Systematic Reviews and Meta-Analyses: The PRISMA Statement. *PLOS Med.* **2009**, *6*, e1000097. [CrossRef]
21. Karasek, R.A.; Theorell, T. *Healthy Work: Stress, Productivity and the Reconstruction of Working Life*; Basic Books: New York, NY, USA, 1990.
22. Lichtenstein, P.; De Faire, U.; Floderus, B.; Svartengren, M.; Svedberg, P.; Pedersen, N.L. The Swedish Twin Registry: A unique resource for clinical, epidemiological and genetic studies. *J. Intern. Med.* **2002**, *252*, 184–205. [CrossRef] [PubMed]
23. Svedberg, P.; Ropponen, A.; Lichtenstein, P.; Alexanderson, K. Are self-report of disability pension and long-term sickness absence accurate? Comparisons of self-reported interview data with national register data in a Swedish twin cohort. *BMC Public Health* **2010**, *10*, 763. [CrossRef]
24. Ludvigsson, J.F.; Svedberg, P.; Olén, O.; Bruze, G.; Neovius, M. The longitudinal integrated database for health insurance and labour market studies (LISA) and its use in medical research. *Eur. J. Epidemiol.* **2019**, *34*, 423–437. [CrossRef]

25. Kaneklin, C.; Gorli, M. "Sustainability at Work" through an Action-Research Perspective: Knowledge Creation and Validity Concerns. *TPM* **2007**, *14*, 185–206.
26. Hansen, V.; Pit, S.W.; Honeyman, P.; Barclay, L. Prolonging a sustainable working life among older rural GPs: Solutions from the horse's mouth. *Rural Remote Health* **2013**, *13*, 2369.
27. Koolhaas, W.; van der Klink, J.J.; Vervoort, J.P.; de Boer, M.R.; Brouwer, S.; Groothoff, J.W. In-depth study of the workers' perspectives to enhance sustainable working life: Comparison between workers with and without a chronic health condition. *J. Occup. Rehabil.* **2013**, *23*, 170–179. [CrossRef]
28. Leider, P.C.; Boschman, J.S.; Frings-Dresen, M.H.; van der Molen, H.F. Effects of job rotation on musculoskeletal complaints and related work exposures: A systematic literature review. *Ergonomics* **2015**, *58*, 18–32. [CrossRef] [PubMed]
29. Vänje, A. Sick Leave—A Signal of Unequal Work Organizations? Gender perspectives on work environment and work organizations in the health care sector: A knowledge review. *Nord. J. Work. Life Stud.* **2015**, *5*, 85–104. [CrossRef]
30. Nilsson, K. Conceptualisation of ageing in relation to factors of importance for extending working life—A review. *Scand. J. Public Health* **2016**, *44*, 490–505. [CrossRef]
31. Eriksson, A.; Orvik, A.; Strandmark, M.; Nordsteien, A.; Torp, S. Management and Leadership Approaches to Health Promotion and Sustainable Workplaces: A Scoping Review. *Societies* **2017**, *7*, 14. [CrossRef]
32. Forslin, M.; Fink, K.; Hammar, U.; von Koch, L.; Johansson, S. Predictors for Employment Status in People With Multiple Sclerosis: A 10-Year Longitudinal Observational Study. *Arch. Phys. Med. Rehabil.* **2018**, *99*, 1483–1490. [CrossRef]
33. Wålinder, R.; Runeson-Broberg, R.; Arakelian, E.; Nordqvist, T.; Runeson, A.; Rask-Andersen, A. A supportive climate and low strain promote well-being and sustainable working life in the operation theatre. *Ups. J. Med. Sci.* **2018**, *123*, 183–190. [CrossRef]
34. GGyllensten, K.; Wentz, K.; Håkansson, C.; Hagberg, M.; Nilsson, K. Older assistant nurses' motivation for a full or extended working life. *Ageing Soc.* **2019**, *39*, 2699–2713. [CrossRef]
35. Thompson, L.; Ford, H.; Stroud, A.; Madill, A. Tortoise or hare? Supporting the chronotope preference of employees with fluctuating chronic illness symptoms. *Psychol. Health* **2019**, *34*, 695–714. [CrossRef] [PubMed]
36. Blomé, M.W.; Borell, J.; Håkansson, C.; Nilsson, K. Attitudes toward elderly workers and perceptions of integrated age management practices. *Int J. Occup. Saf. Ergon.* **2020**, *26*, 112–120. [CrossRef]
37. Gyllensten, K.; Torén, K.; Hagberg, M.; Söderberg, M. A sustainable working life in the car manufacturing industry: The role of psychosocial factors, gender and occupation. *PLoS ONE* **2020**, *15*, e0233009. [CrossRef]
38. Lindmark, U.; Ahlstrand, I.; Ekman, A.; Berg, L.; Hedén, L.; Källstrand, J.; Larsson, M.; Nunstedt, H.; Oxelmark, L.; Pennbrant, S.; et al. Health-promoting factors in higher education for a sustainable working life-protocol for a multicenter longitudinal study. *BMC Public Health* **2020**, *20*, 233. [CrossRef]
39. Nilsson, K. A sustainable working life for all ages—The swAge-model. *Appl. Ergon.* **2020**, *86*, 103082. [CrossRef] [PubMed]
40. Nunstedt, H.; Eriksson, M.; Obeid, A.; Hillström, L.; Truong, A.; Pennbrant, S. Salutary factors and hospital work environments: A qualitative descriptive study of nurses in Sweden. *BMC Nurs.* **2020**, *19*, 125. [CrossRef]
41. Wang, M.; Ropponen, A.; Narusyte, J.; Helgadóttir, B.; Bergström, G.; Blom, V.; Svedberg, P. Adverse outcomes of chronic widespread pain and common mental disorders in individuals with sickness absence—A prospective study of Swedish twins. *BMC Public Health* **2020**, *20*, 1301. [CrossRef] [PubMed]
42. Ropponen, A.; Narusyte, J.; Silventoinen, K.; Svedberg, P. Health behaviours and psychosocial working conditions as predictors of disability pension due to different diagnoses: A population-based study. *BMC Public Health* **2020**, *20*, 1507. [CrossRef]
43. Helgadóttir, B.; Mather, L.; Narusyte, J.; Ropponen, A.; Blom, V.; Svedberg, P. Transitioning from sickness absence to disability pension—The impact of poor health behaviours: A prospective Swedish twin cohort study. *BMJ Open* **2019**, *9*, e031889. [CrossRef] [PubMed]
44. Mather, L.; Ropponen, A.; Mittendorfer-Rutz, E.; Narusyte, J.; Svedberg, P. Health, work and demographic factors associated with a lower risk of work disability and unemployment in employees with lower back, neck and shoulder pain. *BMC Musculoskelet. Disord.* **2019**, *20*, 622. [CrossRef] [PubMed]
45. Björkenstam, E.; Narusyte, J.; Alexanderson, K.; Ropponen, A.; Kjeldgård, L.; Svedberg, P. Associations between childbirth, hospitalization and disability pension: A cohort study of female twins. *PLoS ONE* **2014**, *9*, e101566. [CrossRef]

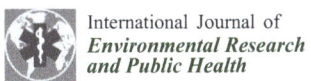

Article

The Complexity of Decreased Work Ability: Individuals' Perceptions of Factors That Affect Returning to Work after Sickness Absence

Ella Näsi [1,2,*], Mikko Perkiö [2] and Lauri Kokkinen [2]

1 Research Unit, The Social Insurance Institution of Finland, Nordenskiöldinkatu 12, 00250 Helsinki, Finland
2 Faculty of Social Sciences, Tampere University, Arvo Ylpön katu 34, 33014 Tampere, Finland; mikko.perkio@tuni.fi (M.P.); lauri.kokkinen@tuni.fi (L.K.)
* Correspondence: ella.nasi@tuni.fi

Abstract: Much of what has been written about decreased work ability is based on quantitative studies and has been written from the perspective of professionals, service providers or authorities. In our qualitative study, we sought to understand how affected individuals themselves perceive and experience the multifaceted factors that are related to their decreased work ability. Sixteen individuals in Finland with musculoskeletal diseases (MSD) participated in semi-structured interviews. The participants were potential clients of a multi-professional service pilot model, the TOIKE Work Ability Centre. Narrative and thematic analyses were utilised. The study found that individuals with decreased work ability have differing perspectives towards returning to work and often complex life situations. Five distinctive groups were identified based on self-assessed health, work ability and orientation towards work or pension: (1) the Successful; (2) the Persevering; (3) the Forward-looking; (4) the Stuck; and (5) the Pension-oriented. Health problems, unemployment, age discrimination, financial difficulties and skill deficits were the major challenges of the interviewees. Furthermore, they perceived the service and benefit systems as complicated. The TOIKE service proved useful to some of them. However, many had not utilised it due to a lack of understanding of its purpose. Identifying the distinctive groups and their needs may improve interventions. Ultimately, this may help to achieve Target 8.5 of the UN Sustainable Development Goals, which advocates the right to employment for all ages and for those with disabilities.

Keywords: decreased work ability; returning to work; counselling; disability pension; partial work ability; rehabilitation; social benefits; musculoskeletal disorders; age discrimination

Citation: Näsi, E.; Perkiö, M.; Kokkinen, L. The Complexity of Decreased Work Ability: Individuals' Perceptions of Factors That Affect Returning to Work after Sickness Absence. *IJERPH* **2022**, *19*, 113. https://doi.org/10.3390/ijerph19010113

Academic Editors: Kerstin Nilsson, Tove Midtsundstad, Peter Lundqvist, Joanne Crawford and Nygård Clas-Håkan

Received: 11 November 2021
Accepted: 20 December 2021
Published: 23 December 2021

Publisher's Note: MDPI stays neutral with regard to jurisdictional claims in published maps and institutional affiliations.

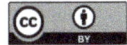

Copyright: © 2021 by the authors. Licensee MDPI, Basel, Switzerland. This article is an open access article distributed under the terms and conditions of the Creative Commons Attribution (CC BY) license (https://creativecommons.org/licenses/by/4.0/).

1. Introduction

The ageing of populations leads to increasing proportions of old-age pensioners and higher morbidity among workers [1–3]. Therefore, many countries in the Global North are concerned about labour productivity and shortages, and worsening dependency ratios [3,4]. In this context, governments are interested in supporting sustainable working life [5] by preventing work disability [2,6,7] and increasing the retirement age [2]. Concurrently, Target 8.5 of the United Nations' Sustainable Development Goals [8] addresses social sustainability, aiming to "achieve full and productive employment and decent work for all women and men." It is of importance to this article that the target particularly notes those with disabilities.

In a perfectly sustainable working life, an individual with an injury or illness always recovers adequately and returns to work smoothly, but in the real world, not everyone can return to work in a timely manner [9,10]. A persistent health issue often is the main obstacle to returning to work or to finding a suitable new job [11–13]. Studies have found that health problems, particularly long-term sickness absences, are strong predictors of filing for disability pensions [2,14,15].

However, abundant research agrees that work disability and returning to work after sickness absence are complex phenomena that encompass many individual, work-related, service-related and environmental challenges [3,9,11,12,14,16–18]. The multifaceted nature of work ability and returning to work is covered under the World Health Organization's biopsychosocial model of disability and functioning [19] and the multidimensional work ability model [7].

When returning to work is not possible, retiring with a disability pension is a way to make a clear early exit from the workforce. However, disability retirement is something that a person cannot resolve independently, as it can be issued only after intense scrutiny, after which it is determined that the individual has a medically confirmed illness, disease or injury that significantly restricts work ability [15]. Consequently, individuals with complex problems may be left "in between," caught within a bureaucratic labyrinth of services waiting for decisions and making recurring claims for rehabilitation, benefits or a pension [12,14,20].

Due to its multifaceted nature, decreased work ability can be viewed as a wicked problem [12,21] because its causes can originate from many sources, its possible solutions are not clearly identifiable nor comprehensive, it keeps evolving and it requires cooperation across different governmental sectors [22]. Alleviating such a wicked problem calls for multi-sectoral and multi-professional collaboration. Concurrently, new kinds of multi-professional interventions and service models have been and are developed in Finland and abroad to alleviate partial work ability using a holistic approach [10,23,24]. This study's underlying assumption is that although many people need individual, holistic support and counselling to return to work and to apply for rehabilitation and other services, suitable advisory services are either not always readily available, or they do not reach those who would benefit from them. Overall, the diversity of social security benefits and services offers support, but their complexity may confuse people and wind up hindering return-to-work efforts [14].

Researchers have expressed a need for more qualitative research to gain a deeper understanding of decreased work ability "from the ground up" [14], particularly individuals' perspectives, thoughts and feelings [10,17,25]. According to Metteri [20], the value of individuals' true-life perceptions is that they challenge and complement official information that authorities provide.

Therefore, this qualitative study's overall purpose was to enhance understanding about the phenomenon of decreased work ability by interviewing affected individuals, with an emphasis on how they perceive this multifaceted societal problem. The aim was to examine sick-listed individuals' experiences regarding decreased work ability, their challenges in returning to work and the services and other factors that help or hinder them in their quest to resolve their situations.

This study's main finding was that individuals with decreased work ability have multifaceted problems, and that five distinctive groups could be identified based on the individuals' self-assessed health and work ability, orientations towards work or pension and perceptions concerning the future. Health issues usually were the main hindrance to returning to work. Age discrimination and a lack of adequate skills or training also emerged as noteworthy challenges. Consequently, the interviewees' needs in terms of support and advisory services varied, implying that services should be tailored carefully according to each group's specific needs.

2. Materials and Methods

This study utilised a semi-structured phone interview method, followed by narrative and thematic analysis, to construct a holistic understanding of subjective human experiences and the meanings that people assign to their experiences with decreased work ability [26,27]. This study was explorative and theory-informed, as the theoretical framework was not determined explicitly a priori [28], but was based instead on a wider comprehension of earlier research on work ability and disability. The rather loosely structured theoretical framework allowed for an inductive, data-driven analysis of the interviews [29]. Määttä [25] previously took a similar approach.

2.1. Study Participants

The interviewees comprised Finnish individuals with decreased work ability who had been receiving a sickness absence benefit for at least six months due to a musculoskeletal disorder (MSD). The 16 participants were recruited from a pool of 24 people whom a social insurance professional (at the Social Insurance Institution of Finland, Kela) advised to utilise a multi-professional pilot service model, called the TOIKE Work Ability Centre, during the first half of 2018. TOIKE aimed to enhance clients' capabilities and opportunities for returning to work at Pirkanmaa and Southern Ostrobothnia hospital districts in Finland [30]. Their multi-disciplinary team included an occupational physician, rehabilitation counsellor, psychologist and social worker, who offered work ability assessments, counselling and guidance, and psychological services. However, only some interviewees contacted the TOIKE Centre. The reason for recruiting individuals from this pool was to acquire rich, qualitative data about decreased work ability and affected individuals' service experiences and needs.

Special attention was paid to guarantee that the data were collected, stored and analysed in a way that keeps informants' identities anonymous because the interviews focussed on sensitive issues, such as the participants' health [27,31]. The Kela ethics committee evaluated and accepted the research plan in June 2018.

Potential interviewees were sent a letter in July 2018 that informed them about the research project and upcoming phone interviews. The recipients were told that participation was voluntary, their identities would not be revealed at any point and their answers would not be used for any other purpose than the current study [32]. Altogether, 16 individuals agreed to participate in phone interviews in August 2018. Each participant was asked specifically for his or her consent to be interviewed and to allow the interview to be audio-recorded for research purposes. Their consent was audio-recorded.

Four interviewees were women and the others men, but gender was not viewed as relevant in this study; therefore, the interviewees were given gender-neutral pseudonyms, such as Sam and Pat. However, their gender can be discerned through the use of the pronouns "he" and "she," which were used for the sake of readability. Instead of exact ages, interviewees' age ranges are reported. Four interviewees were in the "39 years or younger" age group, another four were in the "40–50 years" age group and the final eight were "51 years or older" (see Appendix A for descriptive information in Table A1. Interviewees' profiles). Some of the participants lived in urban areas and some in rural areas, but the exact areas where they lived were not recorded. In Finland, both rural and urban areas have fairly equal access to social and health services.

Most interviewees had done physically demanding work [33] in agriculture, construction, logistics, manufacturing or maintenance. One had done physically demanding work in the hospitality sector, and two had done work that combined physical and mental demands in the health care and transport sectors. One interviewee worked mainly in secretarial work. Only four of the 16 interviewees had returned to their former jobs. One of the younger respondents had been accepted by a study program, where she started her studies for a physically less demanding vocation. Another respondent soon was going to start a work tryout. Most interviewees were receiving temporary financial benefits, such as sickness allowance, unemployment benefits, rehabilitation allowance, rehabilitation subsidy or partial disability pension. Appendix A (Table A1. Interviewees' profiles.) describes each pseudonymised participant using eleven variables and individual summaries.

2.2. Qualitative Interviews

The average interview lasted about 25 minutes, ranging from 15 to 60 minutes. All 16 interviews were conducted in Finnish; only the quotations, which were used to illustrate the results, were translated into English during the reporting phase.

The interviewer encouraged participants to express their honest opinions and original prevailing thoughts, allowing them to emphasise the points that they deemed important. The semi-structured interviews allowed the interviewer to ask open questions to acquire knowledge about the informants' reasoning, opinions and attitudes. The interview guide included 29 questions, of which most were open-ended. The guide also included certain commonly used quantitative questions, such as the interviewee's self-assessment of his or her health on a scale from 1 to 5. The interviewees also were asked to compare their current work ability with their best lifetime work ability with the work ability score, so that 0 represented full work disability and 10 indicated work ability at its best [34]. After each quantitative question, the interviewees were encouraged to explain and elaborate on their numerical answers.

The interview guide included open-ended questions such as: What are the main reasons for you to be outside of working life? What is hindering returning to work? What would help you return to work? Other questions asked how the interviewee felt about the Kela phone call to inform him or her about the TOIKE Work Ability Centre, why individuals either did or did not contact the TOIKE centre and how they perceived the TOIKE service itself.

2.3. Narrative and Thematic Analysis of the Interviews

The interviewees' answers were transcribed verbatim, but without details on intonation, pauses or stuttering. The focus was on content, rather than choice of words or tone of speech [26]. The data were transferred to the Atlas.ti program for analysis.

The analysis primarily was based on inductive coding, used for narrative and thematic analysis, as explained below. However, the data first were organised roughly into a table laying out each interviewee's background. A table of interviewees' profiles (Appendix A, Table A1) was created with each interviewee's age group, employment type and sector and main health concern(s). The table proved useful during the inductive qualitative analysis as a quick reference tool when comparing interviewees with each other. The table was refined further and expanded throughout the entire analytical process to include more specific information, such as the interviewees' labour market situation, future plans, self-assessed health and work ability, success and readiness to return to work and whether they had contacted the TOIKE centre. After narrative and thematic analysis, a summarising column also was added at the end of the analytical process.

Using the Atlas.ti program, a data-based, inductive content analysis was conducted, i.e., the interviews were read carefully several times [29] and thereafter coded with the intention to code each comment without any limiting framework. However, the data collection and analysis processes were theory-informed, as the interview guide was based on previous literature and designed together with work-ability experts. During the open coding stage, "headings" or "labels" were assigned to each meaning unit [29,35]. Following Graneheim and Lundman's [35] guidelines, single sentences usually were identified as meaning units, but sometimes codes were assigned to clusters of sentences or single words. The data were categorised, where appropriate, into positive (+) or negative (−), or onto a numerical scale. For example, the interviewees' answers to whether they successfully had returned to work were coded as positive or negative responses.

In the next step, compiling summarised narratives proved useful as an analytical device [32] to form a clear understanding of each interview and the similarities and differences between interviews. The ontological premise of narrative analysis is that an individual is an active subject who assigns meanings to his or her life and life events [26]. Narrative research aims to understand concrete events and individuals' experiences of their world, actions and endeavours [31].

Therefore, each interview aimed to form a condensed narrative, including the interviewee's vocational background and health issues, and their success in and perceptions of returning to work or orientation towards pension, re-education or rehabilitation. The summarised narratives also included their accounts of their main challenges and experiences with and perceptions of the TOIKE Work Ability Centre and other services. The narratives revealed more or less work-oriented career trajectories that allowed for organising the interviews into five distinctive groups based on the narrative analysis, serving as the core structure for reporting the results. For each group, one narrative was chosen to represent typical stories in the group. Relevant quotes illustrate the interviews' original quiddities.

Concurrent with the narrative analysis, as the interviews were read many times, the initial coding was revised and specified. Codes were combined to form groups [29], termed code families in the Atlas.ti program. The codes and code groups then were organised into themes. The four most relevant emergent themes are reported at the end of the results section.

3. Results

Figure 1 presents the interviewees' self-assessments of their health and work ability, which serves as an introduction for reporting this study's results. Thereafter, the study's main findings are presented by explaining the five distinctive groups that were found to represent decreased work ability (Figure 2). These groups were categorised as a result of the narrative analysis process in which the interviews were rearranged into groups based on the interviewees' orientations towards pension or working life, and their success in returning to work. Furthermore, four main themes emerged from the data in relation to supporting sustainable working lives.

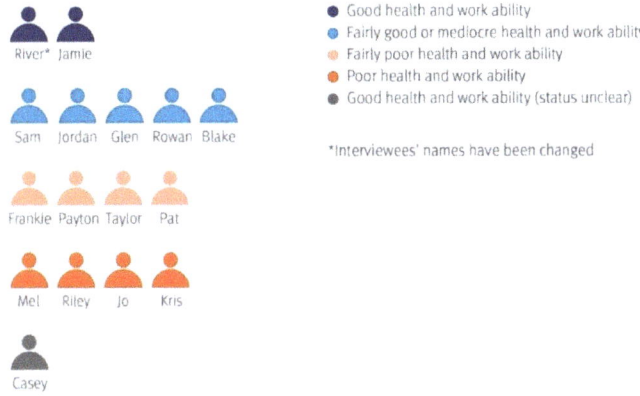

Figure 1. Interviewees' perceived health and work ability.

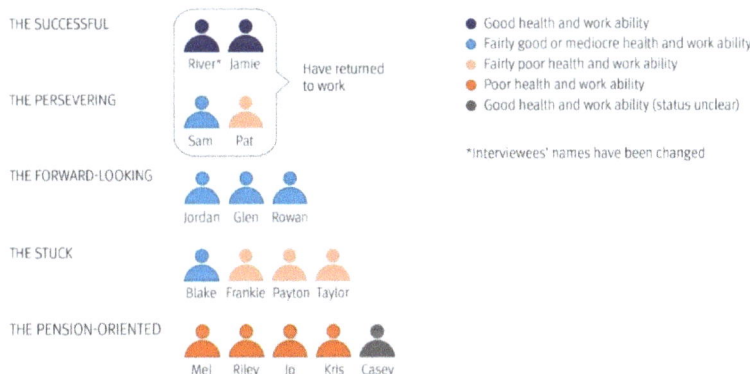

Figure 2. The interviewee groups based on their success in returning to work.

3.1. Perceived Health and Work Ability Predicted Return to Work

The interviewees' self-assessed health correlated rather well with self-assessed work ability. Only two interviewees felt that their health and work ability were good; they were assigned the pseudonyms River and Jamie and are depicted in dark blue in Figure 1. At the opposite end, four other interviewees—Mel, Riley, Jo and Kris—described their health as poor or very poor, and their work ability; they are depicted in orange. Two members in this group, Riley and Kris, itemised a long list of health problems or multiple body parts where they experience pain. Kris' account illustrates the multimorbidity of an interviewee whose health and work ability are poor:

Kris: "My back and right leg are duds. I have had sciatica. There is a problem in my pelvis, and my left bicep is loose. These are all occupational traumas. I am queuing for surgery, and they are saying: 'Aren't you going to work?', even though the orthopaedists have written: 'unfit for work'. Not in my right mind [in reference to not going back to work]! Additionally, then I have type 2 diabetes. Additionally, then I have had a hospital infection [nosocomial infection]. I cannot sit still, cannot sleep... I have medication for high blood pressure."

Those categorised as reporting mediocre or fairly good health and work ability are depicted in light blue in Figure 1, comprising Sam, Jordan, Glen, Rowan and Blake—also pseudonyms. Those reporting fairly poor health and work ability are depicted in light pink and include Frankie, Payton, Taylor and Pat.

One interviewee, given the pseudonym Casey, had a health and work ability status that was difficult to categorise because she provided conflicting information. In the beginning, she assessed her health and work ability as good, but her account of her health is not logical. She claims that she was not ill, but recently went to a physician, complaining about health problems, and was receiving a sickness allowance. She is categorised in her own health and work ability group, called good health and work ability (status unclear) and is depicted in grey.

The narrative analyses revealed certain similarities and consistencies within the participants' narratives, making it meaningful to categorise the individual narratives into five groups, as listed below and illustrated in Figure 2. Success in returning to work and orientation towards work or pension were the main factors in the narratives that shaped these categories. Furthermore, the interviewees' open-ended answers regarding their health issues and recovery, and other factors affecting their motivation regarding returning to work, also impacted the grouping:

1. The *Successful*: work-oriented, returned to work, well-recovered and -motivated: River and Jamie
2. The *Persevering*: somewhat work-oriented, returned to work, not fully recovered, concerned about their work ability: Sam and Pat
3. The *Forward-looking*: work-oriented, have not returned to work, not fully recovered, motivated to find a new job: Jordan, Glen and Rowan
4. The *Stuck*: somewhat pension-oriented, have not returned to work, not recovered, passive: Blake, Frankie, Payton and Taylor
5. The *Pension-oriented*: have not returned to work, not recovered, demotivated: Mel, Riley, Jo, Kris and Casey

In fact, self-assessed health and work ability can be viewed as one of the primary factors affecting an individual's categorisation into a specific group, as demonstrated in Figure 2. Thus, interviewees' better self-assessed health and work ability were associated with a stronger orientation towards and better success in returning to work. Nevertheless, it is worth noting that the correlations were not complete due to the complex nature of decreased work ability. Interviewees who returned to work (the *Successful* and *Persevering* groups) or who were hoping to return to work (the *Forward-looking* group) mostly assessed their health and work ability on the positive side. Accordingly, those who were applying for a disability pension and had difficulties finding a job that would suit their health constraints (the *Pension-oriented* and *Stuck* groups) assessed their health and work ability in most cases as being poor or fairly poor.

However, there were two exceptions to the aforementioned rule. Blake belonged to the Stuck group even though he assessed his work ability as mediocre. He fell and hurt his shoulder, and mentioned having "the blues" occasionally, but otherwise he did not have major health issues. Blake's stagnant situation also was associated with his work history in unstable jobs. He explained that one solution could be re-education, but that his inability to use computers made it difficult for him to access relevant information, and he also was sceptical about the usefulness of studying. In relation to this, he alluded to low self-confidence in his interview answers.

Pat's narrative was a different type of exception to the rule that good health is a precondition for returning to work. He explained that he felt it was necessary to return to work and was also willing to go back, despite his fairly poor health and work ability. Pat's use of the verb "must" when talking about returning to work indicates some level of pressure to return to work, which could be related to him being self-employed, even though he did not use entrepreneurship as an explicit explanation for his prompt return to work. Next, we analyse one by one all main narratives presented in Figure 2.

3.1.1. The Successful Group: Well-Recovered and Returned to Work

Jamie, an entrepreneur, and River, a professional in the health care sector, were placed in the *Successful* group. They recovered well from their illnesses and returned to their old jobs. They were relatively free of pain as well. Jamie's story was chosen to illustrate this group.

Jamie worked in the agricultural sector, in which workloads are seasonally cyclical. He injured his shoulder at work, underwent surgery two months later, then returned to work four months after that. He explained that he himself carried the main responsibility for rehabilitation, actively exercising the injured shoulder under the care of a physiotherapist. Seven months after his operation, Jamie was happy with his recovery and enjoyed work: *"Then it [the shoulder] was operated on, and it feels reasonably good now. It is possible to work [...] It doesn't impede my work tasks in any way."*

When asked about his health, Jamie explained that it was rather good for a man his age, about to turn 60. He assessed his work ability as 8 on a scale of 0–10 and justified it through improved skills: *"My skills have increased, even if my pace has slowed down a bit. Skills have improved in any case."*

One factor that may explain Jamie's eagerness to return to work is that as a self-employed worker in the agricultural sector, he had firm control over his responsibilities, with success or failure having direct consequences on his financial rewards or setbacks. Furthermore, he also pressured the health care professionals to operate on his shoulder promptly to ensure fast recovery. This implied that he was determined to return to work and was motivated and committed to taking care of his work responsibilities: *"I said there is a need to get into surgery as soon as possible because I work in agriculture and the approaching sowing time is putting pressure on me. Additionally, I got [into surgery] very fast then."*

Jamie's quotes above indicate that he felt a desire to return to work, which he found meaningful and important. Both individuals in this group recovered well due to comprehensive medical interventions and personal engagement in their rehabilitation. They did not feel the need to contact the TOIKE Work Ability Centre and were determined to return to their old jobs. Therefore, the following adjectives describe this group: work-oriented; well-recovered; and motivated.

3.1.2. The Persevering: Returned to Work despite Work Ability Concerns

The *Persevering* group included two individuals who returned to work regardless of their prevailing health problems. Sam and Pat both were engaged in physical work in the construction sector. Sam was an employee, and Pat was self-employed; both experienced back pain. Sam added that he was suffering from burnout/fatigue.

Sam's story is provided here as an example to illustrate the situation when an individual returns to work despite not having recovered from a disease or disorder. Sam was in the 40–50 age group. He presumed that his physical and mental health problems, back pain and burnout/fatigue may have been interconnected. To cope, he turned to an occupational health care service for his back problems and a psychiatrist for his mental health problems. He was on medication, did physical exercises and felt a need to rest. Sam also sought and got help from traditional medicine and acupuncture. Despite multiple periods of sick leave, Sam returned to work, which can be interpreted as a sign of being work-oriented. He also assessed his health as mediocre and his work ability as 5.5 on a scale of 0–10, i.e., despite the pain, he felt that he still possessed work capabilities. However, he did not have much choice and said that he had not received much information about rehabilitation: *"The choices that have been available are: 'Be on sick leave or go to work'. 'Take some medicine if you have pain'. This TOIKE is the only thing I've received info about."*

Sam contacted the TOIKE Work Ability Centre. He was confused after not being offered an appointment with them and was told that due to having access to occupational health care services, there would have been little extra benefits available for him from the TOIKE Centre. However, he had some unresolved work-ability issues, so it is likely that he could have benefitted from a holistic advisory service to ensure that his work ability issues were eased, rather than worsened or prolonged.

Both Pat and Sam had many years of potential working life ahead of them, as they were in their 30s and 40s, but they had prolonged health problems that posed a risk of lost work ability in the future. They both worked in the construction sector, which is physically demanding. To sum up, this group of work-oriented individuals can be described as: returned to work; not fully recovered; and having prevailing work-ability concerns.

3.1.3. The Forward-Looking: Searching for New Opportunities

The interviewees in this *Forward-looking* group were seeking a new direction for their careers. They all had musculoskeletal disorders, which inhibited them from returning to their old jobs, but conveyed a strong orientation towards finding suitable work. They include Jordan, who had worked in the hospitality sector; Rowan, who had worked in the transport sector; and Glen, who had worked in logistics. All three were under age 40. They expressed hopefulness, anticipation of recovery and a willingness to find new career paths that would fit their health constraints.

Glen's story illustrates this group. He had been working in a physical job, and his shoulder and clavicle were injured in a violent incident. The injury was rather serious and required two shoulder operations, but the operations were not very successful, and his absence from work due to incapacity lasted a year. His recovery advanced slowly, and he found physiotherapy helpful, but could not return to his old job. He assessed his life satisfaction as mediocre now and envisioned finding a new job or seeking training or education to increase his satisfaction: *"I cannot really do physical work, even though I liked it very much. When I get a job or school [...] or something else, then that will, of course, affect [my life satisfaction] very much in general. I miss working life in a way, going to work and so forth. Even though it is hard, but still."*

Glen recently turned to a nongovernmental organisation (NGO) that offers work tryouts and other types of activities to unemployed people. He hoped to find education or work soon: *"I have tried to make future plans by myself. I have been thinking that I will apply to some college or training in the autumn and try to find a job also at the same time. It is possible that the TOIKE thing would still be useful, but I have not contacted them yet."*

None of the members of this *Forward-looking* group expressed a preference to remain outside of working life. They all were looking forward to finding new directions for their careers, but none had contacted the TOIKE Work Ability Centre. They all had prevailing musculoskeletal disorders, but viewed recovery and regaining work ability as plausible and desirable future trajectories. Thus, this group can be referred to as work-oriented—not fully recovered and not returning to work yet, but looking actively for a new direction.

3.1.4. The Stuck: Having No Clear Exit from Temporary Benefits

The four interviewees in the *Stuck* group—Blake, Frankie, Payton and Taylor—had injury, pain or disease of the upper extremities, and some also had other health problems as well. They had worked in physical jobs to which they had not been able to return. However, they mostly assessed their health and work ability as mediocre or somewhat diminished, rather than highly diminished, and they felt they had some capabilities left. Two were in the 40–50 age group, and two were in the 51+ age group. Taylor and Frankie had been absent from work for six years, Blake for two years and Payton for half a year.

Taylor's story was chosen to represent this group. Taylor lived in a small town, had worked in manufacturing and was unemployed with a shoulder injury. He stated that his decreased work ability was a hindrance to finding new employment: *"I have been trying to look for such a job in which I could work with my arms down. I cannot perform tasks where I need to reach upwards with my arms—that is the kind of work I have always done. My arm just does not work upwards."*

Before injuring his shoulder, he had been unemployed for many years already. When asked about returning to work, he mentioned many factors besides his shoulder injury that have hindered his job search efforts, such as learning difficulties, deterioration of his general health, lack of education or training and ageing. He also cited his place of residence and living conditions as factors that made it more difficult, or even impossible, to find suitable work.

Taylor: Studying doesn't help because I have dyslexia and memory disorders, so that things go in through one ear and out the other. My health condition in general is getting worse. I don't have training for almost anything, and the other thing is that my shoulder is a wreck. These are the two most important reasons. Additionally, then this house—I really cannot go far [...] You know that I am an old bloke already. I do not have such dreams anymore as I had when I was in my 20s."

Taylor had multiple health, social and location-related problems. When asked what he thought about the possibility of contacting the TOIKE Work Ability Centre, he ignored the question at first: *"It is possible that somebody called me [referring to a Kela professional calling and recommending TOIKE]. Sometimes I feel that so many magazine peddlers call me, so I don't care about them [...] Oh, that thing in Tampere [refers to TOIKE]. I did not contact them."*

A common feature of this group was that these individuals did not express a clear preference for retirement, nor much hope for returning to work. For this group, these individuals' prominent health problems were not the only reason for decreased work ability, as they reported a complex mesh of hindrances. Making a living was a challenge for this group. Three out of four cited lack of job opportunities as a major reason for not returning to work.

Another common feature in this group was their unwillingness or inability to acquire new skills. Similar to Taylor, Frankie also claimed that he did not have an adequate, up-to-date education. Frankie also revealed that he had dyslexia in addition to his physical health problems.

Additionally, the following problems came up during the interviews: Their subsistence relied on temporary benefits, they experienced difficulties navigating the benefit and service system, and their financial situations were poor, i.e., they were stuck in a rut of temporary benefits that they could not exit to working life or a disability pension. Overall, a certain level of ineptitude in seeking resolutions to their work disability status was present during these interviews. To summarise, this group comprised people who were somewhat pension-oriented, had not returned to work, had not recovered and were passive and hesitant.

3.1.5. The Pension-Oriented: Inclination towards Early Retirement

Four interviewees given the pseudonyms Mel, Riley, Jo and Kris, who had poor health and work ability, and Casey, who provided contradictory information about her health, comprised the *Pension-oriented* group.

Mel, Jo, Kris and Riley were all over 50 years old, had done physical work and had chronic musculoskeletal problems that caused pain and decreased their functioning. None of them had returned to work and expressed a clear reluctance towards returning, as they viewed themselves as unfit. Jo, Kris and Riley had applied for a disability pension. Mel did not mention any pension application, but did not believe that he could—nor did he want to—return to work. Their main reason for being outside of working life was their poor health. They all mentioned having surgery as an option to recover, but had differing perceptions of surgery's appropriateness for themselves. Kris, Riley and Mel were scared or reluctant to take the surgical route back to work. However, Jo welcomed the prospect of surgery and viewed it as the only solution to his work-ability issues, but as he had assessed his readiness to return to work as zero (on a scale of 0–10) and had applied for a disability pension, it is plausible to categorise him as pension-oriented.

The manifest content of their interviews, including thorough accounts of persisting health problems, affirmed that they were incapable of work; therefore, a disability pension could have been a plausible option for them. It may be worth noting that a risk of justification bias [36] is present in studies that ask participants to self-report their health: Inactive individuals may report poorer health to justify their situation. Kris and Riley aimed to justify staying outside of working life after having worked very hard in the past:

Riley: "Well, I would be happy to return to work if I was healthy. I have always liked to work, but maybe I worked a bit too much because I am a wreck. We pushed night and day then. We did not have any summer holiday or anything. Heavy work. Twelve hours was our shortest day. Then my body started to break up."

Kris' story was chosen as an example to illustrate this group. Kris had worked as an entrepreneur in the construction industry. He ended his business three years earlier due to back and leg pain, and diminishing business opportunities. He also had multiple morbidities and received medical statements from orthopaedists about his decreased work ability. His own assessment of his work ability was zero, and he was applying for a disability pension. However, Kris's pension application was unresolved for the time being, as he was scheduled for surgery in the near future: *"I am a bit [...] multi-handicapped. I should have gone 10–20 years ago to get treated, so maybe something could have been cured. I let myself [get in a bad condition], was stupid and worked too much."*

Kris explained that he did not go to see a doctor immediately after ending his business and implied that this delay was the reason why he had been denied certain benefits that he was expecting to receive from the pension insurance company. Kris relied on basic social assistance to make ends meet. He complained about delays in getting sickness allowance payments, which had aggravated his poor financial situation. He felt frustrated and angry due to these difficulties in accessing social benefits and regretted working too hard, not taking care of his health and not seeking medical care early enough. He felt betrayed and blamed the bureaucracy for his difficult financial situation: *"The last time I received any money was more than a month ago. I am so angry. I am saying I could sue them. I need to visit the hospital often, but I cannot even pay for it [the hospital bills]."*

Casey was a somewhat different case because her health status was hard to determine due to conflicting information. She was over 60 years old, had worked in various secretarial jobs, considered herself fit for work, but could not find work. She explained that she was advised to apply for a sickness allowance in relation to pain that she had experienced and stayed home for many years caring for her husband until he died: *"I had a stomachache, and I pointed out that it stems from here, between my ears. I pointed at my head, and the doctor asked: 'When did the headache start?' Additionally, she made a diagnosis that I have a problem in my head. The problem was in my stomach. So, I have come across these bafflements that I was prescribed medicine for an affective disorder. I did not fetch the pills because it was my stomach that was aching. [...] There is nothing wrong with my health. For two years, I cared for my husband, who had a brain tumour. They just labelled me ill."*

It was difficult to draw reliable and consistent conclusions from Casey's interview transcript. She may have either had a stomach problem or an affective disorder, or both, or her unclear account could have been related to some other physical, mental, cognitive or memory disorder. It is also possible that she intentionally or unintentionally used confusing language at the doctor's appointment and during the interview as a consequence of disappointments or frustration in relation to her difficult life situation.

Casey lived in a small town and mentioned diminishing job opportunities as one reason for not returning to work. However, the employment office required her to participate in activation measures, so they sent her to jobs. For example, she had worked in the city library, where she recalled *"going through books in the storage of the library'*. She felt that the jobs she was assigned were *"nonsense"* because she was given tasks that required fewer skills than what she was capable of doing.

Casey recalled a Kela professional contacting her and stating that she will be *"put into rehabilitation'*. In response, Casey attempted to legitimise her inactivity in the labour market as making space for younger workers: *"There could be an age limit because, you see, I don't see it as useful to try to rehabilitate over-60-year-olds back to work. I am not so young, so is it sensible to employ me? I think, in this situation, it would be more reasonable to hire, for example, someone who is 34 years old."* In accordance with her disdain for rehabilitation, she had not contacted the TOIKE Work Ability Centre.

To summarise, this last group can be called the *Pension-oriented* group because these individuals had not returned to work and were expressing demotivation toward rehabilitation or activation measures and having to return to work.

3.2. Supporting Sustainable Work Ability

In addition to identifying the aforementioned five different groups among the individuals with decreased work ability through narrative analysis (see Figure 2), the following topical themes on supporting sustainable work ability also emerged from the interviews through thematic analysis.

3.2.1. Age and Skills as Factors Affecting Returning to Work

Some interviewees mentioned their age as being a factor even though they were not specifically asked whether they think their age affects their work ability or job opportunities. For example, Blake mentioned age while explaining his difficulties coping with strenuous work and his low motivation to train for a new vocation: *"My work has always been strenuous, and now I cannot move or lift anything with my left arm. I should have this arm treated or then I should change into a different vocation. However, I don't know. I am aged already."*

Casey's main explanation for being outside of working life was age discrimination in the labour market: *"When I became unemployed, I was already too old for the labour market, let alone today. I will be 61 next week. I can tell you that there is nobody in this town who would hire me."*

In addition to Casey, almost all the other interviewees who were over age 50 had given up their hopes and dreams of returning to work. These older individuals had in common that they felt their health and work ability were poor.

Finding work that could be adjusted to accommodate their lighter requirements was difficult, particularly among those over 50 years old. In fact, for the *Stuck* group, difficulties in finding suitable work were equally or an even more serious problem than the health problem itself. Jamie was the only exception among the interviewees over age 50, as he was very motivated to return to work. His case was viewed as an example of *the Successful* group, and his motivation was explained by his well-advanced recovery and meaningful entrepreneurial work.

Having outdated or insufficient training or skills also can be factors that hinder returning to work. For example, Taylor, from the *Stuck* group, attributed his joblessness to a lack of skills, among other things: *'I don't have training for almost anything'*. Another interviewee who had given up hope was Frankie, who had been outside of working life for six years: *"I do not have any vocation at the moment. I have been unemployed for a long time. Actually, I have not been unemployed, but outside of working life."*

On the contrary, those in the *Future-oriented* group, who were all under age 40, were hopeful and eager to find new directions for their careers and motivated to go through re-education if necessary.

3.2.2. The Importance of a Coherent Health Care Service System

The interviewees who reported having easy access to occupational or specialised health care services and who were content with the care and advice that they had received also returned to work. For example, River, who had severe back pain, recovered and returned to her old job due to having a solid doctor-patient relationship. She also was motivated to participate actively in physiotherapy and searched for information about her condition in the literature. Perhaps her background in health care contributed to her ability to search for and comprehend relevant information and commit to the suggested exercise routines. When asked about her own efforts at recovery, River explained: *"I have a very good and close relationship with my doctor. It gave me a lot. Additionally, then I also go to see a private specialist—to get a second opinion. Recovery started and the likelihood of going back to work became clear to me. That I can return, and I will recover. I felt that I don't need anything like that [refers to the TOIKE service]. Active physiotherapy is enough."*

By comparison, Rowan, who had been looking for a new direction independently, recalled incoherence in accessing services. He was a young adult in need of holistic health care services, as he mentioned having "other problems" in addition to his main diagnosis, which was back pain. Rowan's quote illustrates the situation of being "bounced" from one authority or service provider to another: *"I would need a health care service provider who would examine my health as a whole and not consider only one thing at a time. I find it very troublesome because you need to go to different places. With every health issue, you need to have a separate appointment."*

Furthermore, being self-employed and, thus, personally responsible for acquiring occupational health care services may create situations in which potential risks can be anticipated. For example, Pat did not utilise the services of a physiotherapist, but instead tried to manage without, even though he was an entrepreneur doing demanding physical work and suffering from prolonged back pain: *"Perhaps I should think about ergonomics.... I have bought tools that could help."*

3.2.3. The Challenges and Potential of Multi-Professional, Holistic Counselling

In addition to health care services, the interviews indicated that individuals with decreased work ability often needed support from other service sectors, such as social security, rehabilitation and employment services. For example, Rowan also could have benefited from career counselling and vocational rehabilitation because he felt that he was unable to return to his old job due to back pain. These issues were all included in the service package that the TOIKE Work Ability Centre provided. A Kela professional had advised Rowan to contact the TOIKE centre, and he thought that its multidisciplinary counselling could be the kind of holistic service concept that could help him. However, the inconsistency of service paths is disclosed in Rowan's incident: *"In hindsight, I feel that the TOIKE project would have probably helped me. It is probably a service that I would have contacted if these other things had not been around. Maybe the most decisive thing was that there was someone in the health care services who specifically told me that it may not be the right time now, but when things have settled a bit, I should contact them [TOIKE]."*

In addition to Rowan, also other interviewees found the service systems to be fragmented and bureaucratic. The interviewees were not always aware of what kinds of services were available, which kinds they were entitled to and how to apply for them. Sam's quote illustrates the obscurity: *"One expert advised me to do something and then another said the opposite [...] They ask me to provide all kinds of things [forms, applications]. Additionally, then I don't even know what I am supposed to send them, and I send them things without knowing what I am sending. Very unclear. Extremely unclear."*

The interviews indicated that information about new multi-professional services' purpose is not always clear to potential clients, which may lead to avoidance of services designed to help and support clients. For example, Kris and Riley did not want to contact the TOIKE Centre because they anticipated that they would be pressured to go to work.

Riley: "I am on sick leave now. Immediately, they try to activate me. Otherwise, it would be OK, but pain takes away all my strength. I wouldn't mind [contacting the TOIKE], but they immediately started to bombard me with all kinds of requirements. Luckily, I was offered the right to use the gym here. I am content with that. My functionality is low, and the constant pain gets on my nerves."

Payton and River also got the wrong impression from the TOIKE Work Ability Centre. They thought that the primary aim was to guide them toward new vocations, which they wanted to avoid, because they were committed to their current vocations. River's reaction to the Kela phone call, during which she was told she could benefit from career counselling at the TOIKE Work Ability Centre, illustrates the clash between what she thought was offered and what she felt she needed: *"First, I felt confused because I have a permanent job, and I hope they are not trying to direct me somewhere else."*

Despite accessibility challenges, many interviewees mentioned the importance of personal advice that professionals provided. Some received expert guidance and advice from their doctor, occupational health nurse, Kela or the TOIKE Work Ability Centre. For example, Rowan, whose discouragement regarding contacting TOIKE was explained earlier, had received useful advice from a Kela professional. He explained that the Kela phone call gave him a lot of information on vocational rehabilitation and benefits. He was expecting to start a job tryout soon.

Mel and Frankie had visited the TOIKE Work Ability Centre and were satisfied with the multi-professional service there. Mel, who had been outside of working life for six years, said he received good advice from TOIKE. He was advised on how to apply for a partial disability pension and felt that it was best to comply with the advice from professionals to continue receiving benefits: *"I have visited there [TOIKE] a couple of times. I hope Kela is satisfied now that I am doing what they want. I have been in a job tryout through the pension insurance company, but it did not turn out well. They just want to boost their own egos by trying to organise work for me, but they do not consider my situation . . . . I am not fit for work."*

3.2.4. Exits: Justified Career Orientations

The interviews highlighted two desirable *"exit paths"* for individuals from their unresolved life situations (Figure 3). First, for the well-recovered individuals, it is possible to return to work (Exit 1). Second, accessing a disability pension may enhance well-being significantly, particularly among those with the widest disability deficits and advanced age (Exit 2). The analysis demonstrated that the fate of a group with prolonged partial work ability is often—at least temporarily—no exit. These people are left to circulate between service providers and welfare schemes, and may end up applying for and relying on recurring temporary social security benefits, such as unemployment benefits, sickness allowances, rehabilitation allowances and non-permanent disability pensions.

In this study, those in the *Successful* and *Persevering* groups found their way back to work, i.e., Exit 1. However, those in the three other groups were currently in situations with no clear exit yet. Those in the *Pension-oriented* group clearly were yearning for retirement, i.e., Exit 2, and those in the *Future-oriented* group clearly were looking for a new career, i.e., Exit 1. Those in the *Stuck* group were not expressing a clear preference toward either exit, but instead described their personal situations as being awash in confusion and a lack of clarity.

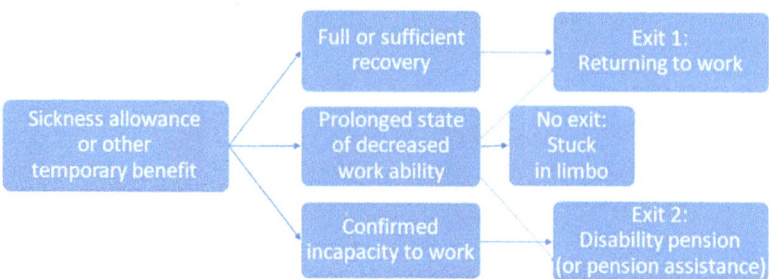

Figure 3. The exit path model. The primary exit from temporary benefits is returning to work. The secondary exit is retiring with a disability pension. (Besides, persons who are over 60 years and unemployed for five years with no or few interruptions, may be eligible for pension assistance, equal in amount to the minimum quarantee pension, in Finland.) If these exits are not available, the individual may be stuck in limbo, circulating between different temporary benefits.

4. Discussion

This qualitative study's results clearly demonstrate that individuals with decreased work ability are a heterogeneous group with complex problems. However, it is possible to identify sub-groups within them. This corresponds with earlier research, e.g., Heikkinen's [37] register-based research on similar study participants in Finland and Lydell et al.'s [17] qualitative study in Sweden. The interviewees in this study expressed many different factors, besides health, that affect returning to work. They revealed individual factors such as advanced age and insufficient skills, work-related factors such as temporary contracts and demanding work tasks, service-related factors such as delayed social benefits or fragmented health care services and environmental and social factors such as remote living areas and family responsibilities.

4.1. Main Findings

This study's main finding is that even though individuals with decreased work ability are a heterogenous group, it is possible to categorise them into distinctive groups based on their orientation and success in returning to work. This study's interviewees provided a collection of unique narratives that included certain similarities in the factors affecting their future career prospects. A comprehensive, data-driven, narrative analysis of the interviews identified five groups among the individuals whose work ability was decreased due to musculoskeletal disorders: (1) the *Successful*; (2) the *Persevering*; (3) the *Forward-looking*; (4) the *Stuck*; and (5) the *Pension-oriented*.

Another clear finding from previous studies and this study alike is that the individual's self-assessed health and work ability is a useful indicator for predicting success in returning to work [38]. Health problems tend to shift individuals towards early retirement, but in addition to health and work ability problems, other individual, work-related, social and environmental circumstances were contributing factors in study participants' success in returning to work.

4.2. Limitations

Using data from 16 interviews to elicit data-driven narrative analysis, this study identified five distinctive groups among individuals with musculoskeletal disorders based on their self-assessed health and work ability, orientations towards work or pension and perceptions concerning the future. All of the potential interviewees had been advised to contact the TOIKE Work Ability Centre due to an MSD and decreased work ability. However, there might have been some differences between those 16 who agreed and those eight who did not agree to participate in the study. Due to lack of data on non-participants we had no means for evaluating whether they had some common characteristics different from the participants, which could have possibly led to finding more categories than we did in the current study. In future studies, these findings should be tested with other conditions, such as mental health disorders, and with larger data sets from different countries to see whether the typology is generalisable to different study designs and populations.

4.3. Interpretation and Implications

The interviews reaffirmed findings from previous literature that advanced age is a factor in increasing pension orientation and obstacles related to returning to work, particularly among individuals with prolonged sickness absences [17,25]. Older people also face difficulties in finding work due to age discrimination within the labour market [2]. Ageing is associated with decreased work ability and increased morbidities [1]; therefore, work can become physically or mentally burdensome at an older age.

The pension orientation conveyed in the interviews usually was derived from negative experiences and delays in rehabilitation or health care, being rejected or discriminated against because of advancing age, or enduring persistent physical pain and feelings of decreased self-efficacy [11]. Furthermore, an interviewee with a stagnant life situation was likely to be associated with a work history comprising unstable jobs [13], and his scepticism about the usefulness of re-education corresponds with Jahoda's [39] argument that the self-confidence of people outside of the workforce often decreases because they feel ashamed and start to question their skills and capabilities [17]. Conversely, those who belonged to the *Successful* group and returned to work described how they had a meaningful job, actively had been seeking medical help and were dedicated to conducting all the exercises recommended to them as rehabilitative measures to support a prompt recovery. This supports the assumption that timely rehabilitation [17,40] should be more readily accessible to all individuals with decreased work ability to stop a possible negative trend of deteriorating health and work ability.

A closer look at the situations of those in the *Pension-oriented* group revealed that their situations were complex: They had multiple morbidities and contextual hindrances, such as outdated professional skills, a history of unstable work contracts, having gone bankrupt or living in a small town where job opportunities were scarce (see [13], for similar circumstances). Additionally, due to their advanced age, they were in the most disadvantaged situation in the current labour market, in which competition for job vacancies is harsh, and age discrimination exists [2]. Consequently, they had given up hope of returning to work and instead clearly were inclined towards retirement. For them, a justified and timely exit with a disability pension could be the difference between a disappointed "in between" life and one of well-being within the limits of their remaining functionality.

The interview data brought up the relevance of labour market dynamics on individuals' career trajectories. Many within the *Stuck* and *Pension-oriented* groups explained that there was a clear lack of job opportunities that accommodated their decreased capabilities, with fewer jobs available in the areas where they lived. Furthermore, they communicated that their skills and education were outdated regarding the current demands of working life. Conversely, interviewees in the *Successful* and *Persevering* groups explained how a desire to work pulled them back into their jobs, which they deemed meaningful, important or necessary.

Therefore, this empirical study's findings are in line with the biopsychosocial approach of the International Classification of Functioning, Disability and Health [19] and the multidimensional work ability model [7]. These holistic models contend that work ability depends not only on the individual's health, but also on their functionality, education and skills, work demands and environment, family and community support, and governmental support and services. This study reinforced the idea that labour market dynamics influence how strongly work pulls the individual back into the workforce or whether current economic situations and stringent competency requirements push employees with decreased work ability or outdated skills out of the workforce [38,41,42].

This study's empirical results, together with previous literature [43], imply that it is important to emphasise enhancing individuals' capabilities through lifelong learning. A requirement for sustainable careers in today´s working life is that everyone's skills are updated regularly. Of course, this would require substantial input from society, employers and individuals themselves.

As this study adds to the existing literature on decreased work ability's complex nature, it is plausible to assert that decreased work ability is a wicked problem. Decreased work ability's wickedness can be elaborated through the concept of the triple burden of decreased work ability, i.e., the complex mesh of problems present in the *Stuck* and *Pension-oriented* narratives in this study. The three main burdens suppressing the partially disabled are: (1) health problems; (2) lack of job opportunities; and (3) financial distress. When these burdens are combined, they create a vicious cycle that is difficult to break (see [25]), in which the individual is not empowered to utilise the capabilities (see [44]) that he or she has left.

The theoretical contribution of this thesis is *the exit path model* based on previous literature [12] and this study's empirical results. The exit path model simplifies the alternative working-life prospects of individuals with decreased work ability into two clear exits—(1) *returning to work* or (2) *retiring with a disability pension*—and an additional unclear option of remaining in limbo between resolutions and having (3) *no exit*. Additionally, other studies [17,25,37] identified this kind of stalemate situations among the participants in their studies. The primary exit from temporary benefits is returning to work, as working supports health and well-being. The secondary exit is retiring with a disability pension, which ends uncertainty and eases the person's stress caused by feelings of enduring a temporary status and related social benefits. However, if a clear exit is not available, the individual may be locked into remaining in limbo, shifting to and from various temporary benefits [12,14,37].

This exit path model proved useful in presenting the different situations and service needs of the five groups found among this study's interviewees. Those in the *Successful* and *Persevering* groups utilised the primary exit and returned to work, but it is likely that those in the *Persevering* group, who returned to work with perpetual work ability concerns, could have benefited from rehabilitative services such as physiotherapy, assistive technologies or psychological methods of pain management. These would be important in ensuring that their work ability improves, rather than declines, in the future. Those in the *Forward-looking* group currently were on temporary benefits, but their focus was on returning to work. They expressed hopefulness and motivation, implying that for them, the preferred exit—finding suitable work—seems plausible. It may be justified to assume that for those in the *Forward-looking* group, perhaps the most essential service would be career counselling to pave their paths towards new careers.

Meanwhile, those in the *Stuck* and *Pension-oriented* groups currently seemed to be stuck "in between" without a clear exit that would have resolved their situations. Some interviewees in the *Stuck* group still could have had a chance to navigate their way back to work. However, as their situations were complex, they would have needed appropriate rehabilitation and new work opportunities in which work demands would have been adjusted to their decreased capabilities (see also [25,45]). They would have also benefited from multi-professional advice in many aspects, such as re-education, health care, pain management and applying for services and benefits.

By comparison, based on the perceptions and narratives of those in the *Pension-oriented* group, it may be justifiable to conclude that their well-being would have been served best by allowing them to utilise the secondary exit of retiring with a disability pension. They conveyed many factors that contribute to substantially decreased work ability: multimorbidity; advanced age; outdated competence; and a lack of job opportunities.

In ideal situations, health care and other services support the returning-to-work process, but some individuals instead felt that they were turned down or passed from one authority or service to another (see also [25]). Health care services in particular were experienced as a fragmented system in which the individual felt like they were being "bounced" from one service provider to another, with overly long waiting times. The TOIKE Work Ability Centre plan viewed this problem as an important issue that needs to be tackled [30].

Furthermore, Määttä's [25] qualitative data analysis of citizens' accounts of their experiences with defects in the social security system uncovered similar situations of delayed access to services or denied benefits and consequent feelings of betrayal and grief. Kris' narrative also could be categorised as an example of an "unfair and unbearable situation" that Metteri [20] uncovered in her analysis of situations in which the promise of the welfare state was not fulfilled for individuals who fell through the security net.

The hesitation and misconceptions that some interviewees had towards the multi-professional TOIKE centre imply that these potential clients had not assimilated the information on the forms of advice available. Thus, it is important that communication and promotion of advisory interventions be adjusted to clients' individual needs. Some clients could benefit from career counselling or re-education, others could benefit more from advice on ergonomics and assistive tools, and some could be better served by helping them apply for a disability pension, rehabilitation or other benefits and services. All these forms of advice would have been available at the TOIKE Work Ability Centre, but not all potential clients were aware of them. These challenges regarding information and communication also have been reported in previous studies. For example, Aalto et al. [46] have suggested that information on available services should be increased in conjunction with the development of integrated care alternatives. Additionally, the findings from a study conducted in the UK [18] stressed the importance of role clarity, particularly clients' needs for sufficient information about the services that they are offered. Therefore, in accordance with acknowledging differentiated service needs and offering individually tailored interventions [17], service providers also should invest in approaching rehabilitation prospects with tailored messages.

Additionally, employment type may play a role in the returning-to-work process. Entrepreneurs do not need to convince their employers of their work ability; thus, the decision to return to work may be mostly in their own hands. Furthermore, entrepreneurs' return to working life may be easier in "work as you wish'-like platform-mediated occupations. Optimally, the platform economy creates new part-time employment for those with partial work abilities (e.g., [47]). However, as social security in many countries largely is based on full-time salaried employment, working part-time poses a risk of falling outside social security schemes because part-time work does not always match requirements and thresholds (e.g., having paid contributions for a certain duration within a specific period) set for accessing social security benefits [48].

On the whole, decreased work ability should not be viewed solely as an individual's attribute or problem. Instead, it is societies' responsibility to build working life, which includes everyone with differing capabilities. However, employers currently are not readily offering jobs to individuals whose work ability has decreased. The interviews in this study demonstrated how age discrimination, health problems and lack of up-to-date skills are common factors hindering a return to work, which may intertwine in a way so that it is not easy to distinguish them. Inclusion of individuals with health problems or disabilities is a question of both equity and provision of preventive and curative health and rehabilitation services. Supporting sustainable careers requires that workers' skills and knowledge get updated continuously to ensure that everyone's work ability is compatible with ever-changing demands throughout their working lives. Consequently, proactive action to support sustainable careers may decrease individuals' feelings of being discriminated against and, thus, their intention to retire prematurely.

5. Conclusions

Previous research has found that individuals with decreased work ability are a heterogeneous group, but this qualitative study's main finding was that five distinctive groups could be identified among those with decreased work ability based on their orientations towards work or pension, their self-assessed health and work ability and their perceptions concerning the future: Those in the *Successful* group had managed to recover well and were motivated to return to their old jobs. Those in the *Persevering* group returned to work despite enduring pain and persistent work ability concerns. Those in the *Forward-looking* group had not recovered, nor returned to work, but were optimistically searching for new vocations in which they could flourish despite their health limitations. Those in the *Stuck* group had not recovered, nor returned to work, but unlike the previous group, they were passive and hesitant about returning to work. Those in the *Pension-oriented* group had complex problems, and they had given up hope of ever returning to work and instead clearly were inclined towards retirement.

The exit path model, constructed primarily on work ability literature, proved congruent with the different work or pension orientations found within the interviewees' narratives. Considering that one-size-fits-all types of service models are not compatible with alleviating the wicked problem of decreased work ability, it may be useful to utilise the exit path model as a guide for designing services and communicating about them to different client groups. Those in the *Future-oriented* group should be guided towards the primary exit, which is returning to working life by finding a new suitable job that matches their decreased capabilities. However, it may be appropriate to help those in the *Pension-oriented* group exit smoothly and secure a pension without unnecessary struggles and stalemate situations related to temporary benefits. A considerable challenge lies in rehabilitating those in the *Stuck* group back into working life because their prolonged and multi-faceted challenges often require long-term collaboration among different sectors, such as health care, rehabilitation, education or training and employment services. Currently, the multi-professional service models being developed still often are fragmented, recounting the difficulty of designing and promoting cross-sectoral services.

This study indicates that in the current labour market climate, in which tough competition and age discrimination exist, it can be difficult for an individual with decreased capabilities to return to work after sickness absence. Therefore, it is important for society to bear responsibility for supporting sustainable careers, and to induce employers and employees to work together towards a more sustainable working life. It appears that a need exists for a systematic societal structure that acknowledges the capabilities of the partially disabled and steers them towards work that is adjusted to their individual needs. This is important for diminishing the current polarisation of the dichotomous working life, in which people viewed as fit for work are welcomed and those who are not 100% fit for work cannot find a place for themselves in the labour market.

Author Contributions: Conceptualisation, E.N. and M.P.; methodology, E.N.; formal analysis, E.N.; investigation, E.N.; data curation, E.N.; writing—original draft preparation, E.N.; writing—review and editing, E.N., M.P. and L.K.; visualisation, E.N.; supervision, M.P. and L.K.; project administration, E.N. All authors have read and agreed to the published version of the manuscript.

Funding: This research received no external funding.

Institutional Review Board Statement: The study was conducted according to the guidelines of the Finnish National Board on Research Integrity TENK, and approved by the Ethics Committee of the Social Insurance Institution of Finland (29 June 2018).

Informed Consent Statement: Informed consent was obtained from all subjects involved in the study.

Data Availability Statement: The data used in this study are managed by the authors. The data are not publicly available due to privacy.

Acknowledgments: We thank Karoliina Koskenvuo and Riitta Luoto (The Social Insurance Institution of Finland) and Tuula Haukka-Wacklin and Miisa Visakorpi (Pirkanmaa Hospital District) for advice and support in designing and conducting this study.

Conflicts of Interest: The authors declare no conflict of interest.

Appendix A

Table A1. Interviewees' profiles.

Pseudonym [1]	Age [2]	Worker/Entrep. [3]	Sector [4]	Health concern [5]	RTW [6]	Situation [7]	Plan [8]	SAH [9] (1–5)	WA [10] (0–10)	Readiness [11] (0–10)	TOIKE [12]	Summary [13]
Jamie	≥51	Entrep.	Agric.	Shoulder injury	Yes	Recovered, returned-to-work	Continues in old job	4	8	10	No.	Work-oriented, well recovered, motivated
River	40–50	Worker	Health	Back pain	Yes	Recovered, returned-to-work	Continues in old job	4	9	10	No.	Work-oriented, well recovered, motivated
Sam	40–50	Worker	Constr.	Back pain and burnout	Yes	Has pain, but returned-to-work	Continues in old job	3	5.5	?	Yes. No visit was booked.	Somewhat work-oriented, not fully recovered, work ability concerns
Pat	≤39	Entrep.	Constr.	Back and leg pain	Yes	Has pain, but returned-to-work	Continues in old job	2	4	?	No.	Somewhat work-oriented, not fully recovered, work ability concerns
Glen	≤39	Worker	Logistics	Shoulder injury	No	Unemployed after sick-leave	Needs a new direction	3	5.5	7.5	No, but considers.	Work-oriented, not fully recovered, hopeful
Jordan	≤39	Worker	Hosp.	Back and leg pain	No	Sick-leave	Going to re-education	4	4.5	2.5	No.	Work-oriented, not fully recovered, hopeful
Rowan	≤39	Worker	Transp.	Back pain + other	No	Sick-leave	Needs a new direction. Going to a work tryout	3	3	3.5	No, but considers.	Work-oriented, not fully recovered, hopeful
Taylor	≥51	Worker	Manuf.	Shoulder injury, dyslexia, memory disorders	No	Prolonged absence: sick-leave/unemployed	Cannot find work	2	5	?	No.	Somewhat pension-oriented, not recovered, hesitant, passive
Blake	≥51	Worker	Manuf.	Arm injury (+ mental health)	No	Unstable work history	Temporary disability pension	3	5.5	6.5	Yes. No visit was booked.	Somewhat pension-oriented, not recovered, hesitant, passive
Frankie	40–50	Worker	Agric.	Arm & knee pain, arthritis, dyslexia	No	Prolonged absence: sick-leave/unemployed	Cannot find work. Applying for partial disability pension	2	4	5	Yes. Has visited.	Somewhat pension-oriented, not recovered, hesitant, passive
Peyton	40–50	Entrep.	Maint.	Arm pain	No	Rehabilitee/partial disability pension	May return to work	1	2.5	3.5	No.	Somewhat pension-oriented, not recovered, hesitant, passive
Kris	≥51	Entrep.	Constr.	Back/leg pain + other	No	Business ceased. Receives sickness allowance	Applying for disability pension	1	0	0	No.	Pension-oriented, disabled, reluctant
Mel	≥51	Worker	Manuf.	Back pain	No	Cannot return to old job due to sickness	Applying for partial disability pension	2.5	0.5	?	Yes. Has visited.	Pension-oriented, disabled, reluctant

Table A1. Cont.

Pseudo-nym [1]	Age [2]	Worker/Entrep. [3]	Sector [4]	Health concern [5]	RTW [6]	Situation [7]	Plan [8]	SAH [9] (1–5)	WA [10] (0–10)	Readiness [11] (0–10)	TOIKE [12]	Summary [13]
Jo	≥51	Worker	Constr.	Knee pain	No	Attended rehabilitation. Receives sickness allowance	Applying for disability pension	2	2	0	Yes. Has a visit booked.	Pension-oriented, disabled, reluctant
Riley	≥51	Entrep.	Maint.	Back/wrist pain + other	No	Business ceased. Receives sickness allowance	Going to rehabilitation. Applying for disability pension	1	2	0	No.	Pension-oriented, disabled, reluctant
Casey	≥51	Worker	Office	Unclear, reports to be healthy	No	Attended rehabilitation and activation measures	Cannot find work	4	9	10	No.	Pension-oriented, health status unclear, reluctant

[1] Interviewee's pseudonym. [2] Interviewee's age group. The interviewees were categorised into three major age groups based on a categorization by Määttä [25]: early career ≤39, active career 40–50, later career ≥51. [3] Interviewee's employment type, i.e., whether he/she was a worker (i.e., employee) or an entrepreneur (i.e., self-employed). [4] The sector in which the interviewee worked: agric. = agriculture, constr. = construction, health = health care, hosp. = hospitality, logistics = logistics, maint. = maintenance, manuf. = manufacturing, office = office work, transp. = transportation. [5] The disease, disorder, injury or other health concern causing decreased capacity (self-reported). [6] Has the interviewee returned to work (RTW)? [7] Current situation (recovered, has pain, returned-to-work, on a sick-leave, unemployed, prolonged absence, unstable work history, business ceased, in rehabilitation, partial disability pension, etc.). [8] Future labour market plan or prospects. [9] Self-assessed health (SAH) on a scale 1–5 (1 = very poor, 5 = very good). [10] Self-assessed work ability (WA) on a scale 0–10 (0 = work ability at its lifetime worst, 10 = work ability at its lifetime best). [11] Concerning returning to work, how ready does the interviewee feel? (0 = not at all ready, 10 = perfectly ready). [12] Has the interviewee been in contact with the TOIKE centre? [13] Summary of the interviewee's profile, based on categorised data in this table and other answers to open-ended interview questions.

References

1. Barnett, K.; Mercer, S.W.; Norbury, M.; Watt, G.; Wyke, S.; Guthrie, B. Epidemiology of multimorbidity and implications for health care, research, and medical education: A cross-sectional study. *Lancet* **2012**, *380*, 37–43. [CrossRef]
2. Riekhoff, A.-J. Retirement Trajectories in the Netherlands and Finland Institutional Change, Inequalities, de-Standardisation and Destabilisation. Doctoral Thesis, Tampere University, Tampere, Finland, 2018.
3. Vornholt, K.; Villotti, P.; Muschalla, B.; Bauer, J.; Colella, A.; Zijlstra, F.; Van Ruitenbeek, G.; Uitdewilligen, S.; Corbière, M. Disability and employment—Overview and highlights. *Eur. J. Work Organ. Psychol.* **2018**, *27*, 40–55. [CrossRef]
4. Adams, G.A.; Beehr, T.A. *Retirement: Reasons, Processes, and Results*; Springer Pub: New York, NY, USA, 2003.
5. Vuori, J.; Blonk, R.; Price, R.H. *Sustainable Working Lives: Managing Work Transitions and Health throughout the Life Course*; Springer: Dordrecht, The Netherlands, 2015.
6. Pekkala, J. Occupational Class Differences in Sickness Absence: Changes over Time and Diagnostic Causes. Doctoral Thesis, University of Helsinki, Helsinki, Finland, 2018.
7. Lmarinen, J.; Gould, R.; Järvikoski, A.; Järvisalo, J. Diversity of work ability. In *Dimensions of Work Ability. Results of the Health 2000 Survey*; Gould, R., Ilmarinen, J., Järvisalo, J., Koskinen, S., Eds.; Finnish Centre for Pensions: Helsinki, Finland, 2008; pp. 13–24.
8. United Nations. Transforming Our World: The 2030 Agenda for Sustainable Development. Available online: https://sustainabledevelopment.un.org/post2015/transformingourworld/publication (accessed on 2 November 2021).
9. Loisel, P.; Durand, M.-J.; Berthelette, D.; Vézina, N.; Baril, R.; Gagnon, D.; Larivière, C.; Tremblay, C. Disability prevention: New paradigm for the management of occupational back pain. *Dis. Manag. Health Outcomes* **2001**, *9*, 351–360. [CrossRef]
10. Pransky, G.S.; Loisel, P.; Anema, J.R. Work disability prevention research: Current and future prospects. *J. Occup. Rehabil.* **2011**, *21*, 287–292. [CrossRef]
11. Ekberg, K.; Wåhlin, C.; Persson, J.; Bernfort, L.; Öberg, B. Is mobility in the labor market a solution to sustainable return to work for some sick listed persons? *J. Occup. Rehabil.* **2011**, *21*, 355–365. [CrossRef] [PubMed]
12. Gjersøe, H.M. Getting sick and disabled people off temporary benefit receipt: Strategies and dilemmas in the welfare state's frontline. *Nord. J. Work. Life Stud.* **2016**, *6*, 129–145. [CrossRef]
13. Kerätär, R.; Taanila, A.; Jokelainen, J.; Soukainen, J.; Ala-Mursula, L. Work disabilities and unmet needs for health care and rehabilitation among jobseekers: A community-level investigation using multidimensional work ability assessments. *Scand. J. Prim. Health Care* **2016**, *34*, 343–351. [CrossRef]
14. MacEachen, E.; Kosny, A.; Ferrier, S.; Chambers, L. The "toxic dose" of system problems: Why some injured workers don't return to work as expected. *J. Occup. Rehabil.* **2010**, *20*, 349–366. [CrossRef] [PubMed]
15. Salonen, L.; Blomgren, J.; Laaksonen, M.; Niemelä, M. Sickness absence as a predictor of disability retirement in different occupational classes: A register-based study of a working-age cohort in Finland in 2007–2014. *BMJ Open* **2018**, *8*, e020491. [CrossRef]

16. Haugli, L.; Maeland, S.; Magnussen, L.H. What facilitates return to work? Patients experiences 3 years after occupational rehabilitation. *J. Occup. Rehabil.* **2011**, *21*, 573–581. [CrossRef] [PubMed]
17. Lydell, M.; Hildingh, C.; Månsson, J.; Marklund, B.; Grahn, B. Thoughts and feelings of future working life as a predictor of return to work: A combined qualitative and quantitative study of sick-listed persons with musculoskeletal disorders. *Disabil. Rehabil.* **2011**, *33*, 1262–1271. [CrossRef]
18. Sanders, T.; Wynne-Jones, G.; Nio Ong, B.; Artus, M.; Foster, N. Acceptability of a vocational advice service for patients consulting in primary care with musculoskeletal pain: A qualitative exploration of the experiences of general practitioners, vocational advisers and patients. *Scand. J. Public Health* **2019**, *47*, 78–85. [CrossRef] [PubMed]
19. World Health Organization. *International Classification of Functioning, Disability and Health: ICF*; World Health Organization: Geneva, Switzerland, 2001; ISBN 978-92-4-154542-6.
20. Metteri, A. Hyvinvointivaltion Lupaukset, Kohtuuttomat Tapaukset ja Sosiaalityö (Promises of a Welfare state, Non-Fulfilment of These Promises and Social Work). Doctoral Thesis, Tampere University, Tampere, Finland, 2012.
21. Lahey, P. From Welfare to Work for People with Disabilities in Receipt of Public Income Benefits: A Wicked Problem for Policy Makers. Doctoral Thesis, McMaster University, Hamilton, ON, Canada, 2019. Available online: http://hdl.handle.net/11375/23823 (accessed on 22 December 2021).
22. Blackman, T.; Greene, A.; Hunter, D.J.; McKee, L.; Elliott, E.; Harrington, B.; Marks, L.; Williams, G. Performance assessment and wicked problems: The case of health inequalities. *Public Policy Adm.* **2006**, *21*, 66–80. [CrossRef]
23. Saikku, P.; Karjalainen, V. Network governance in activation policy—Health care as an emergent partner. *Int. J. Sociol. Soc. Policy* **2012**, *32*, 299–311. [CrossRef]
24. Mattila-Wiro, P.; Tiainen, R. *Involving All in Working Life—Results and Recommendations from OTE Key Project 'Career Opportunities for People with Partial Work Ability'*; Reports and Memorandums of the Ministry of Social Affairs and Health: Helsinki, Finland, 2019; p. 36.
25. Määttä, A. Työkyvytön vai työtön? Työkyvyttömyydestä aiheutuva sosiaaliturvan väliinputoaminen elämänkaaren eri vaiheissa (Unfit for work or unemployed? Falling outside social security schemes due to work disability during different stages of the lifespan). *Kuntoutus* **2011**, *34*, 18–28.
26. Elliott, J. *Using Narrative in Social Research: Qualitative and Quantitative Approaches*; SAGE: London, UK, 2005.
27. Silverman, D. *Doing Qualitative Research: A Practical Handbook*, 3rd ed.; SAGE: London, UK, 2010.
28. Grant, C.; Osanloo, A. Understanding, selecting, and integrating a theoretical framework in dissertation research: Creating the blueprint for your "house". *Adm. Issues J. Educ. Pract. Res.* **2016**, *4*, 12–16. [CrossRef]
29. Elo, S.; Kyngäs, H. The qualitative content analysis process. *J. Adv. Nurs.* **2008**, *62*, 107–115. [CrossRef]
30. Heikkinen, V.; Uitti, J. Osatyökykyisille tie työelämään (OTE), Polut hoitoon ja kuntoutukseen, Projekti 7 (Road to Work for Individuals with Decreased Work Ability, Pathways to Healthcare and Rehabilitation, Project 7). Available online: https://docplayer.fi/48361905-Hallituksen-karkihanke-osatyokykyisille-tie-tyoelamaan-ote-polut-hoitoon-ja-kuntoutukseen-projekti-7.html (accessed on 2 November 2021).
31. Vuokila-Oikkonen, P.; Janhonen, S.; Nikkonen, M. Kertomukset hoitotieteellisen tiedon tuottamisessa: Narratiivinen lähestymistapa (Stories in producing knowledge for nursing science: A narrative approach). In *Laadulliset tutkimusmenetelmät hoitotieteessä (Qualitative Methods in Nursing Science)*; Janhonen, S., Nikkonen, M., Eds.; WSOY: Juva, Finland, 2001; pp. 81–115.
32. Green, J.; Thorogood, N. *Qualitative Methods for Health Research*, 4th ed.; SAGE: Los Angeles, CA, USA, 2018.
33. Tuomi, K.; Ilmarinen, J.; Jahkola, A.; Katajarinne, L.; Tulkki, A. *Work Ability Index*, 2nd ed.; Finnish Institute of Occupational Health: Helsinki, Finland, 1998.
34. Gould, R.; Koskinen, S.; Seitsamo, J.; Tuomi, K.; Polvinen, A.; Sainio, P. Data and Methods. In *Dimensions of Work Ability. Results of the Health 2000 Survey*; Gould, R., Ilmarinen, J., Järvisalo, J., Koskinen, S., Eds.; Finnish Centre for Pensions: Helsinki, Finland, 2008; pp. 25–32.
35. Graneheim, U.H.; Lundman, B. Qualitative content analysis in nursing research: Concepts, procedures and measures to achieve trustworthiness. *Nurse Educ. Today* **2004**, *24*, 105–112. [CrossRef]
36. Dwyer, D.S.; Mitchell, O.S. Health problems as determinants of retirement: Are self-rated measures endogenous? *J. Health Econ.* **1999**, *18*, 173–193. [CrossRef]
37. Heikkinen, V. Pitkäaikaistyötön vai pysyvästi työkyvytön: Tyyppitarinoita 2000-luvun teollisuuskaupungista (Long-Term Unemployed or Permanently Disabled—Types and Narratives from an Industrial Town of the 2000s). Doctoral Thesis, Tampere University, Tampere, Finland, 2016.
38. Harkonmäki, K. Predictors of Disability Retirement from Early Intentions to Retirement. Ph.D. Thesis, University of Helsinki, Helsinki, Finland, 2007.
39. Jahoda, M. *Employment and Unemployment*; Cambridge University Press: Cambridge, UK, 1982.
40. Ministry of Social Affairs and Health. *Kuntoutuksen Uudistamiskomitean Ehdotukset Kuntoutusjärjestelmän Uudistamiseksi (Recommendations of the Rehabilitation Reform Committee for Reforming Rehabilitation)*; Reports and Memorandums of the Ministry of Social Affairs and Health: Helsinki, Finland, 2017; p. 89.
41. Beehr, T.A. The process of retirement: A review and recommendations for future investigation. *Pers. Psychol.* **1986**, *39*, 31–55. [CrossRef]

42. Kohli, M.; Rein, M.; Guillemard, A.-M.; van Gunsteren, H. (Eds.) *Time for Retirement: Comparative Studies of Early Exit from the Labor Force*; Cambridge University Press: Cambridge, UK, 1991.
43. Heslin, P.A.; Keating, L.A.; Ashford, S.J. How being in learning mode may enable a sustainable career across the lifespan. *J. Vocat. Behav.* **2020**, *117*, 103324. [CrossRef]
44. Sen, A. *Development as Freedom*, 1st ed.; Oxford University Press: Oxford, UK, 1999.
45. Tamin, J. *Occupational Health Ethics: From Theory to Practice*; Springer Nature: Cham, Switzerland, 2020; Chapter 5; ISBN 978-3-030-47282-5.
46. Aalto, A.-M.; Elovainio, M.; Tynkkynen, L.-K.; Reissell, E.; Vehko, T.; Chydenius, M.; Sinervo, T. What patients think about choice in healthcare? A study on primary care services in Finland. *Scand. J. Public Health* **2018**, *46*, 463–470. [CrossRef] [PubMed]
47. Poutanen, S.; Kovalainen, A.; Rouvinen, P. (Eds.) *Digital Work and the Platform Economy: Understanding Tasks, Skills and Capabilities in the New Era*, 1st ed.; Routledge: New York, NY, USA, 2019; ISBN 978-0-429-46792-9.
48. Schoukens, P. Digitalisation and social security in the EU. The case of platform work: From work protection to income protection? *Eur. J. Soc. Secur.* **2020**, *22*, 434–451. [CrossRef]

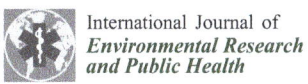

Article

Redefinition and Measurement Dimensions of Sustainable Employability Based on the swAge-Model

Jianwei Deng [1,2], Jiahao Liu [1], Wenhao Deng [1], Tianan Yang [1,2,*] and Zhezhe Duan [3,*]

1. Beijing Institute of Technology, School of Management and Economics, Haidian District, Beijing 100081, China; Dengjianwei2006@163.com (J.D.); bitliujiahao@163.com (J.L.); dwenhao215@163.com (W.D.)
2. Sustainable Development Research Institute for Economy and Society of Beijing, Beijing 100081, China
3. Institute of Urban Governance, School of Government, Shenzhen University, Shenzhen 215123, China
* Correspondence: tianan.yang@bit.edu.cn (T.Y.); duanzz@szu.edu.cn (Z.D.)

Abstract: Objectives: To solve the labour shortage, we clarify the definition and dimensions of sustainable employability, and make it possible to develop sustainable employability scales in the future and lay the foundation for subsequent quantitative research. Finally, people's sustainable employability can be improved. Highly sustainable employability employees can continue to work in the labour market and their working lives can be prolonged. Labour market supply will increase and labour shortage will be partly solved. Methods: We discuss the concept of sustainable employability based on some previous studies. Our conclusion is that the existing definitions and measurement dimensions are problematic. The swAge-model, a tool that helps us understand how to make working life more sustainable and healthier for all ages, can be the basis of sustainable employability. Results: We develop a discussion paper concerning the definition and measurement dimensions of sustainable employability using the swAge-model with an added factor of intrinsic work value and the dynamic chain. Conclusions: Our definition of sustainable employability takes environmental factors into consideration and makes it clear that it is not a solely personal characteristic, but the result of an interaction between individuals and the environment, thus distinguishing employability from work ability. We use the swAge-model as a basis to make the composition of our definition more logical and informed. Our measurement dimensions are clearly described to facilitate the future development of a scale, and our concept may ultimately help to extend the working lives of older and retired workers and thus solve the future labour shortage problem.

Keywords: sustainable employability; definition; measurement dimensions; the swAge-model

1. Introduction

Sustainable employability commonly refers to the ability of employees to participate in work and the labour market during their lifetimes [1]. Because this ability is very important for individuals, organisations, and society, it deserves our attention. For individuals, work provides economic security and social ties, as well as forming an important part of and giving meaning to their daily lives. Organisations need productive employees to improve organisational performance and survive market competition. Society needs as many people as possible to participate in the labour market to maintain economic welfare and social stability [2]. In view of the aging of the global population, there may be a labour shortage in the future [3] and research on sustainable employability is necessary. However, the current definition and framework of sustainable employability are still very confusing, which hinders subsequent research [4]. This article aims to solve this possible labour market crisis through clarifying definition and dimensions of employees' sustainable employability and laying foundation for scales development and quantitative research that can affect this ability. Finally, sustainable employability can be achieved and prolong employees' working lives, and even extend them past the official retirement age.

In the medical sector, for example, the aging of the labour force has led to a continuous decrease in the overall number of medical workers. At the same time, the number of patients has been increasing. This imposes a heavy workload on the medical staff, causing physical, mental, and emotional pressures [5]. More and more healthcare workers encounter mental health problems due to job difficulties, and many choose to change departments or leave their jobs before the official retirement age, thus causing a further reduction in medical staff [6]. Meanwhile, the productivity of medical workers may decline due to their poor physical condition and the instability of the staff caused by resignations and changes. The quality of medical services may decline accordingly [7]. The reduction of medical resources and the increase in demand are very urgent problems for the organisation of medicine as a whole and society. Sustainable employability can prolong the careers of employees in the medical industry, guarantee the working ability of the medical staff, retain trained experts, and maintain their irreplaceable skills and professional knowledge. Helping medical organisations build a stable and healthy workforce will benefit individuals, organisations, and society [8,9].

2. The Development and Deficiencies of the Sustainable Employability Concept

Although sustainable employability is of great significance to individuals, organisations, and society, there are still many gaps and deficiencies in the definition and dimensions used to measure this capacity. It was first defined by van der Klink et al. as follows: 'sustainable employability means that, throughout their working lives, workers can achieve tangible opportunities in the form of a set of capabilities. They also enjoy the necessary conditions that allow them to make a valuable contribution through their work, now and in the future, while safeguarding their health and welfare. This requires, on the one hand, a work context that facilitates this for them and on the other, the attitude and motivation to exploit these opportunities [1]. This definition has been widely used in subsequent studies [9–11]. It describes sustainable employability as a multidimensional concept, acknowledges the importance of employees and job characteristics, and, to a certain extent, acknowledges the longitudinal characteristic, an individual's employability over time, of this concept. However, Fleuren et al. noted that there are omissions in this definition. They argued that: 1. this definition does not specify which dimensions constitute an individual's sustainable employability; 2. sustainable employability cannot be regarded as a characteristic of both the job and the employee simultaneously; 3. based on assumptions that have not been fully verified, we cannot assert that achieving value in work will lead to sustainable employability; 4. the definition of sustainable employability should include unemployed people to make the concept applicable to a larger group; and 5. the definition of sustainable employability should address the inherently longitudinal characteristic, that is, an individual's employability over time [2]. Among the shortcomings proposed, the first is particularly obvious in later studies. For example, Roczniewska et al. and Hazelzet et al. both acknowledged the definition put forward by van der Klink when studying the theoretical background of sustainable employability, but in the quantitative analysis stage their measurement dimensions varied. The former mainly used three dimensions: productivity, physical and mental health, and happiness, while the latter replaced happiness with valuable work and long-term perspective [9,11]. In other words, because there are no clear measurement dimensions in the definition, different studies have different understandings of the same definition. Their measurement methods are biased and cannot be standardised, which makes it impossible to directly compare different research results and form a comprehensive understanding of the concept.

In their later research, Fleuren et al. formulated their own definition according to the points they raised, after integrating and reviewing existing sustainable employability definitions. They argued that sustainable employability refers to the ability of an individual to function in work and the labour market, or that employability is not negatively (and preferably positively) affected by personal employment status. This ability can be captured by combining nine indicators (perceived health status, work ability, recovery needs, fatigue, job satisfaction, job motivation, perceived employability, skill gap, and job performance) to describe the extent to which a person can be employed at different stages of his or her work life [4]. Compared with the deficiencies in the definition proposed by van der Klink et al., this definition clearly sets out nine dimensions of sustainable employability, which facilitates its measurement. The definition also emphasises that sustainable employability is a longitudinal concept with a time dimension. However, it remains unclear whether employability is a personal characteristic or the result of an interaction between the environment and the individual, and whether its definition covers reasonable groups.

Some studies argue that sustainable employability is not a personal concept, but the result of an interaction between the employee and the environment [12,13], while Fleuren et al. consider it a personal characteristic. We are more inclined towards the interactionist point of view, because sustainable employability should take into account labour market characteristics [14]. The concept of employment itself also includes personal and organisational characteristics as input variables, which is the important difference between work and employment [4]. If we simply regard sustainable employability as a personal characteristic rather than resulting from the interaction between the working environment, the labour market, and individuals, we ignore important differences between the similar concepts of sustainable employability and sustainable workability. Furthermore, although the definition of Fleuren et al. applies to some unemployed individuals, it ignores older or retired individuals. Because the authors measure sustainable employability according to the nine aspects listed above, they ignore the role of the individual's opportunity to enter the labour market (an environmental characteristic). The employability of an older or retired individual may be overestimated. Although these groups (for example, medical staff and teachers) may maintain a high working ability due to the accumulation of knowledge and experience [15], organisations might discriminate against older workers by showing them less appreciation and investing fewer resources in them. This would significantly reduce their chances of entering the labour market [16,17]. Therefore, even if older or retired individuals have the ability to work but cannot find employment, their actual employability is relatively low. However, as this variable is not considered in the definition of Fleuren et al., the sustainable employability of these groups according to this definition may be overestimated, suggesting that the definition cannot be widely applied to all groups. As the starting point of the original definition of van der Klink et al., work value has been mentioned many times in subsequent papers as a conceptual dimension of sustainable employability [18]. However, Fleuren et al. did not discuss or mention it in the process of establishing their definition. This has led to doubts about its accuracy. Therefore, there are some indicators missing in the mode of measurement proposed by Fleuren et al. Lastly, although there is a basis for the selection of each of the nine measurement indices proposed by Fleuren et al., the logical connection between the indices is not strong, and it is hard to classify them.

A key feature of recent changes in the labour market is that information and communication technologies (ICT) play an increasingly important role in several aspects of employment [19]. These technologies have affected the nature and employment situation of many industries and occupations, and their use will affect the location and time of work [20]. They underpinned the development in job search, recruitment, and selection practices [21]. Therefore, if employees want to make employability sustainable, they have to consider the impact of the digital age. Whether employees have digital exclusion determines whether they can adapt to this digital age and continue to work. However, the previous definitions of sustainable employability rarely emphasized the background of the times, indicating the importance of ICT.

Therefore, to solve the aforementioned problems, this paper redefines sustainable employability and its measurement dimensions by taking into account environmental factors, broadening its application to retired and elderly employees, incorporating work value, and simplifying the measurement method of Fleuren et al. for greater ease in future research.

This will facilitate the study of intervention measures for sustainable employability and ultimately help resolve the future labour shortage caused by population aging.

3. Establishing a New Sustainable Employability Concept

3.1. Sustainable and Intrinsic Work Value

The adjective sustainable is used to describe something that is 'able to continue at the same level for a period of time' [22]. Finkbeiner et al. also point out that sustainability is at the original level. Specifically, it means that the resources are maintained after use, and the total amount has not decreased or even increased, which implies positive development and added value for the environment and stakeholders [23]. Similarly, PubMed defines sustainable development as 'a process of change in which the exploitation of resources, the direction of investments, the orientation of technological development, and institutional change are all in harmony and enhance both current and future potential to meet human needs and aspirations' [24].

As far as the sustainability of employability is concerned, we define employability to be sustainable if workers perceive that their work or work environment is valuable [1]. Jonathan Holslag's The Strength of Paradise showed that work has become trivial and unattractive to many people in modern society. He advocated paying more attention to the values that are vital to human survival, arguing that values such as meaning and recognition can be satisfied in the workplace and can thus motivate people to continue working [25]. According to the theory of self-depletion, a person must consume resources when performing volitional activities (e.g., process control, active choice, initiation behaviour, and overcoming reactions), but such resources are often limited. The more abundant the resources available to perform volitional activities, the easier it is to succeed. For employees to successfully achieve sustainable employment and maintain a high level of sustainable employability, employees' intrinsic motivation is needed as a resource for consumption [26]. According to self-determination theory, the satisfaction of basic psychological needs is very important for individual intrinsic motivation [27]. A valuable job can satisfy employees' psychological needs of autonomy, competence, and psychological relatedness, thus promoting their intrinsic motivation [28]. In other words, according to the self-determination theory, the intrinsic work value that employees think can bring them intrinsic motivation. Combined with the theory of self-depletion, intrinsic work value, as a motivating factor, can be used as a resource to help employees maintain and even increase the original employability. Intrinsic work value connects self-depletion theory and the self-determination theory and injects 'sustainable' into employability. Studies have shown that when employees consider work as meaningful and can provide them with recognition, they are more likely to maintain their employability to increase their job security [29]. At the same time, empirical research has shown that intrinsic work value has a strong positive correlation with the three indicators of sustainable employment for employees of all ages (i.e., workers' employability, work engagement, and affective commitment) [28].

In summary, by combining self-depletion theory with self-determination theory, we explain the impact of work value on employment sustainability as proposed by Jonathan Holslag and add intrinsic work value into the definition of sustainable employability as the dimension that makes employability sustainable.

3.2. Employability and Dynamic Chain

Employability was originally defined by Hillage and Pollard as a person's ability to obtain and maintain employment and productivity [30]. In fact, from 'maintaining and obtaining', we can infer the concept of sustainability. In subsequent development studies, employability has been defined as individuals' job opportunities in the internal or external labour market [31]. Based on this definition, scholars have examined what constitutes this kind of 'opportunity'. Some have evaluated the realisation of job opportunities from the perspective of mobility (job transitions), others have focused on how personal advantages such as knowledge, skills, and attitudes influence job opportunities (movement capital), while others have explored the personal evaluation of job opportunities (perceived employability). Due to these different approaches, employability has become a vague and catch-all concept. To resolve this confusing situation, Forrier connected different concepts of employability into a 'dynamic chain' of three dimensions, namely job transitions, movement capital, and perceived employability [32]. Job transitions expand a person's movement capital [33], movement capital improves a person's perceived employability [34], while perceived employability encourages employees to achieve further job transitions [35].

3.3. Sustainable Employability and the swAge-Model

The swAge-model is considered to be a tool in the task of understanding how to make working life more sustainable and healthier for all ages, which can be the basis of sustainable employability [36,37]. The swAge-model describe three influence levels of importance for work life participation and to a sustainable extended working life: the individual level, micro level; the organizational and enterprise level, meso level; and the society level, macro level. Based on swAge-model, we have formed a more logical and informed definition of sustainable employability.

At the macro level, as mentioned earlier, the digital age has a huge impact on the labour market. ICT has a profound impact on the sustainability of employability, so digital exclusion should be used as one of the dimensions of sustainable employability. At the meso level, based on the original framework of van der Klink et al., we have selected intrinsic work value' as one of the dimensions of sustainable employability, which makes employees more willing and able to continue employment and achieve sustainability in employability as well. At the micro level, combined with the dynamic chain, the three dimensions are included in the definition of sustainable employability, since they are related by mutual influence and promotion in a way that allows sustainability: through the interactions among the three dimensions, employability can remain unchanged or even increase over a period of time. The dimensions of this definition can be seen in Figure 1. Therefore, we define sustainable employability as follows:

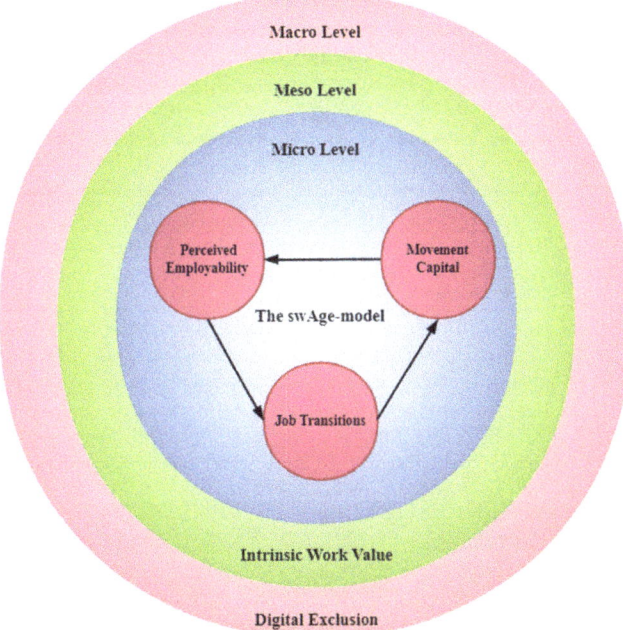

Figure 1. The dimensions of sustainable employability.

'In the digital age, sustainable employability refers to the ability of individuals who pursue work with high intrinsic value and avoid digital exclusion, remain in employment during their lifetimes. They expand personal movement capital through job transitions to improve their perception of employability, which encourages them to further achieve job transitions. The three components of job transitions, movement capital, and perceived employability are constantly promoted in a circular way, such that individuals can maintain or improve their original job opportunities in the labour market'.

First, this definition shows clear measurement dimensions including digital exclusion, intrinsic work value, job transitions, movement capital, and perceived employability, which facilitates the unification of subsequent measurement methods and the horizontal comparison of different studies later. Second, this definition considers that sustainable employability is a characteristic of the interaction between environment and individual, taking into account a person's opportunities in the labour market, and meaning that this definition is better adapted to older or retired employees and prevents overestimation of their employability. Finally, this definition is based on the swAge-model, which takes into account the characteristics of the digital age, and combines the framework of van der Klink et al. and dynamic chain, which is simpler, more logical and more reliable than previous dimensions.

4. Components of Sustainable Employability

4.1. Digital Exclusion

Digital exclusion is broadly defined as being unable to access or use internet-enabled technology and Web-based services [38]. It can be divided into three aspects including access, motivation, and low confidence [19]. Access includes issues of physical access to hardware and software and affordability thereof. Motivation refers to encompassing lack of interest in or lack of perceived need to use ICT. Low confidence mainly means that employees lack confidence to adapt to the digital age and ICT [38].

4.2. Intrinsic Work Value

When the task is regarded as meaningful, challenging, and conducive to personal development, and when employees are recognised for their contributions, the work is regarded as having intrinsic value [28]. Recent research has focused on employees' views on four aspects of work: meaning, recognition, challenge, and learning value. Work is considered meaningful when it provides a sense of accomplishment, purpose, and contribution [39]. Recognition means that a person's contribution to their organisation is acknowledged and is usually regarded as one of the intangible rewards that motivate employees [40]. Challenge refers to when difficult task elements require employees to exert their potential by stimulating their curiosity, creativity, and enjoyment [41]. Learning value refers to the learning experience present in the working environment [42], which leads to the development of employees' abilities [43].

4.3. Job Transitions

Job transitions represent an individual's opportunities in the labour market and include any change in employment situation or substantial changes in job content [44]. These changes can be within the same organisation (internal work transfer), or across different organisations (external work transfer). Specific measurement indices can be divided according to whether internal work transfer or external work transfer is involved [32]. They can also be divided along the line of horizontal work transfer and vertical work transfer [45].

4.4. Movement Capital

Personal advantages increase employees' opportunities in the labour market because they can help individuals effectively cope with labour market changes [46]. Movement capital accounts for these different personal advantages; that is, 'personal skills, knowledge, abilities, and attitudes that affect career mobility' [47]. It is usually divided into four dimensions: human capital, social capital, self-awareness, and adaptability. Human capital refers to an individual's ability to meet specific professional performance expectations [48]. Social capital reflects the value of social networks in one's career [49]. Self-awareness refers to the reflection on one's past and present career and provides direction for future career opportunities [48]. Finally, adaptability refers to the necessary changes in behaviour, emotion, and thought to meet the requirements of the environment [50]. These four dimensions explain employability from the perspective of a person, which has received great attention in previous research [51].

4.5. Perceived Employability

Perceived employability explores employability from the perspective of personal views on existing employment opportunities. Advocates believe that it captures the interaction between personal and environmental factors, because people consider environmental factors such as labour market conditions in addition to personal factors when evaluating their employability [52]. The perception of employability can be determined in relation to current employers (perceived internal employability) or other employers (perceived external employability). These two dimensions are often put forward by other studies and used in empirical studies [53].

5. Discussion

This definition of sustainable employability solves leftover problems from the past. It confirms that sustainable employability is not a personal characteristic, but results from the interaction between individuals and the environment. In recent decades, access to Internet technologies and Web-based services has grown exponentially [19]. Whether employees can adapt to this digital age and avoid digital exclusion determines whether their future employability is sustainable [54]. Therefore, it is very important to emphasize the background of the times in the definition and add relevant dimensions. This further shows that governments can intervene in individuals' sustainable employability through relevant policies, and that organisations should pay attention to the value of employees at work. An individual's sustainable employability may be improved by increasing individual employment opportunities at an environmental level, rather than simply through individual efforts. This broadens the research scope of sustainable employability, develops more ways to increase employees' working years, and solves the problem of future labour market shortages.

In addition, this concept of sustainable employability can apply to retired and older people. These groups are very important part of the medical staff. Some medical staff are relatively old, and their physical functions may have declined, but they are experienced and skilled, and they can still continue to engage in medical-related work [15]. It is important to reactivate the labour force comprising these groups so that we can solve the problem of labour shortages caused by the aging of the current population, especially in the medical sector [8]. To be more precise, our definition and measurement dimensions can evaluate the sustainable employability of these groups to help select relatively high-ability individuals for re-employment, increase their resources for entering the labour market, and ultimately solve the problem of talent shortage.

Furthermore, the new definition provides clear measurement dimensions, thus preventing confusion and incomparability between different studies. Moreover, the establishment of measurement dimensions is conducive to the development of quantitative research, which was called for in a recent qualitative study [55]. Subsequent intervention research on sustainable employability can provide a theoretical reference for enterprises on how to improve employees' sustainable employability and increase their employment years. At the same time, our delineation of measurement dimensions is beneficial to research on sustainable employability in itself, and gives more practical significance to research in this field.

The sWage-model provides three dimensions: the individual level, micro level; the organizational and enterprise level, meso level; and the society level, macro level. We take this model as the basis for the definition and measurement dimensions of sustainable employability. Digital exclusion provides the background for definition at the macro level. Combining with the dynamic chain, we provide employability from the micro level to the definition. Combining self-determination theory and self-depletion theory, we explain the important role of intrinsic work value in the sustainability of employability from the meso level. This not only expands the content of the original theoretical framework, but also broadens their application scope. In other words, we combine different theories and models in our concept of sustainable employability and apply them in the field of management.

6. Limitations and Future Directions

Like all studies, this study has limitations. This article is preliminary work aiming to put forward the definition of sustainable employability and a few measurement dimensions, but cannot determine the specific measurement method. We suggest that descriptive, exploratory, structural, and other research methods can be used for further exploration. To be more precise, first, develop relevant scales based on the dimensions we have established, and verify the reliability and validity of the scales. Then carry out research on the mechanism of sustainable employability to explore its influencing factors and possible impacts. In the end, it will improve the sustainable employability of employees, expand the supply of the labour market, and solve the labour shortage. We have tried our best to review and evaluate and sustainable employability related researches, but there must be other researches that we have not noticed. Subsequent research can expand the scale of literature review and evaluation, and improve our existing definitions and dimensions.

7. Conclusions

We are in a period of population aging during which the labour shortage problem has gradually appeared. Although sustainable employability can prolong the working lives of employees and solve the problem of labour market shortages, the definition and measurement dimensions of this ability are unclear. The latest definition by Fleuren at al. improves on the generality of previous definitions to some extent, but there are still omissions in their conceptualisation. By defining sustainable employability as a personal characteristic, they ignore work value and environmental factors (e.g., labour market, digital age, etc.), which creates confusion with the concept of sustainable working ability and narrows the scope of research. Their neglect of environmental factors also means that retired or older employees are not well considered and measured in the original conceptual framework. Finally, the measurement method proposed by Fleuren et al. comprises nine indicators, but they do not form a logical framework; they are merely a collection of indicators, which is not convincing enough. Therefore, based on the swAge-model, this paper puts forward a new definition of sustainable employability that combines self-depletion theory and self-determination theory to explain the sustainability of employability. This definition makes the measurement dimensions clear and simplifies them as well. It improves the logical connection of the constituent components, helps researchers solve the problems present in the framework of Fleuren et al., facilitates later quantitative research, and provides information and a theoretical reference for future governments and enterprises on how to cope with population aging and labour market shortages.

Author Contributions: J.D., T.Y. and Z.D. conceived and designed the study. J.D., J.L., W.D., T.Y. and Z.D. wrote the draft of this manuscript. All authors have read and agreed to the published version of the manuscript.

Funding: This research was funded by [the National Natural Science Foundation of China] grant number [71974011, 72174022, 71603018, 71804009] and [2020 China National Social Science Foundation Major Project] grant number [Grants 20ZDA024].

Conflicts of Interest: The authors declare no conflict of interest. The funders had no role in the design of the study; in the collection, analyses, or interpretation of data; in the writing of the manuscript, or in the decision to publish the results.

References

1. Van der Klink, J.J.L.; Bültmann, U.; Burdorf, A.; Schaufeli, W.B.; Zijlstra, F.R.H.; Abma, F.I.; Brouwer, S.; Van Der Wilt, G.J. Sustainable employability—Definition, conceptualization, and implications: A perspective based on the capability approach. *Scand. J. Work Environ. Health* **2016**, *42*, 71–79. [CrossRef] [PubMed]
2. Fleuren, B.P.; de Grip, A.; Jansen, N.W.; Kant, I.; Zijlstra, F.R. Critical reflections on the currently leading definition of sustainable employability. *Scand. J. Work Environ. Health* **2016**, *42*, 557–560. [CrossRef] [PubMed]
3. Phillips, D.R.; Siu, O. *Global Aging and Aging Workers*; Oxford University Press: Oxford, UK, 2012; pp. 11–32. [CrossRef]
4. Fleuren, B.P.; de Grip, A.; Jansen, N.W.; Kant, I.; Zijlstra, F.R. Unshrouding the sphere from the clouds: Towards a comprehensive conceptual framework for sustainable employability. *Sustainability* **2020**, *12*, 6366. [CrossRef]
5. Herkes, J.; Churruca, K.; Ellis, L.A.; Pomare, C.; Braithwaite, J. How people fit in at work: Systematic review of the association between person–organisation and person–group fit with staff outcomes in healthcare. *BMJ Open* **2019**, *9*, e026266. [CrossRef] [PubMed]
6. Boumans, N.P.; De Jong, A.H.; Vanderlinden, L. Determinants of early retirement intentions among Belgian nurses. *J. Adv. Nurs.* **2008**, *63*, 64–74. [CrossRef]
7. Bae, S.H.; Mark, B.; Fried, B. Impact of nursing unit turnover on patient outcomes in hospitals. *J. Nurs. Scholarsh.* **2010**, *42*, 40–49. [CrossRef]
8. De Lange, A.H.; Pak, K.; Osagie, E.; Van Dam, K.; Christensen, M.; Furunes, T.; Tevik Lovset, L.; Detaille, S. An open time perspective and social sup-port to sustain in healthcare work: Results of a two-wave complete panel study. *Front. Psychol.* **2020**, *11*, 1308. [CrossRef] [PubMed]
9. Roczniewska, M.; Richter, A.; Hasson, H.; Schwarz, U.V.T. Predicting sustainable employability in Swedish healthcare: The complexity of social job resources. *Int. J. Environ. Res. Public Health* **2020**, *17*, 1200. [CrossRef]
10. Le Blanc, P.M.; Van der Heijden, B.I.; Van Vuuren, T. "I will survive" A construct validation study on the measurement of sustainable employability using different age conceptualizations. *Front. Psychol.* **2017**, *8*, 1690. [CrossRef]
11. Hazelzet, E.; Picco, E.; Houkes, I.; Bosma, H.; de Rijk, A. Effectiveness of interventions to promote sustainable employability: A systematic review. *Int. J. Environ. Res. Public Health* **2019**, *16*, 1985. [CrossRef]
12. Hazelzet, E.; Bosma, H.; de Rijk, A.; Houkes, I. Does dialogue improve the sustainable employability of low-educated em-ployees? A study protocol for an effect and process evaluation of "healthy HR". *Front. Public Health* **2020**, *8*, 446. [CrossRef] [PubMed]
13. Brouwers, L.A.; Engels, J.A.; Heerkens, Y.F.; Van der Beek, A.J. Development of a Vitality Scan related to workers' sustainable employability: A study assessing its internal consistency and construct validity. *BMC Public Health* **2015**, *15*, 551. [CrossRef]
14. De Grip, A.; Van Loo, J.; Sanders, J. The industry employability index: Taking account of supply and demand characteristics. *Int. Labour Rev.* **2004**, *143*, 211–233. [CrossRef]
15. Fleuren, B.P.; Van Amelsvoort, L.G.; de Grip, A.; Zijlstra, F.R.; Kant, I. Time takes us all? A two-wave observational study of age and time effects on sustainable employability. *Scand. J. Work Environ. Health* **2018**, *44*, 475–484. [CrossRef]
16. Truxillo, D.M.; Cadiz, D.M.; Rineer, J.R.; Zaniboni, S.; Fraccaroli, F. A lifespan perspective on job design: Fitting the job and the worker to promote job satisfaction, engagement, and performance. *Organ. Psychol. Rev.* **2012**, *2*, 340–360. [CrossRef]
17. Billett, S.; Dymock, D.; Johnson, G.; Martin, G. Overcoming the paradox of employers' views about older workers. *Int. J. Hum. Resour. Manag.* **2011**, *22*, 1248–1261. [CrossRef]
18. Houkes, I.; Miglioretti, M.; Picco, E.; De Rijk, A.E. Tapping the employee perspective on the improvement of Sustainable Employability (SE): Validation of the MAastricht Instrument for SE (MAISE-NL). *Int. J. Environ. Res. Public Health* **2020**, *17*, 2211. [CrossRef] [PubMed]
19. Green, A.E. Implications of technological change and austerity for employability in urban labour markets. *Urban Stud.* **2017**, *54*, 1638–1654. [CrossRef]
20. Felstead, A. Rapid change or slow evolution? Changing places of work and their consequences in the UK. *J. Transp. Geogr.* **2012**, *21*, 31–38. [CrossRef]
21. De Hoyos, M.; Green, A.E.; Barnes, S.A.; Behle, H.; Baldauf, B.; Owen, D.; Centano Mediavilla, I.; Stewart, J. *Literature Review on Employability, Inclusion and ICT*; Report 2; Institute for Prospective Technological Studies: Brussels, Belgium, 2013.
22. Cambridge Dictionary. Sustainable. Cambridge Dictionary. Available online: https://dictionary.cambridge.org/dictionary/english/sustainable (accessed on 5 September 2021).
23. Finkbeiner, M.; Schau, E.M.; Lehmann, A.; Traverso, M. Towards life cycle sustainability assessment. *Sustainability* **2010**, *2*, 3309–3322. [CrossRef]
24. PubMed. Sustainable Development. PubMed. Available online: https://www.ncbi.nlm.nih.gov/mesh/2027842 (accessed on 5 September 2021).
25. Holslag, J. *De Kracht van het Paradijs [The Strength of Paradise]*; Antwerp: Amsterdam, Holland, 2014.
26. Baumeister, R.F.; Bratslavsky, E.; Muraven, M.; Tice, D.M. Ego depletion: Is the active self a limited resource? *J. Pers. Soc. Psychol.* **1998**, *74*, 1252–1265. [CrossRef]
27. Deci, E.L.; Ryan, R.M. The "what" and "why" of goal pursuits: Human needs and the self-determination of behavior. *Psychol. Inq.* **2000**, *11*, 227–268. [CrossRef]
28. Van Dam, K.; Van Vuuren, T.; Kemps, S. Sustainable employment: The importance of intrinsically valuable work and an age-supportive climate. *Int. J. Hum. Resour. Manag.* **2017**, *28*, 2449–2472. [CrossRef]

29. Van Dam, K. Antecedents and consequences of employability orientation. *Eur. J. Work Organ. Psychol.* **2004**, *13*, 29–51. [CrossRef]
30. Hillage, J.; Pollard, E.; Britain, G. *Employability: Developing a Framework for Policy Analysis*; Department for Education and Employment: London, UK, 1999.
31. Forrier, A.; Sels, L. The concept employability: A complex mosaic. *Int. J. Hum. Resour. Dev. Manag.* **2003**, *3*, 102–124. [CrossRef]
32. Forrier, A.; Verbruggen, M.; De Cuyper, N. Integrating different notions of employability in a dynamic chain: The relation-ship between job transitions, movement capital and perceived employability. *J. Vocat. Behav.* **2015**, *89*, 56–64. [CrossRef]
33. Chudzikowski, K. Career transitions and career success in the 'new' career era. *J. Vocat. Behav.* **2012**, *81*, 298–306. [CrossRef]
34. Wittekind, A.; Raeder, S.; Grote, G. A longitudinal study of determinants of perceived employability. *J. Organ. Behav.* **2010**, *31*, 566–586. [CrossRef]
35. Jiang, K.; Liu, D.; McKay, P.F.; Lee, T.W.; Mitchell, T.R. When and how is job embeddedness predictive of turnover? A meta-analytic investigation. *J. Appl. Psychol.* **2012**, *97*, 1077. [CrossRef]
36. Nilsson, K. A sustainable working life for all ages–The swAge-model. *Appl. Ergon.* **2020**, *86*, 103082. [CrossRef]
37. Nilsson, K. Conceptualisation of ageing in relation to factors of importance for extending working life—A review. *Scand. J. Public Health* **2016**, *44*, 490–505. [CrossRef]
38. Robotham, D.; Satkunanathan, S.; Doughty, L.; Wykes, T. Do we still have a digital divide in mental health? A five-year survey follow-up. *J. Med. Internet Res.* **2016**, *18*, e309. [CrossRef] [PubMed]
39. Fairlie, P. Meaningful work, employee engagement, and other key employee outcomes: Implications for human resource development. *Adv. Dev. Hum. Resour.* **2011**, *13*, 508–525. [CrossRef]
40. Brown, S.P.; Leigh, T.W. A new look at psychological climate and its relationship to job involvement, effort, and performance. *J. Appl. Psychol.* **1996**, *81*, 358–368. [CrossRef] [PubMed]
41. Amabile, T.M.; Hill, K.G.; Hennessey, B.A.; Tighe, E.M. The work preference inventory: Assessing intrinsic and extrinsic motivational orientations. *J. Pers. Soc. Psychol.* **1994**, *66*, 950–967. [CrossRef] [PubMed]
42. Poell, R.F.; Van Dam, K.; Van den Berg, P.T. Organising learning in work contexts. *Appl. Psychol.* **2004**, *53*, 529–540. [CrossRef]
43. Nikolova, I.; Van Ruysseveldt, J.; De Witte, H.; Syroit, J. Work-based learning: Development and validation of a scale measuring the learning potential of the workplace (LPW). *J. Organ. Behav.* **2014**, *84*, 1–10. [CrossRef]
44. Nicholson, N. A theory of work role transitions. *Adm. Sci. Q.* **1984**, *29*, 172–191. [CrossRef]
45. Raemdonck, I.; Tillema, H.; De Grip, A.; Valcke, M.; Segers, M. Does self-directedness in learning and careers predict the employability of low-qualified employees? *Vocat. Learn.* **2012**, *5*, 137–151. [CrossRef]
46. Clarke, M. Understanding and managing employability in changing career contexts. *J. Eur. Ind. Train.* **2008**, *32*, 258–284. [CrossRef]
47. Forrier, A.; Sels, L.; Stynen, D. Career mobility at the intersection between agent and structure: A conceptual model. *J. Occup. Organ. Psychol.* **2009**, *82*, 739–759. [CrossRef]
48. Fugate, M.; Kinicki, A.J.; Ashforth, B.E. Employability: A psycho-social construct, its dimensions, and applications. *J. Vocat. Behav.* **2004**, *65*, 14–38. [CrossRef]
49. Akkermans, J.; Brenninkmeijer, V.; Huibers, M.; Blonk, R.W. Competencies for the contemporary career: Development and preliminary validation of the career competencies questionnaire. *J. Career Dev.* **2013**, *40*, 245–267. [CrossRef]
50. McArdle, S.; Waters, L.; Briscoe, J.P.; Hall, D.T.T. Employability during unemployment: Adaptability, career identity and human and social capital. *J. Vocat. Behav.* **2007**, *71*, 247–264. [CrossRef]
51. Koen, J.; Klehe, U.C.; Van Vianen, A.E. Employability among the long-term unemployed: A futile quest or worth the effort? *J. Vocat. Behav.* **2013**, *82*, 37–48. [CrossRef]
52. De Cuyper, N.; Van der Heijden, B.I.; De Witte, H. Associations between perceived employability, employee well-being, and its contribution to organizational success: A matter of psychological contracts? *Int. J. Hum. Resour. Manag.* **2011**, *22*, 1486–1503. [CrossRef]
53. Van den Broeck, A.; De Cuyper, N.; Baillien, E.; Vanbelle, E.; Vanhercke, D.; De Witte, H. Perception of organization's value support and perceived employability: Insights from self-determination theory. *Int. J. Hum. Resour. Manag.* **2014**, *25*, 1904–1918. [CrossRef]
54. Shao, X.; Yang, Y.; Wang, L. Digital divide or digital welfare? The role of the internet in shaping the sustainable employability of chinese adults. *J. Glob. Inf. Manag.* **2021**, *29*, 20–36. [CrossRef]
55. Van Casteren, P.A.; Meerman, J.; Brouwers, E.P.; Van Dam, A.; Van der Klink, J.J. How can wellbeing at work and sustainable employability of gifted workers be enhanced? A qualitative study from a capability approach perspective. *BMC Public Health* **2021**, *21*, 1–10. [CrossRef]

MDPI
St. Alban-Anlage 66
4052 Basel
Switzerland
Tel. +41 61 683 77 34
Fax +41 61 302 89 18
www.mdpi.com

International Journal of Environmental Research and Public Health Editorial Office
E-mail: ijerph@mdpi.com
www.mdpi.com/journal/ijerph

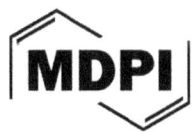

www.ingramcontent.com/pod-product-compliance
Lightning Source LLC
LaVergne TN
LVHW070456100526
838202LV00014B/1731